EXPERT
RAPID
RESPONSE

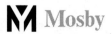 Mosby

St. Louis Baltimore Boston Carlsbad Chicago Minneapolis New York Philadelphia Portland
London Milan Sydney Tokyo Toronto

Publisher: Stanley Loeb
Editorial Director: Stephen Daly
Clinical Director: Cindy Tryniszewski, RN, MSN
Editors: Beth Adams, Catherine E. Harold
Clinical Editors: Marlene Ciranowicz, RN, MSN, CDE; Maryann Foley, RN, BSN; Colleen Seeber-Combs, RN, MSN, CCRN; Beverly A. Tscheschlog, RN
Designer: Guy Jacobs
Illustration Manager: Philip Ashley
Illustrators: Kristin Mount and Graphic World Illustration Services
Senior Composition Specialist: Pamela Merritt
Manufacturing Manager: William A. Winneberger, Jr.
Cover Illustration: Doree Loschiavo

Printed in the United States of America
Composition by Mosby Electronic Production, Philadelphia
Printing/binding by R.R. Donnelley and Sons, Inc.

Mosby, Inc.
11830 Westline Industrial Drive
St. Louis, Missouri 63146

Library of Congress Cataloging-in-Publication Data

Expert rapid response.
p.   cm.
Includes index.
ISBN 0-323-00377-X
1. Emergency nursing—Handbooks, manuals, etc.   I. Mosby, Inc.

[DNLM: 1. Nursing Care handbooks. 2. Emergencies—nursing handbooks. 3. Acute Disease—nursing handbooks. WY 49 E96 1998]
RT120.E4E97 1998
610.73'61—dc21
DNLM/DLC
for Library of Congress   98-20962
                                CIP

98 99 00 01 02/9 8 7 6 5 4 3 2 1

Contents

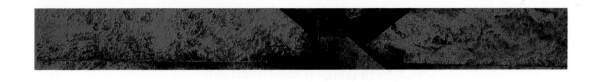

Contributors and Consultants

Contributors

Heatherlee Bailey, MD
Instructor of Emergency Medicine
Allegheny University of the Health Sciences
Department of Emergency Medicine
Philadelphia, Pennsylvania

Cynthia A. Blank-Reid, RN, MSN, CEN
Trauma Nurse Coordinator
Allegheny University of the Health Sciences
Medical College of Pennsylvania Division
Philadelphia, Pennsylvania

Sally A. Brozenec, RN, PhD
Assistant Professor
Rush University College of Nursing
Chicago, Illinois

Heather A. Butler, RN, MSN, CNS, CCRN
Clinical Instructor
River College School of Nursing
Nashua, New Hampshire
Clinical Nurse, PACU and ICU
Southern New Hampshire Medical Center
Nashua, New Hampshire

Marcy Caplin, RN, MSN, CS
Independent Consultant
Hudson, Ohio

Kay Coulter, RN, CRNI
Founder and Principal Instructor
Intravenous Therapy Consultation and Education Company
Clearwater, Florida

Kendra Stastny Ellis, RN, MS, CCRN
Staff Nurse-Surgical and Trauma ICU
Parkland Memorial Hospital
Harry Hines
Dallas, Texas

Ellie Franges, RN, MSN, CNRN, CCRN
Director Neuroscience Services
Sacred Heart Hospital
Allentown, Pennsylvania

JoAnne Konick-McMahan, RN, MSN, CCRN
Clinical Nurse Specialist, Heart Failure Study
University of Pennsylvania School of Nursing
Philadelphia, Pennsylvania

Susan McGann, RN, BSN, CEN
President
Delaware Valley Latex Allergy Support Network, Inc.
Philadelphia, Pennsylvania

Heather Boyd-Monk, SRN, BSN, CRNO
Assistant Director of Nursing for Ophthalmic Education Programs
Wills Eye Hospital
Philadelphia, Pennsylvania

Lewis J. Kaplan, MD
Assistant Professor of Surgery
Allegheny University of the Health Sciences
Division of Trauma and Surgical Critical Care
Philadelphia, Pennsylvania

Chris Platt Moldovanyi, RN, MSN
Registered Nurse Medical Consultant
Phillips and Mille Co., LPA
Middleburg Heights, Ohio

Sally S. Russell, RN, MN, RNC
Coordinator of Programs, Educational Services
St. Elizabeth Medical Center
Lafayette, Indiana
Instructor
St. Elizabeth School of Nursing
Lafayette, Indiana

Laureen M. Tavolaro-Ryley, RN, MSN, CS
Geriatric Psychiatric Clinical Nurse Specialist-Private Practice
Clinical Instructor University of Pennsylvania
Philadelphia, Pennsylvania

Consultants

Karen E. Burgess, RN, MSN
Nurse Consultant and Educator
Neuroscience and Medical Surgical Nursing
Sierra Madre, California
Instructor and Consultant, Neuroscience Nursing
UCLA School of Nursing
Educational Outreach Program
Los Angeles, California

Catherine Dowling, RN, MSN, CCRN, CS
Clinical Nurse Specialist
Neurosurgery
Detroit Receiving Hospital
Detroit, Michigan

Andrea Rothman Mann, RN, MSN
Third Level Chairman
Instructor, Nursing Education
Frankford Hospital School of Nursing
Philadelphia, Pennsylvania

Marilyn Sawyer Sommers, RN, PhD, CCRN
Professor, College of Nursing and Health
University of Cincinnati
Cincinnati, Ohio

Foreword

As you know, an expert nurse doesn't simply wait for directions. In today's fast-paced health-care settings, you need to assess, anticipate, evaluate, and respond to your patients within minutes, delivering care in the most efficient, coordinated, and effective manner possible. That's a difficult challenge for even the most experienced nurse, particularly when a patient's condition is urgent and you're under tremendous pressure to do exactly the right thing at exactly the right time.

Rarely have I come across a book that can actually help you meet that goal, one that's both practical and yet focused enough to provide the kind of real-life support nurses need to perform at the highest level in urgent clinical situations. But you're holding one in your hands, and that's why I'm happy to recommend *Expert Rapid Response*, a book that offers features and benefits you can translate immediately into improved patient care—and greater peace of mind.

Expert Rapid Response guides you step-by-step through more than 100 of the most urgent, time-sensitive clinical challenges you'll ever face. And using this book, you'll know how to respond quickly and decisively to every one of them—recognizing key warning signs and symptoms, prioritizing your actions, and delivering the complete ongoing care your patients need.

Expert Rapid Response is easy to use. It's organized A-to-Z by topic. And for each of the more than 100 urgent patient-care situations covered in the book, you'll find the key points that every nurse wants and needs to know, including:
- What to look for
- What to do immediately
- What to do next
- Follow-up care you need to perform
- Special considerations to be aware of.

Throughout *Expert Rapid Response*, you also find dozens of detailed illustrations and charts, as well as special timesaving features that offer valuable, up-to-date clinical insights and information that will help bolster your clinical skills and round out your knowledge. For example—

- **Danger Signs and Symptoms:** Points you to critical assessment findings and what they mean.
- **Tips and Techniques**: Describes and shows you how to perform key procedures.
- **NurseALERT:** Provides important advice and warnings.
- **Diagnostic Tests:** Reviews normal and abnormal ranges and prepares you for pre- and post-test intervention and teaching.
- **Pathophysiology:** Highlights functional abnormalities that accompany various diseases and disorders.
- **Treatment of Choice:** Explains the latest and most preferred treatment.

Did you ever wish you had an always-reliable clinical expert walking with you from patient to patient—helping you prioritize your actions, confirming your suspicions about a patient's illness, and guiding you step-by-step through complex patient care? *Expert Rapid Response* is the closest you'll come to that reliable clinical expert, and it's available any time you need it.

Expert Rapid Response will help you become that expert nurse you're constantly striving to be—one who knows exactly what to do and when to do it, particularly when the situation is life-threatening and your patient needs you most.

Cynthia A. Blank-Reid, RN, MSN, CEN
Trauma Nurse Coordinator
Allegheny University Hospitals -
Medical College of Pennsylvania
Philadelphia, PA

ABDOMINAL PAIN

Although common and usually minor, abdominal pain sometimes warns of a serious—even life-threatening—problem. When it does, your patient's condition may quickly deteriorate if you don't detect and treat the underlying problem promptly. That's why any time a patient complains of abdominal pain—especially pain that's sudden and severe—your response must be rapid, yet thorough.

By understanding the common causes of abdominal pain and the clues that can help you differentiate among them, you'll have the basic tools you need to respond appropriately. (See *Common causes of abdominal pain*, page 2.)

Types of abdominal pain

When assessing abdominal pain, remember that the features you uncover can help you isolate the problem. That's because there are three general types of abdominal pain—visceral, parietal, and referred—and each type produces a different clinical picture.

Visceral pain arises from damage to hollow abdominal organs, such as the stomach. Regardless of the organ involved, symptoms commonly begin as a dull, diffuse, intermittent pain at the abdominal midline. Over time, the pain localizes at a site specific to the affected organ. For example, the pain of appendicitis may start in the periumbilical region and then localize to the right lower quadrant.

Parietal pain results from inflammation or irritation of the parietal peritoneum. It may warn that intestinal contents or blood has spilled into the peritoneal cavity. Patients typically describe the pain as steady, aching, and severe. Parietal pain localizes at the site of the underlying problem and can be aggravated by palpation, movement, coughing, or sneezing.

Referred pain is experienced at a cutaneous site removed from the affected organ. In the spinal cord, pain stimuli from the viscera travel through some of the same neurons that carry pain messages from the skin. As a result, the patient experiences the pain in the skin, even though the pain originates in the viscera. For example, pain produced by pancreatitis is commonly referred to the left shoulder. An injured spleen

COMMON CAUSES OF ABDOMINAL PAIN

Although abdominal pain usually results from a GI disorder, it can also stem from a disorder of another body system, such as the genitourinary, musculoskeletal, or immune system. Or it may warn of a complication, such as GI hemorrhage from peptic ulcer disease.

Common causes of abdominal pain include:

- appendicitis
- cholecystitis
- Crohn's disease
- diverticulitis
- endometriosis
- intestinal obstruction
- intestinal perforation
- ovarian cyst
- pancreatitis
- pelvic inflammatory disease
- peptic ulcer disease
- peritonitis
- pyelonephritis
- renal calculi
- ruptured ectopic pregnancy.

or perforated ulcer may affect the left shoulder as well. Subphrenic abscess pain commonly refers to the right shoulder. Cholecystitis and pancreatitis pain is often experienced in the midback.

WHAT TO LOOK FOR

For all types of abdominal pain, remember that your patient's description will be subjective, leaving you to gauge its severity on a relative scale. Also, because abdominal pain is often generalized, the patient may have trouble pinpointing its exact location. Be sure to investigate carefully, using the full range of assessment techniques.

Clinical findings for a patient with abdominal pain may include the following:

- verbal reports of pain in the abdominal area or, possibly, the shoulders or back
- nonverbal indications of pain, such as grimacing, assuming a fetal position, or guarding the abdomen
- visible abnormalities, including distention, a noticeable mass, visible peristalsis, or vasculature around the umbilicus
- hyperactive or absent bowel sounds
- percussion of air or a solid mass in an inappropriate location
- rigid abdominal muscles during palpation
- tenderness with light or deep palpation
- rebound tenderness (see *Eliciting rebound tenderness*)
- nausea, vomiting, diaphoresis, tachycardia, pallor, and restlessness.

WHAT TO DO IMMEDIATELY

If your patient complains of abdominal pain, start by trying to determine whether it's visceral, parietal, or referred. Begin by asking the patient questions, and then proceed with physical assessment as follows:

- Document the patient's description of his pain. Note whether he describes it as sharp or stabbing (which suggests parietal pain) or as dull, cramping, or aching (which suggests visceral pain).
- Ask the patient to point to the exact location of the pain. If he can do this, suspect parietal pain. If the pain is diffuse and difficult to pinpoint, suspect visceral pain.
- Find out if the pain involves the shoulders or back. If it does, suspect a pancreatic or gallbladder disorder.
- Ask the patient when the pain began, what started it, and what, if anything, relieves it. Also ask about associated symptoms, such as nausea, vomiting, diarrhea, constipation, and changes in stool color and frequency. Also, find out when he had his last bowel movement.
- Inquire about a history of abdominal injuries and surgery and a recent history of peptic ulcer disease, GI cancer, or inflammatory bowel disease. Also ask him if he has recently started taking aspirin, nonsteroidal anti-inflammatory agents, corticosteroids, or warfarin.

TIPS AND TECHNIQUES

ELICITING REBOUND TENDERNESS

To help determine the cause of your patient's abdominal pain, you may want to palpate for rebound tenderness—a cardinal sign of peritoneal irritation. Follow these steps.

With your patient in a supine position, hold your hand at a 90-degree angle to his abdomen. Keeping your fingers straight and extended, press them gently but deeply into an abdominal area far removed from the tender site (see illustration at left).

Now quickly pull your hand straight up, away from the abdomen (see illustration at right). Quick withdrawal allows the abdominal organs to rebound to their previous positions. If the patient has peritoneal irritation, release of pressure will cause intense abdominal pain at the site of the irritation. The pain may be localized, as with an abscess, or generalized, as with a perforated organ.

IMPORTANT PRECAUTION
Because this test can cause severe pain, avoid performing it except to clarify or rule out specific problems. If you must assess for rebound tenderness, wait until the end of your examination to avoid interfering with other aspects of assessment.

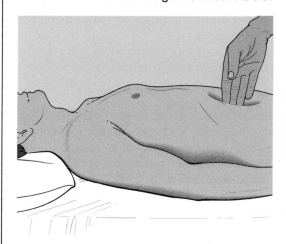 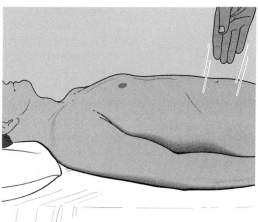

Inspection

- Inspect the skin over the abdomen. Look carefully for scars, which may indicate previous abdominal trauma or surgery. Also look for striae (stretch marks), bruising, and angiomata (visible vascularization, commonly around the umbilicus).
- ➡ NurseALERT Remember that visible vasculature around the umbilicus usually signals liver disease or an obstructed vena cava.
- Inspect the abdominal contour for visible masses, asymmetry, and distention. Keep in mind that generalized distention may stem from obesity, a solid mass, gas, or fluid. With an inverted umbilicus, distention usually suggests gas or obesity; with an everted umbilicus, distention usually suggests ascites or a mass. Localized distention may result from a full bladder, pregnancy, or a large mass in a specific abdominal organ.

Auscultation

- Using the diaphragm of your stethoscope, auscultate the abdomen in all quadrants.
- Listen for bowel sounds. *Hyperactive* bowel sounds are high pitched and occur more frequently than normal; you'll hear them if the patient has increased peristalsis, as with diarrhea or obstruction. *Hypoactive* or *absent* bowel sounds indicate that bowel activity has slowed or stopped, commonly from peritoneal irritation caused by an injury to the abdomen or from surgery. Especially if the patient has hypoactive bowel sounds, you may need to listen to each quadrant for 2 to 5 minutes to assess them fully.
- ➡ **NurseALERT** Always perform auscultation of the abdomen before percussion and palpation, both of which can affect bowel sounds by increasing intestinal activity. Don't conclude that bowel sounds are absent unless you've listened for a full 5 minutes in each quadrant. Also, don't forget that bowel sounds normally are reduced in elderly patients due to aging-related changes.
- Listen carefully for bruits arising from an aortic aneurysm or from turbulent flow in the renal or mesenteric arteries.

Percussion

- Percuss all abdominal quadrants. Be aware that tympany is normal in most locations because the bowel contains a small amount of air. Expect to hear dullness over a stool-filled bowel, areas of ascites, solid organs, and solid or fluid-filled masses. Dullness in the suprapubic area may result from a full bladder or an enlarged uterus.

Palpation

- Perform light palpation in each quadrant, using the pads of your fingers. Press gently with your fingers together to check for muscle tenderness, resistance, and superficial masses. If the patient has a painful area, palpate it last. If his abdomen is rigid and boardlike, he may have acute peritonitis. Ask him to breathe through his open mouth; if his abdomen stays rigid even during exhalation, stop the examination and notify the physician at once.
- After light palpation, perform deep palpation to check for deeper masses and tender areas. Be especially alert for rebound tenderness.
- ➡ **NurseALERT** If your patient has a very tender area or exhibited vigorous guarding during auscultation and light palpation, don't perform deep palpation in that area. He may have peritonitis or a highly inflamed visceral organ, and deep palpation could cause injury or worsen the underlying problem. Also, never perform deep palpation on a pulsatile abdominal mass, which may be an abdominal aortic aneurysm. Fragile aneurysmal walls may rupture under pressure.

WHAT TO DO NEXT

If your patient develops abdominal pain or if his abdominal pain increases, notify the physician. Then take the following steps:
- Establish an I.V. line and administer fluids, as indicated.
- Withhold all oral intake.
- Insert an indwelling urinary catheter, if indicated, and monitor fluid intake and output closely.
- Assess vital signs, watching carefully for hypotension, tachycardia, and fever.
- Administer prescribed analgesics, unless otherwise contraindicated. If the physician has instructed you to withhold pain medications until the health-care team has confirmed the source of the pain, explain the order to the patient and his family.
- Depending on the probable cause of the pain, prepare for insertion of a nasogastric or an intestinal tube as well as for X-rays, laparoscopy, or surgery.

FOLLOW-UP CARE
- Help the patient into a position that's as comfortable as possible.
- Once the treatment plan has been established, instruct the patient and his family about impending diagnostic or treatment procedures.

SPECIAL CONSIDERATIONS
- Watch the patient's facial expressions during your abdominal assessment for nonverbal clues to a tender area.
- If your patient tenses his abdominal muscles when you attempt to palpate, try using your stethoscope instead. When auscultating the abdomen, apply steady downward pressure with the stethoscope's diaphragm as a form of palpation. This maneuver works especially well with anxious children.
- Keep equipment available for insertion of a nasogastric or an intestinal tube. If the patient needs a long intestinal tube, such as a Miller-Abbott or Cantor tube, fill the mercury bag with air before insertion to check for leaks.
- Prepare the patient for any necessary diagnostic tests or surgery, and explain what will happen during these procedures.

ACUTE RESPIRATORY DISTRESS SYNDROME

Acute respiratory distress syndrome (ARDS) imperils a patient's life by inducing acute respiratory failure. The pulmonary capillary endothelium becomes increasingly permeable, causing proteins and intravascular fluid to flood the interstitial spaces and alveoli. Pulmonary edema then develops, lung compliance diminishes, gas exchange deteriorates, and the patient becomes hypoxemic. Not all forms of ARDS have pulmonary edema as a prominent feature. Many forms have intestinal inflammation, abnormal pulmonary air flow, or fibrosis as the primary feature. Keep in mind that the pulmonary edema associated with ARDS, unlike that associated with heart failure, is noncardiac in origin.

With reduced lung compliance, ventilation requires increased airway pressure. Taking the path of least resistance, the increased pressure first travels across uninjured lung segments. This creates increased air volume, which may injure these segments through overdistention, or volutrauma. Alveoli may then rupture and pneumothorax may develop.

Critically ill, the ARDS patient eventually requires mechanical ventilation and may have multisystem organ involvement or organ failure. Early onset of ARDS commonly indicates widespread organ injury and early multisystem failure. It also means that ARDS has developed as a result of underlying organ dysfunction, rather than as a later consequence. Early recognition of ARDS and immediate intervention may help preserve normal organ function.

Causes of ARDS
ARDS can result from direct lung injury or from an indirect cause. The following conditions can lead to ARDS through *direct injury*:
- pneumonia
- lung contusion
- fat embolism
- aspiration
- inhaled toxins or massive smoke inhalation
- exposure to high oxygen concentrations
- near-drowning.

Indirect causes of ARDS include:
- systemic conditions, such as sepsis, shock, multisystem trauma, pancreatitis, and anaphylaxis
- massive blood transfusions
- prolonged cardiac surgery
- disseminated intravascular coagulation.

WHAT TO LOOK FOR
Lung injury in ARDS progresses through four distinct phases. With each stage, clinical findings become more severe and lung function becomes increasingly impaired. (See *How ARDS progresses*.)

WHAT TO DO IMMEDIATELY
If you suspect your patient has ARDS, ensure a patent airway and adequate breathing and circulation and notify the physician. Then take the following actions:
- Bring a manual resuscitation bag to the bedside in case the patient develops respiratory distress (indicated by worsening hypoxemia, tachypnea, tachycardia, and use of accessory muscles for respiration).

HOW A.R.D.S. PROGRESSES

The pathophysiologic events of acute respiratory distress syndrome (ARDS) occur in four distinct phases. As the patient progresses through each phase, lung function grows increasingly impaired.

Pathophysiologic events	Effect on lungs	Clinical findings
PHASE 1 • Lung injury (direct or indirect) • Systemic release of mediators, including tumor necrosis factor, complement fragments, protease, prostaglandins, and endotoxins • Release of toxic by-products, causing microvascular injury • Fluid leakage into interstitial spaces	• Disruption of capillary endothelium • Decreased lung compliance • Onset of interstitial edema • Increased ventilation-perfusion mismatch	• Slight tachypnea • Dyspnea, especially on exertion • Mild hypoxemia • Breath sounds normal or slightly diminished • Decreased Pao_2 • Tachycardia • Apprehension, restlessness
PHASE 2 • Continued fluid leakage into interstitial spaces • Increased lung stiffness, reducing compliance • Poor alveolar ventilation • Increased hypoxemia	• Worsening of interstitial edema, causing further decrease in lung compliance, increase in ventilation-perfusion mismatch	• Pallor • Cool, clammy skin • Increased tachypnea and accessory muscle use • Fine, diffuse crackles • Decreased Pao_2
PHASE 3 • Fluid leakage into alveoli • Alveolar shunting (perfusion without ventilation) • Surfactant damage from fluid in alveoli	• Disruption of alveolo-capillary membrane • Increased alveolar edema, causing further decrease in lung compliance, increase in ventilation-perfusion mismatch	• Severe respiratory distress, with respiratory rate above 30 beats/minute • Worsening hypoxemia • Coarse crackles • Increased tachypnea, possibly with arrhythmias • Labile blood pressure • Decreased Pao_2
PHASE 4 • Alveolar collapse from fluid buildup • Increased alveolar shunting • Fibrosis (from inflammation), with further impairment of gas exchange • Increased $Paco_2$	• Widespread atelectasis, leading to decreases in total lung volume and residual capacity, with continued reduction in lung compliance	• Severe hypoxemia with acute respiratory failure; lack of spontaneous respirations • Increased $Paco_2$ • Pulmonary hypertension • Hypotension with bradycardia and arrhythmias • Metabolic and respiratory acidosis • Deteriorating mental status • Diminishing Pao_2 • Diffuse bilateral and rapidly progressing interstitial or alveolar infiltrates (shown on chest X-ray)

A

- If the patient's respiratory status continues to decline, prepare for endotracheal intubation and mechanical ventilation with positive end-expiratory pressure (PEEP), as ordered. Institute continuous pulse oximetry.
- Check arterial blood gas (ABG) results as indicated, and notify the physician of abnormal values.

➡ **NurseALERT** Keep an adjustable PEEP valve in line with the manual resuscitation bag. PEEP oxygenates the patient more effectively because it makes more alveoli available for gas exchange and increases the lungs' functional residual capacity. To minimize volutrauma and increase mean airway pressure (an important determinant of oxygenation when using a PEEP valve), give slower, longer breaths rather than fast, forceful breaths.

- Administer bronchodilators, such as albuterol (Proventil), as prescribed, to decrease airway resistance and promote airflow.

➡ **NurseALERT** Administer albuterol with caution if your patient has tachycardia but isn't wheezing or hypoxemic. A beta agonist, albuterol increases both the heart rate and myocardial oxygen consumption.

- Be prepared to give analgesics, sedatives, and, if necessary, paralytic agents, as prescribed, to prevent the patient from resisting the mechanical ventilator. These drugs maximize the benefits of ventilation, reducing airway pressure and oxygen consumption during respiration.

WHAT TO DO NEXT

Once the initial crisis passes, carry out the following measures:

- To augment mean airway pressure and diminish peak airway pressure, decrease the tidal volume and maximal flow rate on the mechanical ventilator, as ordered, to help prevent peak airway pressure from exceeding 35 cm H_2O. Check the inspiratory flow waveform; it should be decelerating rather than square.
- Elevate the head of the bed 45 degrees (up to 90 degrees if tolerated) to promote optimal breathing. Also, begin lateral rotation therapy (such as kinetic therapy) or prone positioning, as indicated and ordered.
- Auscultate frequently for wheezes and crackles.
- Perform suctioning carefully, always preoxygenating with 100% oxygen. Limit suctioning to 5 seconds per suctioning episode and no more than four episodes per minute. Remember that excessive suctioning causes loss of mean airway pressure and PEEP and may interfere with alveolar expansion—especially if the patient doesn't have a closed, in-line suction system.
- Continue to give medications, such as bronchodilators, as prescribed, and to assess for adverse drug effects, including tremors, tachycardia, and restlessness.

- Obtain routine laboratory tests, as indicated, to check for infection. Obtain samples for blood cultures, Gram stain of sputum specimens, sputum culture and sensitivity, urinalysis, and urine culture and sensitivity.
- Administer antibiotics to combat a presumed or known source of infection, as prescribed. If the infection source is unknown, expect to give antibiotics that eradicate such nosocomial organisms as methicillin-resistant *Staphylococcus aureus* and *Pseudomonas*.
- Monitor all physiologic parameters, keeping in mind that ARDS commonly involves multisystemic or multiorgan failure. Carefully evaluate urine output, blood coagulation, and GI function.
- Be alert for worsening hypoxemia, which may indicate that your patient's lung compliance is continuing to decrease despite treatment.
- Throughout your care, provide emotional support and clear, concise explanations to the patient and family.

FOLLOW-UP CARE
- Continuously monitor the patient's vital signs, checking for tachycardia, hypertension, hypotension, tachypnea, and apnea.
- Monitor the rate, depth, and quality of respirations.
- Auscultate breath sounds frequently for wheezes and crackles.
- Assess sputum for quantity, color, odor, and consistency.
- Monitor pulmonary function studies and oxygen saturation or pulse oximetry values.
- If the patient experiences adverse effects of PEEP, such as hypotension, prepare for the insertion of a pulmonary artery catheter.
- Check for jugular vein distention.
- Give I.V. fluids, as prescribed, to maintain adequate hydration.
- Administer total parenteral nutrition or enteral tube feedings, as prescribed, to maintain optimal nutrition.
- Assess fluid intake and output at least every 8 hours.
- Evaluate neurologic status, noting any changes in level of consciousness, orientation, and behavior.
- Routinely evaluate skin color and capillary refill.
- Monitor ABG values, complete blood count, albumin and electrolyte levels, and urine, sputum, and blood culture tests, as indicated.

SPECIAL CONSIDERATIONS
- If the patient's oxygenation fails to improve despite volume- or pressure-controlled ventilation, anticipate the need to increase the inspiratory cycle so that it's equal to or exceeds the expiratory cycle, known as inversed I:E ratio. By increasing the inspiratory cycle, you'll allow more time for the alveoli to expand and for gas exchange to occur. Or you may administer inhaled nitric oxide to lower pulmonary vascular resistance and pressure, reduce airway and pulmonary artery pressures, and enhance the elimination of carbon dioxide.

A

AIRWAY OBSTRUCTION, ACUTE

Acute airway obstruction occurs when some object or condition blocks the normal flow of air through the tracheobronchial tree. Generally, the more proximal and complete the occlusion, the more dire the threat to the patient's life.

A complete airway obstruction must be cleared immediately by abdominal thrusts, emergency tracheotomy, or needle cricothyrotomy. Otherwise, it rapidly progresses to respiratory arrest and death. Even a partial airway obstruction can be fatal if it prevents adequate breathing and gas exchange or progresses to complete obstruction (as in epiglottitis).

Causes of airway obstruction
Common causes of acute airway obstruction include:
- blockage caused by the tongue (especially if the patient is unconscious)
- aspiration of foreign bodies (coins and toy parts in children, partial dentures in adults)
- epiglottitis
- pharyngeal abscess
- allergic reactions (from angioedema of the tongue)
- tracheal displacement (such as by a large goiter, lymphoma, or lung tumor)
- trauma (such as laryngeal fracture, an expanding neck hematoma, or tracheal or bronchial disruption)
- central nervous system disorders (for instance, cerebrovascular accident)
- postoperative swellings (as with anterior cervical surgeries).

WHAT TO LOOK FOR
Clinical findings in airway obstruction include:
- inability to speak, breathe, or cough (with complete obstruction)
- dyspnea and tachypnea accompanied by tachycardia and hypertension (classic signs of partial obstruction)
- emotional distress or panic (with partial and complete obstruction)
- agitation and restlessness progressing to loss of consciousness (from hypoxia and hypercapnia, with partial and complete obstruction)
- stridor (with partial obstruction; see *Stridor: The sound of acute distress*)
- nasal flaring (with partial and complete obstruction)
- diaphoresis (with partial and complete obstruction)
- cyanosis (with partial and complete obstruction)
- clutching of the throat, known as the universal distress signal (with complete obstruction)
- decreased diaphragmatic excursion and increased use of accessory muscles (with partial obstruction)

STRIDOR: THE SOUND OF ACUTE DISTRESS

A loud, harsh sound that occurs during breathing, stridor signals passage of air through a partially obstructed or narrowed upper airway. Stridor warns of and immediately precedes an acute upper respiratory tract obstruction. For instance, it may follow extubation, accompany an anaphylactic or anaphylactoid reaction, or arise during a severe pharyngeal infection.

RECOGNIZING STRIDOR
Usually, stridor occurs on inspiration. With severe obstruction, you also may hear it on expiration.

To evaluate for stridor, listen for a high-pitched, harsh, raspy sound as the patient breathes. Be aware, however, that it may sound like whistling or wind blowing instead.

If you detect stridor, assess the patient further for signs of an airway obstruction. Take special note of stridor that stops abruptly. Be aware that inspiratory chest movements and absent breath sounds may be an ominous sign of complete airway obstruction.

RESPONDING TO STRIDOR
If you detect stridor, you'll need to intervene quickly as follows:
- Attempt to clear an obvious airway obstruction by using the abdominal thrust maneuver or your finger, if appropriate.
- Prepare for endotracheal intubation or cricothyroidotomy and mechanical ventilation, as indicated.
- Administer 100% humidified oxygen by way of a nonrebreather mask, as ordered. Evaluate and monitor the patient's oxygen saturation level.
- Administer epinephrine, 0.3 ml in 3 ml of normal saline solution, using a nebulizer, if prescribed to treat laryngospasm. Repeat every 3 to 5 minutes as needed.
- Reassess the patient's vital signs regularly.
- Institute continuous cardiac monitoring to evaluate for life-threatening arrhythmias.

A

- decreased respiratory effort (as partial obstruction progresses to complete obstruction)
- diminished breath sounds (with partial obstruction)
- absent breath sounds (with complete obstruction).

WHAT TO DO IMMEDIATELY
If you suspect acute airway obstruction, activate your institution's emergency call system. Then follow these steps:
- If the patient is conscious and sitting or standing, perform the abdominal thrust maneuver until the foreign body is expelled or the patient becomes unconscious.
- If the patient becomes unconscious, place him in a supine position. Open the airway with the head-tilt, chin-lift maneuver, and perform five abdominal thrusts followed by a finger sweep to remove a possible foreign object. If you're unsuccessful in removing the foreign object, repeat the sequence of abdominal thrusts and finger sweep, and attempt to ventilate.
- Check for a carotid pulse. If absent, start cardiopulmonary resuscitation according to the American Heart Association's basic cardiac life support guidelines.
- Prepare for endotracheal intubation and mechanical ventilation, if indicated. Anticipate the need for a tonsil-tip suction device to clear secretions from the oropharynx and a suction catheter to clear secretions from the endotracheal tube.

- Establish I.V. access and begin I.V. fluid infusions, as prescribed, with normal saline solution. These agents help combat hypoperfusion in a patient who has progressed from respiratory to cardiac arrest.
- Initiate continuous cardiac monitoring to evaluate the heart rate and rhythm.
- Prepare to transport the patient to a monitored setting, such as the intensive care unit, if he's on a general medical-surgical unit or in the emergency department. If he has undergone a needle cricothyrotomy, prepare for transport to the operating room. As appropriate and ordered, bring emergency airway equipment, resuscitation drugs, and I.V. fluids along during transport.
- ➡ **Nurse ALERT** Don't transport a patient alone after needle cricothyrotomy. Insist that a physician, anesthesiologist, or other health-care worker skilled in airway management accompany you.
- If indicated, assist with nasogastric tube insertion for gastric decompression.

WHAT TO DO NEXT
Once the patient's condition has stabilized, take the following steps:
- Maintain airway patency.
- Administer supplemental oxygen, as prescribed.
- Keep the patient in a position that promotes optimal airway clearance, such as high Fowler's or semi-Fowler's.
- Continue to monitor vital signs, especially blood pressure and pulse rate, at least every hour.
- Monitor arterial blood gas (ABG) values, as ordered, and report abnormal results. Assess oxygen saturation with continuous pulse oximetry or ABG values.
- Monitor breath sounds and respiratory rate and depth at least every hour.
- Suction the endotracheal tube and oropharynx as often as needed to maintain a patent airway.
- Prepare the patient for diagnostic tests (such as chest X-ray, bronchoscopy, or thoracic computed tomography) to verify the cause of airway obstruction.
- Throughout your care, tell the patient what's happening and explain the purpose of all medical equipment and procedures. Offer emotional support to him and his family.

FOLLOW-UP CARE
- After endotracheal extubation, encourage hourly coughing, deep breathing, and incentive spirometry.
- Continue to monitor the patient's oxygen saturation levels, using pulse oximetry or ABG values, as ordered.

SPECIAL CONSIDERATIONS

- Keep emergency airway equipment, such as a tracheotomy tray, at the bedside in case airway obstruction recurs.
- ➡ **NurseALERT** If you're caring for a child with known or suspected epiglottitis, don't attempt to examine his throat or obtain a throat culture. Doing so may trigger laryngospasm. Keep emergency resuscitation equipment readily available.
- If your patient's airway obstruction resulted from foreign body aspiration, teach him appropriate safety measures to prevent future aspiration.

A

ANAPHYLAXIS

Anaphylaxis represents an extreme and potentially fatal systemic allergic response. Anaphylaxis can occur as true anaphylaxis or as an anaphylactoid reaction. With either, the most common triggering substances include medications, hormone preparations, serum products, certain foods (especially fruits, nuts, and shellfish), venoms (especially from bees), I.V. contrast media that contains iodine, hydroxyethyl starch, and ABO-group incompatible blood and blood products.

True anaphylaxis

In true anaphylaxis, a specific substance (or antigen) to which the patient previously was exposed interacts with antibodies created at the time of initial exposure. With subsequent exposure, these antibody-antigen complexes activate mast cells, eosinophils, or basophils, which release powerful chemicals. The chemicals include histamine, heparin, and platelet activating factor as well as other proteins that cause bronchoconstriction, increased microvascular permeability, and vasodilation. Unchecked, this reaction may progress to cardiovascular collapse, seizures, diffuse intravascular coagulation, hemorrhage, pulmonary edema, and death. (See *How anaphylaxis develops,* page 14.)

Anaphylactoid reaction

Unlike true anaphylaxis, an anaphylactoid reaction isn't mediated by preformed antibodies. It is a severe idiosyncratic allergic reaction to an agent (such as morphine) to which the patient has never previously been exposed. This reaction leads to release of the same mediators from mast cells and basophils and to the same clinical signs and symptoms seen in true anaphylaxis. The consequences of true anaphylaxis and anaphylactoid reaction are equally serious and, possibly, life-threatening.

WHAT TO LOOK FOR

Besides a recent history of exposure to an inciting agent, such as a bee sting, the patient experiencing anaphylaxis may have:

- feelings of uneasiness or impending doom

HOW ANAPHYLAXIS DEVELOPS

Anaphylaxis occurs on reexposure to a specific inciting agent, or antigen. The illustrations below show the chain of events that take place in anaphylaxis.

With the first exposure, the antigen sensitizes B lymphocytes. The B lymphocytes respond by producing immunoglobulin E (IgE) antibodies specific to the offending antigen. The IgE antibodies bind to mast cells and basophils, leaving the antigen-binding portion of the antibodies exposed to react to the allergen.

On subsequent exposure, the antigen binds to the exposed portion of the IgE antibody. This binding activates basophils, eosinophils, and mast cells, causing release of mediators such as histamine, kinins, chemotactic factor, and other vasoactive factors (including leukotrienes, prostaglandins, and thromboxanes).

Release of these substances causes vasodilation, smooth-muscle contraction, enhanced vascular permeability, and increased mucus production. Further chemical release—along with spreading of these chemicals throughout the body by basophils—triggers the systemic responses that lead to signs and symptoms.

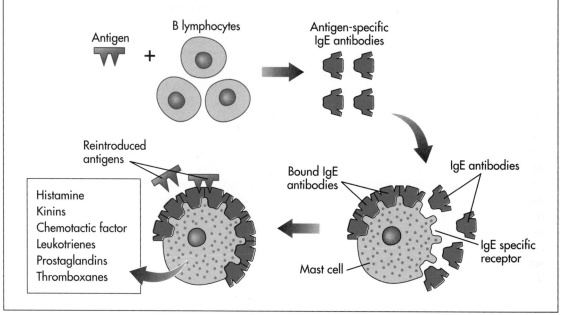

- sensation of a lump in the throat
- hoarseness, stridor, coughing, dyspnea, and tightness of the chest
- angioedema (acute swelling of the eyelids, lips, tongue, hands, and feet)
- headache
- dizziness
- diffuse wheezing and a prolonged expiratory phase (heard on auscultation)
- copious, watery nasal secretions
- nasal congestion and sneezing
- tachycardia, a weak and thready pulse, and hypotension (with impending shock)
- tachypnea

- severe anxiety
- flushed skin
- pruritus, urticaria
- cool extremities
- disorientation progressing to loss of consciousness
- nausea, vomiting, and abdominal pain (from GI tract edema).

WHAT TO DO IMMEDIATELY

Call for help—anaphylaxis is always an emergency. Establish and maintain a patent airway, and check for breathing and circulation. Then intervene as follows:

- If necessary, remove the suspected cause of anaphylaxis—a blood transfusion, for example.
- Call for emergency resuscitation equipment and a crash cart.
- Establish I.V. access and begin infusing fluid volume expanders with normal saline or lactated Ringer's solution, as prescribed, to maintain circulatory volume.
- To reverse bronchospasm and hypotension, give epinephrine subcutaneously, as prescribed. Expect to inject 0.3 to 0.5 ml of 1:1,000 solution every 5 to 10 minutes, as needed, until symptoms abate, blood pressure is adequate, and breathing is no longer labored. (For severe anaphylaxis, the physician may order 3 to 5 ml of 1:10,000 solution I.V.)
- Check the patient's vital signs every 5 minutes.
- Draw blood samples for arterial blood gas (ABG) analysis, as ordered, and monitor oxygen saturation through pulse oximetry.
- Using a nonrebreather face mask, administer supplemental 100% oxygen, as prescribed.
- If the patient has laryngeal edema, administer epinephrine nebulization therapy, as prescribed.
- Give an inhaled beta agonist, such as albuterol (Proventil), as prescribed, to help relieve bronchospasm.
- If the patient remains unstable, prepare to administer a bolus of I.V. epinephrine followed by a continuous infusion, as prescribed. If indicated, assist with insertion of an endotracheal tube to maintain a patent airway and allow mechanical ventilation. Keep suction equipment on hand, including supplies for suctioning the endotracheal tube and the oropharynx (tonsil-tip catheter).
- Administer prescribed I.V. histamine-receptor antagonists. The physician may prescribe a histamine$_1$ (H$_1$)-receptor antagonist, such as diphenhydramine hydrochloride (1 mg/kg), and an H$_2$-receptor antagonist, such as ranitidine, famotidine, or cimetidine. If these agents are readily available, expect to administer them along with epinephrine. (Commonly, H$_1$-receptor antagonists are available as emergency medications, whereas H$_2$-receptor antagonists must come from the pharmacy.)

A

➡ **NurseALERT** When administering histamine-receptor antagonists (especially diphenhydramine), stay alert for hypotension—the most common adverse effect. Assess the patient's blood pressure continuously, and notify the physician if it drops or if the patient shows signs or symptoms of hypotension.

➡ **NurseALERT** Keep in mind that laryngeal edema or severe bronchorrhea during anaphylaxis may prevent endotracheal access. If this happens, the emergency team will have to create alternate airway access. Expect to notify a surgeon immediately, and obtain 14G and 16G needles, over-the-needle catheters, and oxygen extension tubing for a needle cricothyrotomy.

- As indicated, institute continuous cardiac monitoring to evaluate changes in cardiac status, such as life-threatening arrhythmias or a heart rate faster than 140 beats/minute.
- Throughout your care, reassure the patient because she's likely to be anxious and frightened. Remember that anxiety increases oxygen demand.

WHAT TO DO NEXT
Once your patient is stable, take these actions:
- Continuously monitor her vital signs, oxygen saturation, hemodynamic parameters (such as blood pressure and mean arterial pressure), and response to therapy.
- Assess lung sounds and respiratory rate and depth at least every hour to verify relief of bronchospasm and assess lung inflation. Watch for signs and symptoms of airway obstruction, such as agitation, an altered level of consciousness, and hypoxemia. As needed, suction the airway.
- Obtain serial ABG readings, as ordered, to check for hypoxemia and acid-base imbalances.
- Keep the patient positioned for maximum chest expansion and to decrease airway swelling, as in high Fowler's position.
- Assess for adverse drug effects, including tremors, tachycardia, arrhythmias, and hypertension—especially if the patient is receiving I.V. epinephrine.
- If indicated, insert an indwelling urinary catheter. Monitor hourly urine output. Notify the physician if the output drops below 30 ml/hour.
- Provide emotional support for the patient and family.
- Continue to monitor the patient closely for at least 24 hours after the anaphylactic episode.

➡ **NurseALERT** Be aware that cardiovascular collapse (as evidenced by hypotension or cardiopulmonary arrest) may recur up to 8 hours after initially successful therapy. To prevent or treat this dire complication, the physician may prescribe corticosteroids (100 mg of I.V. hydrocortisone every 8 hours). Because exogenous corticosteroids may cause hyperglycemia, you'll need to monitor fingerstick blood glucose levels.

FOLLOW-UP CARE
- If the patient was intubated, upper airway (laryngeal) edema may complicate her ventilatory efforts immediately after extubation. To combat this problem, expect to administer epinephrine nebulization therapy.
- After endotracheal extubation, continue to monitor the patient's respiratory status closely. For instance, auscultate her breath sounds and monitor her oxygen saturation with pulse oximetry or ABG analyses. To maximize lung expansion, encourage hourly coughing, deep breathing, and incentive spirometry.
- Monitor her vital signs continuously, as indicated.
- Inform the patient and family about her condition and the treatments she's receiving.
- Document the agent or condition that triggered anaphylaxis, if known, and urge the patient to avoid it to prevent future reactions.

SPECIAL CONSIDERATIONS
- Advise the patient to obtain medical alert identification that lists the agent or condition that triggered her anaphylaxis.
- Teach the patient how to use an emergency anaphylaxis treatment kit. Instruct her to carry the kit at all times.
- Urge the patient to inform all health-care providers, including dentists, that she has experienced anaphylaxis and to tell them the agent or condition that triggered it (if known).
- Anticipate the need for skin testing to identify other possible anaphylaxis-inducing agents. Also be aware that the patient may need to undergo immunotherapy for hyposensitization.

ANGINA PECTORIS

Defined as transient chest pain associated with myocardial ischemia, angina pectoris typically starts in the chest and may radiate to the back, jaw, arm, or neck. With prolonged ischemia, myocardial infarction (MI) may occur, posing a threat to the patient's life.

Angina pectoris reflects an oxygen supply that is insufficient to meet the needs of myocardial tissue. As the flow of blood and oxygen to the heart diminishes, cells change from aerobic to anaerobic metabolism. Lactic acid then builds up in the cells, altering the permeability of cell membranes and releasing such substances as histamine, kinins, and enzymes. These chemicals stimulate terminal nerve fibers in the cardiac muscle, which send pain impulses to the central nervous system. The patient experiences these impulses as angina.

A

Classifying angina

Angina pectoris is classified as stable, unstable, or Prinzmetal's. *Stable* angina occurs intermittently over a long period, with each episode having a similar onset, duration, and intensity. Often referred to as exertional angina, stable angina occurs when myocardial oxygen demand rises, usually on exertion or with emotional stress.

With *unstable* angina (also called crescendo, progressive, and preinfarction angina), chest pain lasts longer and occurs more frequently than in stable angina. Usually, the pain occurs at rest. Sometimes seen in patients with no history of stable angina, unstable angina may progress to acute MI.

Prinzmetal's, or variant, angina typically occurs at rest and results from coronary artery spasm.

Tracing the causes

Most often, angina pectoris results from atherosclerotic heart disease, which narrows coronary arteries and decreases coronary blood flow. Angina also can occur from other conditions that reduce coronary blood flow even when the coronary arteries are normal—for instance, aortic stenosis, hypotension, low blood volume, and hypertrophic cardiomyopathy.

WHAT TO LOOK FOR

If you suspect that your patient's chest pain is cardiac in origin, you'll need to intervene quickly to prevent a potentially life-threatening complication of myocardial ischemia. (See *Identifying the origin of chest pain,* pages 20 and 21.)

When assessing the patient, look for these general signs and symptoms of angina pectoris:

- substernal chest pain or discomfort, which may radiate to the neck, jaw, arms, or back; the patient may describe the pain as a squeezing, aching, or burning sensation or as heaviness, pressure, tightness, or even indigestion
- anxiety
- dyspnea
- weakness
- cold, clammy skin
- diaphoresis.

Other signs and symptoms vary with the type of angina. For instance, a patient with *stable angina* may have:

- mild to severe chest pain with a predictable pattern—usually brought on by meals, exertion, or stress—that lasts for 1 to 3 minutes but may persist up to 15 minutes; the pain may radiate to other areas of the body
- relief of pain with rest, removal of the provoking factor, or administration of a sublingual vasodilator, such as nitroglycerin

- ST-segment depression or T-wave changes on the ECG.

With *unstable angina*, the patient may have:
- more severe, longer-lasting chest pain than in stable angina
- chest pain that occurs at rest or with little exertion
- ST-segment elevation or T-wave changes on the ECG
- pain unrelieved by rest or medication.

Clinical findings in *Prinzmetal's* angina may include:
- chest pain at rest that isn't associated with increased physical demands and isn't relieved by nitroglycerin; pain usually resolves spontaneously
- transient ST-segment elevation.

WHAT TO DO IMMEDIATELY

If your patient's signs and symptoms suggest angina pectoris, follow these steps:
- Assess her pain using the PQRST approach. (See *PQRST approach to assessing chest pain*, page 22.)
- Check the patient's vital signs before and after administering prescribed nitrates.
- Obtain serial 12-lead ECGs and assess for ST-segment and T-wave changes.
- Begin continuous ECG monitoring for ischemia and arrhythmias.
- Enforce complete bed rest, and administer supplemental oxygen, if prescribed.
- Establish I.V. access and administer medications, as prescribed.
- Give prescribed nitrates, such as nitroglycerin sublingually (one tablet every 5 minutes to a maximum of three tablets, as needed) or I.V. nitroglycerin. Titrate the dosage to the patient's blood pressure and symptom relief.
- Administer morphine sulfate for pain relief and to reduce myocardial oxygen consumption, as prescribed.
- ➡ **NurseALERT** If your patient is receiving morphine, monitor her respiratory rate and depth carefully. Remember that morphine is a respiratory depressant.
- Administer calcium channel blockers, as prescribed, to reduce myocardial oxygen demands, enhance myocardial oxygen supply, and prevent coronary artery spasm.
- Administer beta blockers, if prescribed, to reduce myocardial oxygen needs.
- Give aspirin or other antiplatelet agents, as prescribed, to help prevent thrombus formation or further progression of a coronary artery thrombus.
- If your patient has unstable angina, expect to administer a continuous I.V. heparin infusion.

IDENTIFYING THE ORIGIN OF CHEST PAIN

Chest pain may signal a life-threatening emergency or reflect a less serious condition. If your patient complains of chest pain, focus your assessment on identifying the underlying cause so you can intervene immediately, if necessary. Use this chart to correlate the types of chest pain with clinical findings and probable causes.

Pain characteristics	Clinical findings	Alleviating factors	Probable cause
• Substernal heaviness, pressure, burning, or chest pain • May be severe • May radiate to shoulders, neck, jaws, arms, or back	• Dyspnea • Diaphoresis • Weakness • Anxiety • ECG changes (depressed or elevated ST segments, elevated T-wave changes)	• Rest • Nitroglycerin • Oxygen • Morphine • Calcium channel blockers	Angina pectoris
• Substernal heaviness, pressure, burning, or chest pain • May be severe • May radiate to shoulders, neck, jaws, arms, or back	• Diaphoresis • Nausea • Weakness • Anxiety • Pallor • Cardiac enzyme elevations • ECG changes (Q waves, inverted T wave, elevated ST segment)	• Nitroglycerin • Morphine • Thrombolytics • Rest • Oxygen	Myocardial infarction
• Substernal chest, abdominal, or back pain (depending on location of aneurysm)	• Hoarseness • Dysphagia • Cough • Distention of neck veins • Dyspnea • Pulsatile abdominal mass or bruit	• Blood pressure control • Surgery	Aortic aneurysm
• Severe stabbing, ripping, or tearing pain in anterior chest • May radiate to shoulders, neck, abdomen, back, or legs as it progresses	• New aortic murmur • Diminished or absent peripheral pulses • Tachycardia • Bilateral blood pressure differential • Altered level of consciousness • Paralysis • Paresthesias • Decreased bowel sounds • Oliguria	• Blood pressure control • Surgery • Analgesics	Aortic dissection
• Sharp, severe, substernal or left-sided chest pain • May radiate to shoulders, arms, neck, and back • Worsens with inspiration, lying down, coughing, swallowing, and trunk movement	• Fever • Friction rub • Dyspnea • Shallow respirations • ECG changes (elevated ST segment, inverted T wave)	• Leaning forward • High Fowler's position • Analgesics • Anti-inflammatory drugs • Antibiotics	Pericarditis

Pain characteristics	Clinical findings	Alleviating factors	Probable cause
• Severe, sharp chest pain	• Severe dyspnea • Hemoptysis • Anxiety • Diaphoresis • Accentuated P_2 (pulmonic component of S_2) • Tachycardia • Tachypnea • Decreased breath sounds	• Analgesics • Oxygen • Anticoagulants • Thrombolytics • Surgery	Pulmonary embolus
• Mild to severe, sharp or tearing unilateral chest pain	• Decreased breath sounds and impaired chest expansion on affected side • Dyspnea • Cyanosis • Tachycardia • Anxiety	• Chest tube insertion	Pneumothorax
• Sudden onset of severe sub-sternal chest pain at rest; may awaken patient from sleep at night • Pressure, burning, tightness, or squeezing sensation • May radiate to left arm, neck, jaws, or back	• Dyspnea • Vomiting	• Nitrates • Sedatives • Small, frequent feedings of soft foods • Surgery	Esophageal spasm
• Burning in chest or mid-epigastric area • May radiate upward • May occur with stress, consumption of food or alcohol, smoking, bending over, or lying down	• Heartburn • Regurgitation • Diaphoresis	• Antacids • Antisecretory agents • Sitting up • Avoidance of alcohol and smoking • Surgery	Hiatal hernia
• Severe to excruciating pain in lower chest around right rib margin • May radiate to back • May follow heavy meal or occur when lying down	• Tachycardia • Diaphoresis • Prostration • Fever • Nausea • Vomiting	• Analgesics • Surgery • Lithotripsy • Cholesterol solvents	Biliary colic in cholelithiasis
• Sharp, stabbing pain or sore-ness in rib cage or sternum • Worsens with deep inspira-tion or palpation • Does not radiate	• Shallow respirations • Diaphoresis • Possibly redness or swelling at pain site	• Analgesics • Steroids • Position changes	Costochondritis

PQRST APPROACH TO ASSESSING CHEST PAIN

Using a systematic approach can expedite your assessment of a patient's chest pain. The PQRST method described below groups major pain characteristics alphabetically by their first letter. When questioning the patient about her pain, focus on the key words denoted by the letters in this acronym.

P: PROVOCATIVE AND PALLIATIVE FACTORS
Find out what activities seem to *p*rovoke your patient's chest pain—for instance, physical exertion, rest, sleep, deep breathing, or coughing. Ask if a particular factor, such as rest, nitroglycerin use, or changing position, seems to *p*alliate (relieve) the pain.

Q: QUALITY
Next, elicit specific pain *q*ualities by asking the patient to describe the pain. Document her description in her own words, such as "sharp," "heavy," "burning," "aching," or "tightness." Ask if the pain is associated with other symptoms, such as sweating, nausea, shortness of breath, coughing, palpitations, and light-headedness.

R: REGION AND RADIATION
Hone in on the *r*egion of the pain and its *r*adiation pattern (if any). Ask the patient to point to the area where she experiences the pain. Inquire if she also experiences pain in her neck, jaws, back, or arms.

S: SEVERITY
Have your patient rank the *s*everity of her pain on a scale of 0 to 10, with 0 being no pain and 10 being the worst pain imaginable.

T: TIMING
Help your patient pin down the precise *t*iming of her chest pain by asking when the pain began, whether it came on suddenly or gradually, and if this is the first time she's ever had it.

WHAT TO DO NEXT
Once your patient's condition had stabilized, take these steps:
- Initiate long-acting nitrate therapy, as prescribed.
- Prepare your patient for cardiac catheterization or other diagnostic tests, if ordered, to determine the location and severity of heart disease and to guide treatment.
- If indicated, prepare your patient for a revascularization procedure to restore blood flow to coronary arteries. (See *Revascularization procedures.*)

FOLLOW-UP CARE
- Continue to assess your patient for chest pain and to evaluate the effectiveness of medications.
- Help the patient identify her risk factors for coronary artery disease and develop a plan for risk modification, such as weight loss, a low-cholesterol diet, exercise, smoking cessation, diabetes control, blood pressure reduction, and stress modification.
- If chest pain recurs, promptly evaluate its characteristics, check vital signs, and obtain a 12-lead ECG. Then notify the physician and administer nitroglycerin, as prescribed.

SPECIAL CONSIDERATIONS
- Check the expiration dates on nitroglycerin bottles on your unit, and discard expired bottles. Keep nitroglycerin tablets in their original light-resistant bottle; close the bottle tightly after each use.

TREATMENT OF CHOICE

REVASCULARIZATION PROCEDURES

If your patient has coronary artery disease, the physician may recommend a revascularization procedure to restore blood flow through the arteries to the myocardium. Such procedures include percutaneous transluminal coronary angioplasty (PTCA), coronary stent placement, atherectomy, laser angioplasty, and coronary artery bypass grafting (CABG). The choice of procedure depends on the patient's medical status and the extent of coronary artery blockage and accompanying myocardial tissue damage.

If your patient is scheduled for revascularization, be sure to explain the purpose of the procedure and tell her what to expect. After she returns from the procedure, assess her closely for signs and symptoms of possible complications.

PERCUTANEOUS TRANSLUMINAL ANGIOPLASTY

In PTCA, a balloon-tipped catheter is introduced through an artery (usually the femoral artery), advanced to the left side of the heart, and threaded into an artery narrowed by an atherosclerotic lesion. Then the balloon is inflated and the stenotic artery dilated.

PTCA can be done under local anesthetic, avoiding the need for chest incision, cardiopulmonary bypass, and a long hospital stay. Potential complications include coronary artery dissection, rupture, spasm, and restenosis (which may lead to infarction). Serious complications may necessitate emergency CABG.

CORONARY STENT PLACEMENT

A self-expanding, scaffold-like structure, a stent is inserted into a coronary artery with the aid of a balloon-tipped catheter. (In some cases, the artery is predilated by PTCA to prevent acute closure.) As the balloon inflates, the stent expands, compressing the atherosclerotic plaque and intimal flaps against the arterial wall. The balloon then is deflated and removed, leaving the stent in place.

Possible complications of coronary stent placement include stent thrombosis (which warrants anticoagulation therapy), reocclusion, hemorrhage, myocardial infarction, arrhythmias, arterial injury, and coronary artery spasm.

ATHERECTOMY

In atherectomy, a rotary cutter is used to remove an atherosclerotic plaque from a coronary artery. The plaque material may be dispersed into the circulation, collected and removed, or aspirated. Afterward, angioplasty may be done to smooth the intima.

Risks associated with atherectomy include hemorrhage, peripheral vascular complications, and acute coronary artery closure.

LASER ANGIOPLASTY

Laser angioplasty uses a laser-tipped catheter to vaporize an atherosclerotic plaque in a coronary artery. Vaporization makes the plaque less thrombogenic and welds together any fractures in the intimal wall. Laser angioplasty is still being perfected.

CORONARY ARTERY BYPASS GRAFTING

In CABG, one or more occluded coronary arteries are bypassed using grafts from the saphenous vein or internal mammary or radial arteries. CABG relieves symptoms and improves the quality of life for patients who have angina that's unresponsive to medical therapy.

- Understand that nitrate tolerance can develop. As prescribed, provide a nitrate-free period each day—preferably at night, unless your patient has a history of nocturnal angina.
- Discuss each prescribed medication with the patient, including its indications, dosage, administration schedule, and possible adverse effects.
- Teach your patient how to use and store nitroglycerin properly.

APPENDICITIS

Just below the cecum, at the start of the large intestine, extends a worm-like process called the vermiform appendix. Although its role is unknown, this small structure can create serious consequences if it ruptures or becomes inflamed.

Irritation of the appendix—typically from a kink, a stool pellet (fecalith), or some other obstruction—causes it to become inflamed, edematous, and ischemic. If the condition goes untreated, the appendix may become gangrenous.

If the appendix ruptures, it may cause potentially deadly peritonitis or sepsis. For 8 to 36 hours after the rupture, local vascular dilation, hyperemia, and increased capillary permeability lead to decreased vascular and intestinal fluid volume. To offset the fluid deficit, the body engages a systemic response that involves catecholamine release, increased secretion of antidiuretic hormone, and shunting of blood away from the GI and urinary systems. Eventually, bowel activity ceases.

An intestinal contaminant can spread throughout the entire peritoneum in 3 to 6 hours, aided by diaphragmatic movements and small changes in body position. Within 72 hours, the untreated patient typically develops septicemia, circulatory or respiratory failure, fluid and electrolyte imbalances, and renal failure. These complications may prove fatal.

Clearly, the inflamed appendix must be treated as quickly as possible before it ruptures. If rupture occurs, the treatment of choice is surgical removal with vigorous use of antibiotics and nasogastric and intestinal tubes to decompress and rest the GI tract.

WHAT TO LOOK FOR
Clinical findings for the patient with appendicitis may include:
- epigastric or periumbilical pain (earliest sign), later localizing to McBurney's point (midway between the right anterior iliac crest and the umbilicus)
- abdominal rigidity and guarding
- pain increased by movement, respirations, and coughing
- rebound tenderness
- anorexia
- nausea
- fever.

After rupture of the appendix, clinical findings may also include:
- abdominal pain more diffuse and less severe than before rupture
- hypoactive or absent bowel sounds
- vomiting
- temperature above 101° F (38.3° C)
- abdominal distention with bacterial peritonitis
- tachycardia with a weak pulse.

WHAT TO DO IMMEDIATELY
If you suspect your patient has appendicitis, notify the physician. Then take the following measures:
- Watch carefully for changes in the pain pattern and location, a sudden increase in temperature, and onset of vomiting.

➡ **NurseALERT** Keep in mind that a change in the location or character of the pain may suggest that the appendix has ruptured. Specifically, the patient may experience sharp, localized pain at the time of rupture. After rupture, the pain may become generalized and even subside completely. In addition to noting a change in the patient's description of his pain, you'll notice postural changes, increased guarding, and abdominal rigidity.

- Monitor the patient's vital signs (especially temperature, pulse rate, and blood pressure) to help track his hemodynamic status.
- Administer pain medication, as prescribed.
- Establish and maintain an I.V. access site, and prepare to administer isotonic fluid replacement, as prescribed, to maintain fluid and electrolyte balance. Don't give the patient anything by mouth.
- Prepare the patient for surgery, if indicated.
- If the appendix has ruptured, watch for signs and symptoms of hypovolemic shock and septicemia, including hypotension, tachycardia, fever, dyspnea, and diaphoresis.

WHAT TO DO NEXT
Once the initial crisis has passed, take these steps:
- Continue to monitor your patient's vital signs and temperature every 1 to 2 hours.
- Monitor hemodynamic parameters, as indicated.
- If rupture has occurred, elevate the head of the bed to help localize the infection and maximize chest excursion.
- Maintain a patent I.V. access site and replace fluids, as prescribed. Anticipate giving I.V. antibiotics to treat infection, as ordered.
- Prepare for possible placement of a nasogastric or an intestinal tube for gastric decompression. Assist with tube insertion, and connect the tube to a suction source, as indicated.
- Continue to assess the patient's pain level and pattern. Notify the physician right away if the pain changes.

FOLLOW-UP CARE
- After the patient returns from surgery, provide routine postoperative care. To reduce the risk of complications, encourage coughing, deep breathing, frequent turning, and early ambulation.
- Monitor the patient's vital signs at least every 4 hours; report a temperature above 100.4° F (38° C).
- Watch carefully for complications. For example, if the patient continues to have a fever, localized pain, and redness or warmth at the incision site, suspect an abscess around the site.
- Monitor bowel sounds, and routinely ask the patient if he has passed flatus or stool.
➡ **NurseALERT** Know that peristalsis stops when the appendix ruptures or the patient undergoes surgery. Also, fluid exudate secreted during the inflammatory process may promote the formation of fibrous adhe-

sions, which contribute to intestinal obstruction. Before discharge, monitor the patient carefully to make sure the bowel has resumed normal function.

SPECIAL CONSIDERATIONS

- Be sure to document the patient's condition carefully throughout his illness. Use a flowsheet to track vital signs, pain intensity, level of consciousness, and fluid intake and output.
- Because this patient may be rushed into surgery, you may have little time for patient teaching. Do your best to prepare the patient for surgery; describe the procedure, if possible.

ARTERIAL OCCLUSION

Acute arterial occlusion typically comes on abruptly, giving little or no warning of the tissue compromise to follow. If arterial blood flow is occluded, distal tissues become oxygen-deprived, ischemic, and infarcted. The extent of the ischemia and infarction depends on the organs and tissues involved.

A common cause of arterial occlusion is embolization of thrombi that form in the heart as a result of infective endocarditis, atrial fibrillation, myocardial infarction, heart failure, mitral valve disease, prosthetic heart valves, or cardiomyopathy. Emboli can also develop from atherosclerotic plaque, which breaks off and travels through the arterial circulation until it lodges in a smaller blood vessel. Arterial thrombosis causes acute occlusion at the site of atherosclerotic plaque. Procedures such as arteriography and arterial catheter insertion can also result in arterial occlusion.

How an embolus occludes an artery

Traveling through the arterial circulation, an embolus eventually lodges in an artery whose diameter is smaller than its own. Most often, it comes to rest at the point where the artery branches or has become narrowed from atherosclerosis. Arteries most commonly affected include the cerebral, coronary, mesenteric, and renal arteries and those of the extremities (such as the femoral artery).

Usually, an acute arterial occlusion can be reversed—at least to some extent. For instance, if the femoral artery becomes acutely occluded after cardiac catheterization, the surgeon can remove the clot and restore circulation to the extremity. With cerebrovascular accident (CVA) caused by an embolus, administering thrombolytic therapy within 3 to 6 hours of symptom onset is likely to restore some functions in the affected body area.

Thus, your keen awareness of signs and symptoms—and swift and accurate interventions—may help preserve your patient's body function or even save her life.

WHAT TO LOOK FOR

Signs and symptoms of acute arterial occlusion have a sudden onset and vary with the occlusion site. For instance, with an occlusion producing ischemia in an extremity, expect the classic "five Ps" in that extremity:

- pain (usually severe)
- pulselessness
- paresthesias
- pallor (and coldness)
- paralysis (see *Five Ps of neurovascular assessment,* page 28).
- ➡ **NurseALERT** Be aware that paralysis is a *late* sign of ischemia. By the time it appears, nerve damage may be irreversible. Even after blood flow is restored, the patient may continue to experience paralysis and ischemic neuropathy.

With an embolic CVA caused by acute occlusion of a cerebral artery, clinical findings may include sudden onset of:

- hemiparesis
- hemiplegia
- speech impairments, such as aphasia
- altered level of consciousness.

With a coronary artery embolism, you may detect characteristic evidence of acute myocardial infarction, such as:

- severe substernal chest pain
- anxiety
- dyspnea
- diaphoresis
- nausea
- vomiting.

Occlusion of the renal artery may lead to decreased urine output and elevated blood urea nitrogen and serum creatinine levels. If the mesenteric artery is involved, look for abdominal pain and vomiting.

WHAT TO DO IMMEDIATELY

If you suspect an acute arterial occlusion, notify the physician. Then take these immediate measures:

- Place the patient on bed rest.
- Administer heparin by continuous I.V. infusion, as prescribed, to prevent thrombus growth and inhibit embolization. Remember that the faster the ischemia resolves, the greater the chances for preserving function in the affected area. Typically, the physician prescribes a bolus dose of heparin I.V., followed by an infusion titrated to keep activated partial thromboplastin time (APTT) at $1\frac{1}{2}$ to 2 times the control level.

A

FIVE *Ps* OF NEUROVASCULAR ASSESSMENT

Acute arterial occlusion of an extremity can lead to permanent nerve and muscle damage—or even loss of the limb—unless the problem is detected and corrected promptly.

Remember to assess limbs bilaterally, comparing the affected limb to the unaffected one, and to evaluate above and below the occlusion site. Assess the unaffected limb first to establish a baseline.

To maintain an organized approach to neurovascular assessment, use the "five Ps" approach:

- *Pain.* If your patient complains of pain, ask her to describe its location, quality, and intensity. Have her rank its intensity on a scale of 0 to 10, with 0 representing no pain and 10 indicating the worst pain imaginable.
- *Pulses.* Check all pulses in the affected limb to identify those that are palpable. This establishes a baseline for determining if the patient's condition is deteriorating or improving with therapy. Be sure to note the rate and quality of the pulses.
- *Paresthesia.* Ask if the patient has experienced numbness, tingling, or decreased or absent sensa-

tion in an extremity. Tell her to report such symptoms immediately. Lightly touch her extremities and ask her to tell you when she feels your touch.
- *Pallor.* Assess the color and temperature of the extremities. Expect pallor and coolness below an arterial occlusion. To evaluate skin temperature, use the back of your hand. Check capillary refill by pressing on the nail bed firmly enough to produce blanching. Normally, the color returns to the nail bed within 3 seconds; a longer interval signifies reduced circulation in the extremity, possibly from an arterial occlusion.
- *Paralysis.* When assessing range of motion, note any deficits that may indicate nerve damage affecting motor function. To test extremity strength, ask the patient to push and pull against your resistance at each joint. If you suspect arterial occlusion of an upper extremity, test her grip strength too.

REPORT ABNORMALITIES
Document your assessment findings, and report any abnormalities or ominous trends to the physician immediately.

- As prescribed, administer a thrombolytic agent, such as urokinase (Abbokinase) or streptokinase (Kabikinase), to dissolve or lyse a newly formed clot. (See *Caring for your patient during thrombolytic therapy*.)
- ➡ **NurseALERT** Be aware that after successful thrombolytic therapy in an extremity, reperfusion can cause local tissue swelling. This in turn may lead to compartment syndrome, a condition in which severe swelling within a confined space cuts off blood flow and presses on nerves around the affected area. To avoid tissue necrosis, immediately report any pain, edema, or weakness in the affected limb. Also, remember that reperfusion arrhythmias may occur after thrombolytic therapy for coronary artery occlusion. To detect such arrhythmias, monitor your patient's heart rate and rhythm continuously and be prepared to administer an antiarrhythmic.

WHAT TO DO NEXT
After the initial crisis passes, follow these guidelines:
- If indicated, prepare your patient for an embolectomy or a thrombectomy. The surgeon may perform balloon angioplasty or an atherectomy under local anesthesia to treat embolic occlusions. In some cases, a thrombus is removed by a percutaneous endovascular technique, in which a wire is threaded through the occlusion during

TIPS AND TECHNIQUES

CARING FOR YOUR PATIENT DURING THROMBOLYTIC THERAPY

To lyse or dissolve a thrombus, the physician may order a thrombolytic agent, such as streptokinase or urokinase, which can be given I.V. or administered directly into the thrombus.

For direct administration, a catheter is inserted percutaneously into an artery during angiography. Once the catheter advances into the thrombus, the physician infuses the thrombolytic drug. Complete thrombus dissolution may take 24 to 48 hours.

During thrombolytic therapy, keep the patient on complete bed rest. As indicated, prepare her for angiography performed at specific intervals to assess therapeutic effectiveness.

Be aware that the thrombolytic agent lyses the thrombus but doesn't prevent new thrombi from forming. Therefore, the physician will probably prescribe heparin as well. Because thrombolytics carry the risk of hemorrhage, they may be contraindicated in some patients—for example, those with cerebral hemorrhage, severe hypertension, aortic dissection, active bleeding, or acute pericarditis and those who have recently undergone major surgery.

PROMOTING A SUCCESSFUL OUTCOME
If your patient will be receiving a thrombolytic agent, you can help promote therapeutic effectiveness and safety by taking the following steps.

Assess and monitor the patient closely
- Before therapy begins, obtain baseline activated partial thromboplastin time, prothrombin time, thrombin time, hematocrit, and platelet count. Monitor these values frequently throughout therapy.
- Obtain baseline vital signs. Monitor vital signs frequently during the course of therapy.
- Perform a baseline neurologic assessment, and monitor for changes that may signal intracranial hemorrhage.
- Assess for signs and symptoms of hemorrhage in other sites—tarry stools, hematuria, altered level of consciousness, lowered blood pressure, tachycardia, hematuria, back pain, epistaxis, bruising, petechiae, and decreasing hematocrit. Test all stools and emesis for occult blood.

Guard against trauma and bleeding
- Take steps to prevent trauma and bleeding, such as avoiding venous and arterial punctures and injections and avoiding taking rectal temperatures.
- Instruct the patient to brush her teeth gently with a soft-bristled toothbrush and to use an electric shaver rather than a razor.

Watch for allergic reactions
- Assess for allergic reactions to the thrombolytic agent, such as itching, rash, bronchospasm, fever, and chills. Remember that streptokinase is strongly antigenic and can induce anaphylaxis, especially in a patient who previously received the drug or had a recent streptococcal infection. Such a reaction can occur up to several days after streptokinase therapy.

A

angiography and laser atherectomy, atherectomy, or balloon angioplasty is performed.
- Assess your patient's clinical status, paying special attention to the organ or tissue involved in the occlusion. For instance, with femoral artery occlusion, perform frequent neurovascular checks of the legs, including pulses, paresthesia, paralysis, pallor, and pain.
- After an embolic CVA, perform frequent neurologic assessments, checking level of consciousness, pupillary response to light, reflexes, and motor and sensory functions.
- Monitor APTT if your patient's receiving I.V. heparin. Report any value outside the therapeutic range ($1\frac{1}{2}$ to 2 times control). If she's receiving thrombolytic therapy, monitor coagulation studies and report any values outside the desired therapeutic levels.

- If the patient has received heparin or thrombolytics, assess for signs and symptoms of bleeding, including blood in the stool or urine, decreased blood pressure, tachycardia, back pain, and changes in level of consciousness. Also monitor APTT, prothrombin time (PT), and hematocrit; report abnormal values.
- If your patient continues to be at risk for embolus formation, give oral anticoagulants (such as warfarin [Coumadin]), as prescribed. Adjust the dose, as prescribed, to achieve a PT of 1½ to 2 times control or an international normalized ratio of 2 to 3½. Discontinue heparin, as prescribed, when blood levels of oral anticoagulants become therapeutic.

FOLLOW-UP CARE

- Continue to monitor your patient's neurovascular, neurologic, renal, and cardiovascular status.
- Monitor laboratory test results and report abnormal values.
- If the patient has undergone surgery, restrict her activities, as appropriate.
- Assess the surgical incision for hemorrhage and signs and symptoms of infection.

SPECIAL CONSIDERATIONS

- Once arterial blood flow has been restored, stay alert for signs and symptoms of reocclusion.
- Know that after acute arterial occlusion caused by thrombosis of an atherosclerotic vessel, the patient may need more complicated arterial surgery, such as endarterectomy or bypass grafting, to improve blood flow. Explain the ordered procedure.
- Tell the patient and her family what has happened, and explain the treatments she has received. Help her identify risk factors for atherosclerosis (such as smoking, hyperlipidemia, and poorly controlled diabetes mellitus) and devise a plan for risk modification.
- Teach the patient about signs and symptoms of arterial occlusion, and tell her to report these immediately.
- If the patient will be discharged on oral anticoagulants, stress the importance of having frequent blood tests to determine the appropriate dosage. Provide instruction on such topics as oral anticoagulant therapy, dietary restrictions, bleeding prevention strategies, and monitoring for bleeding. Urge her to carry medical identification at all times.

ASTHMA ATTACK

A person with asthma experiences recurrent episodes of dyspnea, wheezing, coughing, and excessive mucus production. Triggered by such factors as allergens, infection, cold air, exercise, and emotional stress, acute asthma attacks are the most common reason asthmatic patients seek urgent medical treatment.

Although the exact mechanism underlying asthma is unknown, researchers have identified important features of the disease. For example, patients with asthma tend to have a family history of allergic signs and symptoms and an immunoglobulin E response to environmental antigens.

Features of the disease include:
- an allergen, such as mold spores, or a nonallergen, such as cold air, which causes an airway inflammation response
- histamine and leukotrienes that are released from mast cells and a bronchospasm
- abnormal levels of cyclic adenosine monophosphate that accumulate in smooth muscles of bronchioles (an important intracellular trigger for muscle activation)
- an increase in the number of immunomodulator cells in the airways, which contributes to inflammation.

In an acute asthma attack, these and other features combine to constrict the bronchioles, promote mucosal edema, impede expiratory airflow, and cause production of mucous plugs that further obstruct airflow. (See *Inside an asthmatic bronchiole*, page 32.)

Over time, the work of breathing becomes increasingly difficult, intrathoracic pressure increases, and venous return diminishes. These changes may lead to cardiac instability, respiratory acidosis, and respiratory failure. Hypercapnia and hypoxemia (both late signs of asthma) cause a decreased level of consciousness and loss of airway protection.

Usually, acute asthma attacks subside when the patient receives inhaled or nebulized beta agonists. For severe attacks, treatment also may include glucocorticoids and inhaled anticholinergics to reduce inflammation and open spastic airways. By responding rapidly with the most appropriate treatment, you can help minimize the impact of an acute asthma attack.

WHAT TO LOOK FOR
Typically, the asthmatic patient has a history of previous treatment for acute attacks. During an acute asthma attack, clinical findings may include:
- severe dyspnea, tachypnea
- intercostal muscle retractions and nasal flaring
- loss of chest and abdominal synchrony with respirations
- anxious, fearful, wide-eyed facial expression
- difficulty speaking more than a few words between breaths
- diaphoresis
- diminished peak expiratory flow rate (PEFR)

A

PATHOPHYSIOLOGY

INSIDE AN ASTHMATIC BRONCHIOLE

In a normal bronchiole, the unobstructed airway allows gas to pass to the lungs without effort or awareness.

During an asthma attack, contact with an allergen results in release of histamine and related substances in the bronchiole. These chemicals cause bronchial smooth muscles to contract, leading to swollen mucous membranes and copious mucus buildup in the bronchiole.

This process causes epithelial injury and edema, changes in mucociliary function, reduced clearance of respiratory tract secretions, and greater airway responsiveness. As expiratory airflow diminishes and gas is trapped in the airways, alveoli become hyperinflated. Increased airway resistance then induces labored breathing.

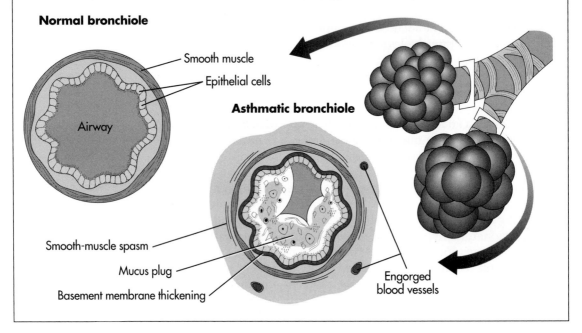

Normal bronchiole

Smooth muscle

Epithelial cells

Airway

Asthmatic bronchiole

Smooth-muscle spasm

Mucus plug

Basement membrane thickening

Engorged blood vessels

- pulsus paradoxus
- cyanosis (peripheral, progressing to central)
- respiratory distress, wheezing, and sensation of chest tightness increase as attack progresses
- ➡ **NurseALERT** Know that cessation of wheezing during an acute asthma attack may indicate worsening distress. The patient's airways may have narrowed even more, allowing so little air to pass that he stops wheezing.

WHAT TO DO IMMEDIATELY
If you think that your patient is having an acute asthma attack, maintain an adequate airway and notify the physician. Then carry out the following interventions:
- Continue to assess and maintain the patient's airway, breathing, and circulation.

- Connect the patient to a cardiac monitor, noninvasive blood pressure cuff, and arterial oxygen saturation (SaO$_2$) device for continuous monitoring.
- Administer supplemental oxygen by face mask, as prescribed, to keep SaO$_2$ above 95%.
- ➡ **NurseALERT** Use caution when giving oxygen to an asthmatic patient. Administering 100% oxygen to increase SaO$_2$ may promote absorption atelectasis. In this state, all oxygen is absorbed, leaving little or no nitrogen to keep alveoli open.
- Position the patient with the head of the bed elevated at least 45 degrees to promote optimal chest expansion.
- Establish I.V. access and administer fluids, as ordered and indicated. Be sure to give fluids slowly—overhydration can increase interstitial fluid buildup and worsen small-airway obstruction.
- Perform a baseline assessment of the patient's respiratory effort, speaking ability (sentence length), and PEFR, as ordered. Auscultate lungs for breath sounds and obtain a blood sample for arterial blood gas (ABG) analysis, as indicated.
- As prescribed, administer a nebulized or an inhaled beta agonist, such as albuterol (Proventil), if your patient doesn't show severe respiratory distress and appears alert, oriented, and hemodynamically stable.
- After each treatment, reassess the patient's vital signs, breath sounds, speech pattern, PEFR, respiratory pattern, wheezing, and general appearance.
- ➡ **NurseALERT** During therapy, check closely for indications of acute respiratory failure, which can emerge rapidly from mucous plugging and diaphragmatic fatigue. Also watch for cardiac arrhythmias caused by beta agonists or worsening hypoxemia.
- After the first nebulized or inhaled treatment, prepare for glucocorticoid administration, if indicated. For mild to moderately severe asthma, anticipate giving oral steroids (prednisone, 0.5 to 1.0 mg/kg for adults; 2 mg/kg for children), as prescribed. For severe asthma, anticipate giving I.V. steroids (methylprednisolone, 125 mg initially for adults; 2 mg/kg for children).
- If the patient doesn't improve, expect the physician to order another bronchodilator treatment as soon as you finish giving the first one. Prepare to give a beta agonist and an anticholinergic, such as atropine or ipratropium bromide (Atrovent), especially if the patient has significant mucus. Repeat the anticholinergic dose every 4 to 6 hours.
- If your patient hasn't improved after three treatments, expect to obtain repeat ABG values to assess pH and partial pressure of arterial carbon dioxide (PaCO$_2$). Look for metabolic and respiratory acidosis, and continue to monitor serial ABG values, as indicated.
- ➡ **NurseALERT** Anticipate intubation if your patient continues to wheeze and have difficulty breathing even as a low PaCO$_2$ begins to rise and a high pH begins to fall. Persistence of these problems means that he's in respiratory failure and heading for respiratory arrest as muscles grow increasingly fatigued.

WHAT TO DO NEXT

Once the patient's condition stabilizes, take these steps:

- Continue to check vital signs, respiratory pattern, breath sounds, speech pattern, PEFR, wheezing, and general appearance after each treatment.
- Remember that inability to breathe is a terrifying experience. Throughout your care, provide the patient with plenty of reassurance and emotional support and stay with him during an acute attack.
- Continue to monitor the patient's fluid balance by assessing fluid intake and output and skin turgor. Be sure to include insensible fluid losses in your calculation.
- If bronchospasm doesn't resolve or if metabolic or respiratory acidosis occurs, assist with endotracheal intubation. Expect this situation to occur in about 1 of every 100 asthmatic patients.
- Watch carefully for the development of status asthmaticus, and intervene appropriately as needed. (See *Responding to status asthmaticus with medications*.)

FOLLOW-UP CARE

- If indicated, obtain a sputum specimen (for Gram stain and culture and sensitivity) to assess whether bacteria may have caused the asthma attack and to guide antibiotic therapy.
- In severe asthma with sputum containing many white cells, expect to give an antibiotic even if no bacteria are present. Immunodeficient patients (such as patients who test positive for the human immunodeficiency virus and recipients of solid organ transplants) also may receive antiviral therapy, antifungal therapy, or both until culture results are available.
- Continue giving medications, as prescribed, to reverse bronchospasm. As the patient improves, anticipate switching from nebulized drug forms to inhaled forms given by way of a metered-dose inhaler.
- Obtain fingerstick blood glucose levels if the patient is on steroid therapy.
- Expect to switch from I.V. to oral corticosteroid therapy. Before discharge, give prednisone, 0.5 to 1.0 mg/kg/day, as prescribed.

SPECIAL CONSIDERATIONS

- As prescribed and after your patient is stabilized, be prepared to give ancillary agents, such as cromolyn sodium nasal spray or inhaler (Intal Aerosol Spray), to reduce your patient's responsiveness to inhaled allergens. Cromolyn sodium stabilizes mast cell and eosinophil membranes.
- Before discharge, teach the patient and family about asthma, including possible triggers and ways to avoid them, signs and symptoms of an impending attack, and measures to minimize the severity of an attack.
- Show the patient how to evaluate PEFR at home.
- Reinforce the need to comply with therapy to prevent future acute asthma attacks.

A

TREATMENT OF CHOICE

RESPONDING TO STATUS ASTHMATICUS WITH MEDICATIONS

If your patient's acute asthma attack continues or worsens despite standard treatment, he's probably in status asthmaticus—an emergency that can lead to acidosis, respiratory failure, and, possibly, death.

In most cases, the treatment of choice for status asthmaticus involves the administration of combined medications, such as those described below.

MEDICATIONS
Bronchodilators
If an inhaled beta agonist doesn't halt bronchospasm, expect to give albuterol (Proventil; most common), isoetharine (Bronkosol), isoproterenol (Isuprel), or metaproterenol (Alupent) by continuous nebulization.

Epinephrine
For a patient under age 35 who has persistent, severe bronchospasm, expect the physician to order epinephrine (0.3 ml of 1:1,000 epinephrine) subcutaneously. (In older patients, this treatment can increase the risk of cardiac arrhythmias.)

Glucocorticoids
In addition, the physician may prescribe I.V. glucocorticoid therapy—typically, methylprednisolone (Solu-Medrol; 125 mg as a loading dose, followed by 60 mg every 6 to 8 hours, until the physician prescribes a tapering dose) or hydrocortisone (Solu-Cortef; 100 mg every 8 hours, until the physician prescribes a tapering dose). Remember to check the patient's blood glucose levels by fingerstick while he's receiving steroids.

Magnesium
Even for patients without a magnesium deficiency, the physician may prescribe a loading dose of magnesium as adjunctive therapy. Magnesium may help reverse refractory bronchospasm by relaxing bronchial smooth muscle.

Methylxanthines
As prescribed, give methylxanthine agents, such as theophylline (Bronkodyl). The patient may receive a loading dose of 5.6 mg/kg, followed by a continuous I.V. infusion at 0.5 to 0.9 mg/kg/hour, titrated to relieve bronchospasm and reduce airway pressure. Be sure to check serum theophylline levels daily, and watch for adverse neurologic reactions, especially tremors, anxiety, and seizures.

Keep in mind that certain antibiotics (erythromycin, clarithromycin, azithromycin), histamine-2 blockers, and anticonvulsants raise theophylline levels and pose the danger of toxicity by decreasing hepatic metabolism of theophylline.

ENDOTRACHEAL INTUBATION
If drug therapy proves ineffective or the patient deteriorates into respiratory failure, he may need endotracheal intubation and mechanical ventilation. If prescribed, administer sedatives, a neuromuscular blocker, or both to support ventilation.

CAREFUL MONITORING OF PATIENT
Throughout treatment, monitor the patient closely for changes in respiratory status and lung function. Stay especially alert for adverse effects of treatment, including tachycardia, arrhythmias, tremors, and hyperglycemia. Also, because the patient will be receiving multiple drugs, watch for possible drug interactions and incompatibilities.

ATRIAL FIBRILLATION

Normally, the sinoatrial node in the wall of the right atrium acts as the heart's pacemaker. This specialized group of cells depolarizes rhythmically, causing the heart muscle to contract at a steady, normal rate.

In atrial fibrillation, abnormal impulses arise from many atrial sites, causing disorganized electrical activity rather than steady, rhythmic beating. The atria fibrillate, or quiver, rather than contract normally. In some cases of atrial fibrillation, more than 350 atrial impulses may reach the atrioventricular (AV) node. The AV node can conduct only 100 to 180 impulses per minute (beats/minute) to the ventricles. The AV node selectively blocks many of the excessive atrial impulses from reaching the ventricles. Because the AV node blocks these impulses in an unpredictable and irregular pattern, the ventricles in turn respond in an irregular rhythm. Also, because the atria don't contract when they fibrillate, they can't provide an atrial kick to force remaining blood from the atria into the ventricles. As a result, stroke volume declines and cardiac output may drop by up to one-third.

Atrial fibrillation can be acute or chronic; patients with chronic atrial fibrillation are able to maintain normal or near normal cardiac output, provided their heart rate remains controlled (usually less than 100 beats/minute). When atrial fibrillation is acute, or when the heart rate is higher than 100 beats/minute, cardiac output may drop precipitously. Depending on the length of time in atrial fibrillation and the size of the atrial chambers, treatment should be started to establish a normal sinus rhythm.

Atrial fibrillation is associated with a high risk for embolic stroke. That's because blood pools in the atria, increasing the risk of thrombus formation and embolization—especially to the cerebral and pulmonary vasculature.

If your patient has atrial fibrillation, be prepared to intervene to help her cope with the effects of decreased cardiac output and hypotension. Without prompt treatment to slow the ventricular rate, restore atrial contractions, and establish a normal sinus rhythm, she could become severely hypotensive and progress to shock and even death.

Risk factors
Patients with cardiomyopathy, coronary artery disease, heart failure, hypertensive heart disease, pericarditis, rheumatic heart disease, Wolff-Parkinson-White (WPW) syndrome, and thyrotoxicosis are prone to atrial fibrillation. You may also see atrial fibrillation in patients with healthy hearts who are fatigued or under unusual stress and in those who are heavy users of alcohol, caffeine, cigarettes, or cocaine.

WHAT TO LOOK FOR
Clinical findings for a patient with atrial fibrillation may include:
- characteristic ECG findings (see *Recognizing atrial fibrillation*)
- irregular pulse
- abnormal pulse rate, usually elevated
- complaints of palpitations, skipped heartbeats, and dizziness
- peripheral pulse slower than the apical pulse, known as pulse deficit
- hypotension
- confusion
- reduced cardiac output
- decreased urine output.

WHAT TO DO IMMEDIATELY
If your patient is experiencing intolerable symptoms from atrial fibrillation, follow these steps:
- Check her vital signs and watch for hypotension.

RECOGNIZING ATRIAL FIBRILLATION

In atrial fibrillation, several sites of atrial irritability trigger a rapid succession of abnormal impulses. These impulses take over the role of the sinoatrial (SA) node as the heart's pacemaker. The atrioventricular (AV) node usually blocks enough atrial impulses to maintain a normal ventricular rate.

The illustration below shows how atrial fibrillation affects electrical conduction in the heart. The normal atrial conduction pathway appears in black; the abnormal atrial conduction pathways appear in color.

The waveform shows ECG features of atrial fibrillation, which include irregular QRS complexes, a wavy baseline, and indiscernible P waves. Typically, the atrial rate is 350 to 500 beats/minute, although indiscernible P waves make this rate impossible to measure on an ECG strip.

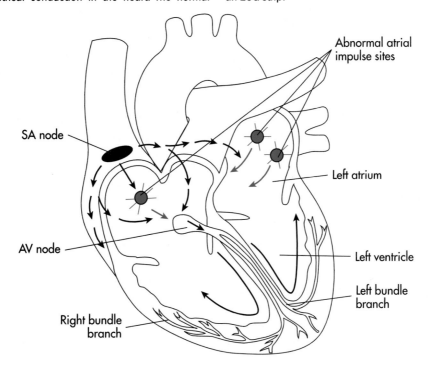

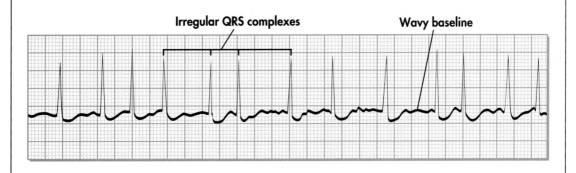

- Begin continuous ECG monitoring.
- Obtain a 12-lead ECG, as indicated.
- Insert an I.V. line and maintain I.V. access.
- Administer supplemental oxygen, as indicated.
- If your patient's ventricular rate exceeds 150 beats/minute and she is symptomatic, prepare her for synchronized cardioversion. (See *Caring for your patient during synchronized cardioversion.*)

➡ **NurseALERT** Because of the increased risk for embolism, a patient with chronic atrial fibrillation is likely to begin anticoagulant therapy before undergoing cardioversion.

- Administer drugs, such as digoxin (Lanoxin), procainamide (Pronestyl), propranolol (Inderal), or quinidine (Quinora), as prescribed.

➡ **NurseALERT** If your patient has WPW syndrome along with atrial fibrillation, *don't* administer digoxin to treat a rapid ventricular rate. In WPW, atrial impulses are conducted to the ventricles through an accessory pathway. This puts the patient at risk for reentrant tachycardia because the pathway can conduct impulses back to the atria and allows impulses to travel faster through it to the ventricles. In this patient, digoxin may induce ventricular fibrillation by decreasing conduction through the AV node and increasing it across the accessory pathway.

WHAT TO DO NEXT
Once the patient is stable, take the following steps:

- Assess for signs and symptoms of cerebral embolism (such as an altered level of consciousness, hemiplegia, hemiparesis, and aphasia) and pulmonary embolism (such as dyspnea, chest pain, hemoptysis, and crackles).
- Monitor your patient's heart rate and rhythm. As ordered, adjust antiarrhythmic drug doses to maintain a ventricular rate between 60 and 100 beats/minute.
- Continue to assess your patient's hemodynamic status, vital signs, breath sounds, skin color and temperature, and complaints of dyspnea, chest pain, and dizziness.
- Keep in mind that a hemodynamically stable patient may receive anticoagulants for 2 to 3 weeks before undergoing pharmacologic or electrical cardioversion. As needed, teach her how and why to take these medications.
- As prescribed, give other antianginals and antiarrhythmics, possibly including verapamil (Isoptin), diltiazem (Cardizem), and amiodarone (Cordarone).
- If your patient has chronic atrial fibrillation, she may need catheter ablation therapy, in which a catheter with an electrode tip destroys the AV node or bundle of His. If so, you'll need to teach her about the permanent ventricular pacemaker she'll receive after the procedure.

TIPS AND TECHNIQUES

CARING FOR YOUR PATIENT
DURING SYNCHRONIZED CARDIOVERSION

If your patient has symptomatic atrial fibrillation that doesn't respond to chemical cardioversion or that causes hemodynamic instability, the physician may use electrical synchronized cardioversion to restore a normal sinus rhythm. This procedure also may be useful in other tachyarrhythmias, such as paroxysmal supraventricular tachycardia and atrial flutter.

HOW SYNCHRONIZED CARDIOVERSION WORKS

Synchronized cardioversion delivers an electrical shock to the myocardium at the peak of the R wave, depolarizing it so that the sinoatrial node can take over as the heart's pacemaker when myocardial cells repolarize.

Although it has the potential benefit of restoring a sinus rhythm, cardioversion can also increase the risk of embolization in patients who have atrial fibrillation once a normal rhythm is restored. The physician may recommend 2-D echocardiography to assess for the presence of thrombus within the atrial chambers.

In addition, delivering a shock on the T wave would interrupt repolarization, possibly triggering ventricular tachycardia or fibrillation.

PREPARING FOR CARDIOVERSION

In most cases, you'll assist the physician in performing cardioversion. In an emergency, nurses with specialized training may perform this procedure at the bedside in a monitored setting.

- Explain the procedure to the patient and family. Encourage them to express their concerns.
- Make sure the patient has signed a consent form.
- If possible and if appropriate, withhold oral intake for 6 to 8 hours before cardioversion.
- Have the crash cart with resuscitation equipment in the patient's room.
- Obtain a 12-lead ECG.
- Insert an I.V. line.
- Give supplemental oxygen, if indicated and prescribed, before the procedure, but remove it during the procedure.
- Monitor the patient's blood pressure with an automatic device. Monitor oxygen saturation by pulse oximetry, if appropriate.
- Check the patient's vital signs.

- Withhold medications before the procedure, as ordered.
- Give sedatives, such as diazepam (Valium) or midazolam (Versed), as indicated and prescribed.
- Place the patient in a supine position.

DURING THE PROCEDURE

- Turn on the defibrillator and set it to the synchronous discharge mode.
- Apply the leads to your patient's chest. Find a lead that allows you to see tall QRS complexes on the oscilloscope. Make sure that the defibrillator senses each QRS complex and that the sync indicator flashes with each beat.
- Apply paste liberally to the paddles, or apply conductive gel pads to the patient's chest.
- Set the energy level as ordered. You'll use the lowest amount of energy (joules) first (usually 50 joules), followed by higher levels if the initial shock doesn't convert the rhythm.
- Place the paddles on your patient's chest, to the right of the sternum in the second intercostal space and on the left midclavicular line in the fifth intercostal space.
- Make sure everyone is clear of the patient's bed before discharging the paddles.
- Hold the paddles in place and press the discharge button. Keep the paddles on the patient's chest until the machine discharges the shock. The machine will wait until it synchronizes with the R wave.

AFTER THE PROCEDURE

- Assess your patient's ECG, level of consciousness, respiratory status, and vital signs frequently.
- Obtain a 12-lead ECG.
- Know that even when successful, synchronized cardioversion may increase the risk of embolization in a patient with atrial fibrillation. Therefore, be sure to evaluate your patient for signs and symptoms of systemic and pulmonary emboli. As prescribed, administer anticoagulants.
- Administer antiarrhythmic medications, as indicated.
- Check the patient's chest for signs of electrical burns, and if present, notify the physician and discuss treatment options.

FOLLOW-UP CARE
- Monitor serum drug levels to avoid toxicity. Closely assess for signs and symptoms of digitalis toxicity.

- Continue to administer antiarrhythmic drugs, as prescribed, and assess and report any adverse effects.
- Monitor your patient's prothrombin time (PT) if she's receiving an oral anticoagulant. Adjust the dose, as prescribed, to maintain the PT at 1½ to 2 times the control or an international normalized ratio of 2 to 3.

SPECIAL CONSIDERATIONS
- Be aware that an increased PT puts elderly or hypertensive patients at increased risk for cerebral hemorrhage and other injuries. Monitor such patients carefully.
- Instruct your patient how to take her pulse at home, and urge her to report changes in heart rate or rhythm. Caution her to notify the physician if her heart rate is less than 60.
- Teach the patient how to identify the signs and symptoms of digitalis toxicity. Instruct her to forgo her daily dose and notify the physician at once if any of those signs or symptoms develops. Urge her to have her serum digoxin levels monitored on the schedule established by the physician.
- Explain the importance of taking potassium supplements, if prescribed.
- Teach your patient how to take oral anticoagulants at home and how to prevent and detect bleeding. Review the signs and symptoms to report immediately, such as blood in the stool or urine.
- Discuss factors that may trigger atrial fibrillation. As needed, help the patient reduce her risk for this arrhythmia by stopping smoking, restricting her intake of alcohol and caffeine, and reducing stress. Also discuss the dangers of cocaine use; if this is a problem, refer her to a substance abuse rehabilitation program.

AV BLOCK, THIRD-DEGREE

In third-degree atrioventricular (AV) block, also called complete heart block, the atria and ventricles beat independently. Although impulses form in the sinoatrial (SA) node, they are not conducted from the atria to the ventricles.

The conduction block may occur in the AV node, bundle of His, or right or left bundle branches. Usually, a ventricular escape rhythm is present; in this situation, the ventricle assumes control because the rate set by the SA or AV node is blocked. Depending on where the escape rhythm arises, the QRS complex may be narrow, as in a junctional rhythm, or wide, as in a ventricular rhythm.

A block that originates above the bundle of His may result from increased parasympathetic tone, such as from:
- inferior-wall myocardial infarction (MI)
- drugs, such as digoxin (Lanoxin), propranolol (Inderal), or verapamil (Isoptin)

- hypoxia
- rheumatic fever
- postoperative complications of mitral valve surgery.

A block originating at or below the bundle of His usually stems from an extensive anterior-wall MI or a diseased conduction system.

The seriousness of the patient's condition depends on his response to a slow ventricular rate and the stability of the escape rhythm. With a junctional escape rhythm, for example, he may have no symptoms. This rhythm usually is stable, with the block in the AV node. A ventricular escape rhythm, on the other hand, tends to be slow and less stable. This places the patient at high risk for decreased cardiac output, especially if he already has compromised output from MI, heart failure, or shock.

WHAT TO LOOK FOR
Regardless of the type of escape rhythm present, the patient may be unable to tolerate a slower-than-normal heart rate or a decrease in cardiac output. Be alert for the following clinical findings:
- slow peripheral pulse rate (typically below 40 beats/minute)
- regular pulse
- decreased cardiac output
- hypotension, syncope, dizziness
- decreased urine output
- altered level of consciousness
- chest pain
- decreased cardiac output
- Adams-Stokes attacks (sudden, recurrent episodes of loss of consciousness, possibly accompanied by seizures)
- characteristic ECG findings (see *Recognizing AV blocks*, pages 42 and 43).

WHAT TO DO IMMEDIATELY
If your patient has a third-degree heart block and is symptomatic, establish and maintain a patent airway and ensure adequate breathing and circulation. Then notify the physician and take these measures:
- Begin continuous ECG monitoring.
- Obtain a 12-lead ECG.
- Administer supplemental oxygen, as needed and prescribed.
- Assess your patient's hemodynamic status, including vital signs, heart and breath sounds, skin color and temperature, capillary refill, level of consciousness, and urine output.
- If the patient is hypotensive, position him flat.
- Establish and maintain I.V. access for emergency drug administration.
- Administer atropine, epinephrine, and dopamine, as prescribed, to support the patient's heart rate and blood pressure until temporary pacemaker insertion. Be aware that transcutaneous pacing may be used until a transvenous pacemaker can be inserted.

RECOGNIZING AV BLOCKS

Your patient with first-degree atrioventricular (AV) block could progress to more serious degrees of AV block. Use the information below to help track his condition.

FIRST-DEGREE AV BLOCK

Rate: 60 to 100 beats/minute
Rhythm: Regular
P wave: Always followed by a QRS complex
PR interval: Greater than 0.20 second
QRS complex: Normal (0.06 to 0.10 second)

Possible causes: Acute inferior myocardial infarction (MI), beta blockers, digitalis toxicity, encainide, flecainide, hyperthyroidism, myocarditis, rheumatic heart disease, verapamil (I.V.)
Usual treatment: None required; physician may reduce dosage of or discontinue beta blocker, flecainide, encainide, or verapamil

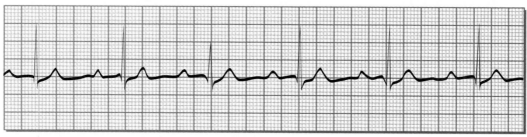

First-degree AV block with prolonged PR interval. Note that a QRS complex follows each P wave.

SECOND-DEGREE AV BLOCK, MOBITZ TYPE I (WENCKEBACH)

Rate: Atrial rate 60 to 100 beats/minute; ventricular rate slower
Rhythm: Irregular
P wave: Not always followed by a QRS complex
PR interval: Lengthens until P wave isn't conducted; cycle repeats after dropped QRS complex

QRS complex: Normal
Possible causes: Beta blockers, digitalis toxicity, inferior MI, ischemic cardiac disease
Usual treatment: None required for asymptomatic patient; for symptomatic patient, physician may stop digoxin, prescribe atropine, or insert pacemaker

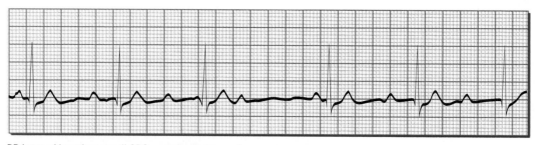

PR interval lengthens until QRS complex is dropped.

SECOND-DEGREE AV BLOCK, MOBITZ TYPE II

Rate: Atrial rate 60 to 100 beats/minute; ventricular rate slower

Rhythm: Irregular

P wave: Intermittently nonconducted, occurring in ratios (2:1, 3:1, and so on)

PR interval: Constant; conducted beats 0.12 to 0.20 second or longer

QRS complex: Normal or prolonged, from bundle branch block

Possible causes: Acute anterior MI, atherosclerotic heart disease, digitalis toxicity, Lenègre's disease, Lev's disease, rheumatic heart disease

Usual treatment: ECG monitoring to detect progression to complete heart block. Symptomatic patient requires pacemaker; physician may prescribe atropine, epinephrine, isoproterenol, or dopamine to increase heart rate until pacemaker can be inserted

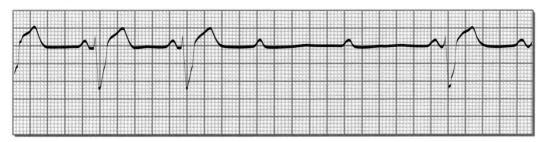

Nonconducted P waves without lengthening of PR interval. Note normal PR interval on conducted beats.

THIRD-DEGREE (COMPLETE) AV BLOCK

Rate: Atrial rate 60 to 100 beats/minute; ventricular rate usually 20 to 60 beats/minute, depending on location of escape rhythm

Rhythm: Regular, but with asynchronous atrial and ventricular rhythms

P wave: Not related to QRS complex

PR interval: No association between atrial and ventricular rhythms

QRS complex: Normal if from AV junction, wide (greater than 0.12 second) if from below bundle of His

Possible causes: Amyloidosis, cardiomyopathy, coronary artery disease, fibrosis or calcification of cardiac conduction system, myocarditis, open-heart surgery, Lenègre's disease, Lev's disease, scleroderma

Usual treatment: Emergency temporary pacemaker insertion; physician may prescribe atropine, epinephrine, or dopamine to increase heart rate and blood pressure until pacemaker can be inserted

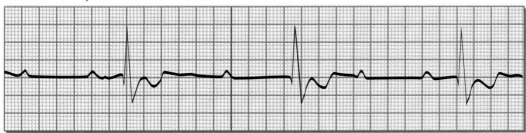

PR interval varies, and P waves are unrelated to QRS complexes.

➡ **NurseALERT** Use caution if administering isoproterenol (Isuprel). Although included in the advanced cardiac life support algorithm for bradycardia, this drug may worsen myocardial ischemia and heart failure by increasing myocardial oxygen demands and causing peripheral vasodilation. Also avoid giving isoproterenol with epinephrine; this combination can be fatal. Finally, remember that atropine, epinephrine, and isoproterenol are contraindicated in patients with narrow-angle glaucoma because these drugs may increase intraocular pressure and lead to vision loss.

- Prepare your patient for temporary pacemaker insertion. (See *Understanding temporary pacemakers.*)
- Keep the emergency cart nearby.

WHAT TO DO NEXT

Once the initial crisis eases, take the following steps:

- Continue to monitor your patient's ECG. Be sure to assess heart rate and rhythm, P waves, PR interval, and QRS complex.
- If your patient has received a temporary pacemaker, assess for appropriate sensing, capture, and pacing.
- Monitor the patient's vital signs, heart and breath sounds, level of consciousness, and urine output frequently. Ask him to tell you if he has shortness of breath, palpitations, chest pain, or dizziness.
- Monitor the patient's oxygen saturation using pulse oximetry or arterial blood gas analysis.

FOLLOW-UP CARE

- If indicated, prepare your patient for permanent pacemaker insertion—even if he's stable and asymptomatic—to prevent Adams-Stokes syndrome. Remember that Adams-Stokes syndrome results from a drop in cardiac output during transitory episodes of heart block or bradycardia. In this syndrome, the patient experiences sudden attacks of altered level of consciousness, syncope, or seizures.
- If the patient has a temporary pacemaker, continue to assess for proper sensing, capture, and pacing. Observe the pacemaker insertion site for signs and symptoms of infection, and provide appropriate care for the site. Take measures to prevent conduction of electric current to the pacemaker.
- If your patient complains of a dry mouth after receiving atropine, provide sugarless hard candy or gum or have him rinse and moisten his mouth with water.

SPECIAL CONSIDERATIONS

- If your patient has had Adams-Stokes attacks or is at risk for them, institute seizure precautions according to your facility's policy. During a seizure, intervene to prevent injury.

UNDERSTANDING TEMPORARY PACEMAKERS

A patient who has a cardiac conduction problem or whose heart can't initiate an impulse on its own may need a temporary pacemaker. Patients who may be candidates for temporary pacemakers include those with second-degree type II atrioventricular (AV) block (symptomatic or asymptomatic), third-degree AV block, symptomatic bradycardia, sick sinus syndrome, and tachyarrhythmias that produce rapid ventricular rates.

Several types of temporary pacemakers (for example, transvenous, transcutaneous, transthoracic, and epicardial pacemakers) are available to treat conditions of varying urgency. A patient with an arrhythmia is likely to receive a transvenous pacemaker. With this type of pacemaker, electrodes are threaded through a vein and advanced to the right atrium, ventricle, or both (see illustration).

NURSING CARE

When caring for a patient with a transvenous pacemaker, follow these guidelines:

- Monitor your patient's vital signs, level of consciousness, skin color and temperature, capillary refill, urine output, and heart and breath sounds.
- Know which pacing mode your patient should have. In the *asynchronous* mode, the pacemaker generates an impulse, regardless of the patient's own rhythm. In the *synchronous* mode, it generates an impulse only when needed, based on the patient's own rhythm.
- Obtain a chest X-ray to verify lead placement and to check for pneumothorax and other complications of pacemaker insertion.
- Care for the insertion site according to your facility's policy.
- Frequently assess the insertion site for signs and symptoms of infection, including drainage, swelling, redness, and tenderness. Also assess the patient's vital signs.
- Watch for indications of myocardial perforation, such as hiccups, and signs and symptoms of cardiac tamponade, such as pulsus paradoxus, narrow pulse pressure, jugular vein distention, and muffled heart sounds.
- Remember that conduction of electric current to the pacemaker electrode and the patient's heart can

cause a life-threatening arrhythmia. Always take appropriate precautions, such as wearing disposable gloves when touching the pacemaker wires, showing the patient how to shave with a rechargeable razor, insulating the ends of unused pacing wires with special caps or a disposable glove, and making sure the patient's bed is properly grounded.

- Place your patient on continuous ECG monitoring, and evaluate the pacemaker's ability to sense, pace, and capture your patient's heart rhythm.
- Keep in mind that even though your patient has a temporary pacemaker, you'll still need to follow advanced cardiac life support algorithms for arrhythmias, if they should occur.
- Provide patient education and emotional support.

IMPORTANT PRECAUTION

If your patient requires defibrillation, disconnect the pacemaker from the pulse generator before delivering a shock. If you don't, you could damage the pacemaker.

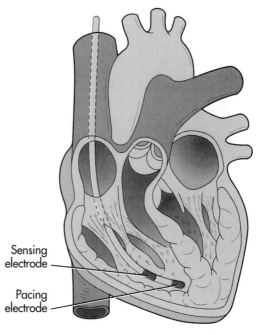

Sensing electrode

Pacing electrode

- If your patient has had a heart transplant, remember that his heart is denervated and may not respond to atropine. He may be more likely to benefit from temporary pacing or I.V. catecholamines, such as epinephrine or dopamine.
- If possible, give epinephrine, dopamine, and isoproterenol through a central line. These vesicant drugs can cause serious damage if they extravasate. If you must give them peripherally, monitor the insertion site frequently and report signs of extravasation immediately. If extravasation occurs, give a local injection of phentolamine, as prescribed, or follow your institution's extravasation protocol.
- If your patient has a temporary pacemaker and requires defibrillation, disconnect the pulse generator before delivering the shock. Otherwise, you may damage the pacemaker unit.

B, C

BOWEL SOUNDS, ABNORMAL

Produced by air, gas, and fecal matter moving through the intestines, bowel sounds reflect intestinal activity and offer important information about your patient's intestinal health and function.

Normally, the intestines produce soft clicking and gurgling sounds about every 5 to 15 seconds. A change from that pattern—such as hyperactive, hypoactive, or absent bowel sounds—may indicate a serious problem. If you find that your patient has abnormal bowel sounds, you'll need to know how to respond promptly and accurately.

Hyperactive bowel sounds

Hyperactive bowel sounds result from abnormally rapid passage of air and fluid through the intestines. Usually, these sounds are high-pitched, metallic, and tinkling. They may correlate with your patient's complaints of abdominal cramping. You may be able to hear loud, gurgling, hyperactive bowel sounds (called borborygmi) even without a stethoscope. Hyperactive bowel sounds may warn of early or partial intestinal obstruction, gastroenteritis, or GI hemorrhage.

Hypoactive bowel sounds

Decreased bowel activity causes bowel sounds with reduced tone, regularity, and loudness. Hypoactive sounds reflect inhibited GI motility, which commonly follows abdominal trauma, including trauma caused by surgery. In fact, after abdominal surgery, the colon typically takes 3 to 5 days to resume normal function. Failure to resume normal activity is termed *ileus*—short for paralytic ileus. Other causes of hypoactive bowel sounds include certain drugs, radiation therapy, and intestinal obstruction. (See *Conditions that alter bowel sounds*, page 48.)

Keep in mind that hypoactive bowel sounds are normal for some people, especially when they're asleep. For others, reduced sounds may precede absent bowel sounds, which warn of a life-threatening problem.

Absent bowel sounds

If you hear no bowel sounds after listening carefully for 5 minutes in each quadrant of the abdomen, your patient has absent bowel sounds (silent abdomen). Abrupt cessation of bowel sounds accompanied by abdominal pain and rigidity suggests a mechanical, vascular, or neuro-

CONDITIONS THAT ALTER BOWEL SOUNDS

Diseases and disorders associated with *hyperactive* bowel sounds include:
- diarrhea
- Crohn's disease
- irritable bowel syndrome
- food hypersensitivity
- gastroenteritis
- GI hemorrhage
- intestinal obstruction (early)
- peritonitis (early)
- ulcerative colitis.

Diseases and disorders that may cause *hypoactive* bowel sounds include:
- inflammatory bowel disease
- intestinal obstruction
- mesenteric artery occlusion
- pancreatitis
- abdominal trauma
- paralytic ileus (early)
- peritonitis (early).

Absent bowel sounds may result from:
- paralytic ileus
- intestinal obstruction (early)
- mesenteric artery occlusion
- abdominal trauma.

genic intestinal obstruction. Gases and intestinal contents back up behind the blockage, expanding the intestinal lumen and raising pressure within the intestine. Eventually, the intestinal wall may perforate, putting the patient at risk for peritonitis, sepsis, and shock. Without immediate treatment, this condition could lead to death.

WHAT TO LOOK FOR

Although significant, abnormal bowel sounds on their own don't indicate a specific diagnosis or justify a particular treatment. If you detect abnormal bowel sounds, check your patient's vital signs and investigate for associated signs and symptoms to help determine a diagnosis.

If the patient has *hyperactive* bowel sounds, ask her if she has:
- a history of abdominal surgery or inflammatory bowel disease
- experienced a recent episode of gastroenteritis
- recently traveled outside the United States
- a history of food allergy.

Clinical findings may include:
- loud, gurgling, splashing, or rushing bowel sounds on auscultation
- high-pitched sounds occurring more often than normal
- fever
- abdominal pain or cramping
- abdominal distention
- rebound tenderness
- abdominal guarding
- nausea and vomiting
- excessive watery or bloody diarrhea.

If she has *hypoactive* bowel sounds, ask her if she has:
- a history of abdominal surgery, pancreatitis, inflammatory bowel disease, or a gynecologic disorder that may cause peritonitis
- a history of a tumor or hernia that may cause a mechanical obstruction
- a history of recent abdominal trauma
- a history of constipation
- a history of use of peristalsis-reducing drugs, such as codeine.

Clinical evidence may include:
- infrequent bowel sounds that are softer and lower in tone than normal
- acute, colicky abdominal pain
- diffuse abdominal pain and distention
- nausea and vomiting
- irregular bowel movements
- fever
- abdominal bruit.

With *absent* bowel sounds, signs and symptoms may include:
- silent abdomen after auscultating for 5 minutes in each quadrant
- acute, colicky abdominal pain
- abdominal distention
- nausea and vomiting (emesis of fecal material suggests complete intestinal obstruction)
- rebound tenderness and abdominal rigidity
- abdominal bruit
- fever
- constipation.

WHAT TO DO IMMEDIATELY

If you detect abnormal bowel sounds, notify the physician. Then carry out these measures:
- Assess the patient's vital signs for changes.
- Evaluate her for associated signs and symptoms, such as abdominal pain, nausea, vomiting, and a change in bowel habits.
- If the patient is vomiting or has signs of complete bowel obstruction, withhold oral food and fluids.
- Establish an I.V. line, if necessary, and give I.V. fluids, electrolytes, or blood, as prescribed.
- Prepare to insert a nasogastric (NG) or an intestinal tube, as indicated, to decompress the intestine.
- Expect to administer antibiotics, as prescribed.
- If the abdomen is distended or complete obstruction is possible, measure abdominal girth to establish a baseline and then remeasure it every 4 to 8 hours.

WHAT TO DO NEXT

After taking initial steps, carry out the following interventions:
- Assess the patient's fluid balance and hydration; monitor intake and output at least every hour.
- Monitor bowel sounds every 1 to 4 hours, depending on the patient's status, history, and the urgency of the presenting situation.
- ➡ **NurseALERT** Know that bowel sounds cease suddenly when an abdominal organ is perforated.
- Prepare the patient for diagnostic testing and, possibly, surgery, as indicated.
- Watch for evidence of shock, such as hypotension, tachycardia, and diaphoresis.

FOLLOW-UP CARE

- Continue to maintain NG or intestinal decompression and suction, as ordered. If the patient has an NG tube, verify correct tube placement at least every 8 hours and before instilling fluid into it. Irrigate the tube every 2 hours with normal saline solution to maintain its patency. Be sure to include suction drainage when calculating fluid output.

B

- Continue to assess vital signs frequently; report any changes, including fever, tachycardia, and hypotension.
- Assess the patient's abdomen, including bowel sounds, for changes. Watch for distention, and track abdominal girth, as indicated.
- Continue I.V. fluid replacement, as prescribed.
- If the patient has undergone surgery, provide routine postoperative care, including measures to minimize the risk of complications (coughing, deep breathing, frequent turning, and early ambulation). Maintain the patency of all drainage tubes. Provide wound care, as ordered.

SPECIAL CONSIDERATIONS
- Warm your stethoscope before auscultating your patient's abdomen; a cold instrument could cause voluntary guarding. Talk to your patient in a reassuring tone to help her relax. Listen for at least 2 minutes in each quadrant of the abdomen. Gently palpating the abdomen with a finger during auscultation may stimulate peristalsis.
- If you hear breath sounds or heartbeats while listening to the abdomen, loops of distended bowel may have invaded the space between the diaphragm and anterior abdominal wall. This finding suggests paralytic ileus, in which the entire intestine becomes distended.
- Remember that the frequency of bowel sounds relates to the patient's last meal. If possible, find out how long ago she ate.

BURNS

A tissue injury resulting from contact with heat, chemicals, electricity, or gas, a burn can be fatal if it's severe or extensive. With a major burn, the patient's chances for survival hinge on stabilizing her condition within the first few hours.

A *thermal* burn, the most common burn injury, is associated with fire, flash flames, scalding, or contact with a hot object. A major thermal burn can cause extensive systemic alterations.

A *chemical* burn results from ingesting, inhaling, or coming into contact with a corrosive substance. Acidic substances that can cause chemical burns include battery acid and toilet bowl cleaner; dangerous alkaline substances include lye, drain cleaner, electric dishwasher detergent, and low-phosphate laundry detergent. Generally, an alkaline burn is more serious than an acid burn because alkalis penetrate more deeply into the skin. With either type of agent, the burning process continues until the substance is removed or inactivated.

An *electrical* burn is caused by intense heat from passage of an electric current through the body. Electricity enters the body at the point of contact and takes the path of least resistance. This path may involve internal structures and deeper tissues before the electrical charge exits the body.

An *inhalation* burn (smoke inhalation), which results from inhaling noxious fumes or irritating particles, is the leading cause of death in the first 24 hours after a burn injury. Smoke inhalation and inhalation burns usually occur when a person is trapped in an enclosed space, exposed to heavy smoke, or unconscious during a fire.

Burn classifications
Burns can be classified in different ways:
- according to depth, as superficial partial thickness (first degree), deep partial thickness (second degree), full thickness (third degree), or full thickness with involvement of underlying structures (fourth degree; see *Gauging the severity of a burn*, page 52)
- according to the extent of body surface area (BSA) involved, as major, moderate, or minor.

Types of *major burns* include:
- partial-thickness burns involving more than 25% of BSA in adults or 20% of BSA in children under age 10 or adults over age 50
- full-thickness burns involving more than 10% of BSA
- burns of the face, eyes, ears, hands, feet, or perineum that could lead to functional or cosmetic impairment
- chemical burns
- high-voltage electrical burns
- burns complicated by inhalation injury or major trauma.

Moderate burns include:
- partial-thickness burns involving 15% to 25% of BSA in adults or 10% to 20% of BSA in children or older adults
- full-thickness burns involving 2% to 10% of BSA that don't cause serious functional or cosmetic impairment of the eyes, ears, face, hands, feet, or perineum.

Minor burns include:
- partial-thickness burns of less than 15% of BSA in adults or less than 10% of BSA in children or older adults
- full-thickness burns involving less than 2% of BSA that don't pose a serious threat or cause serious functional or cosmetic impairment of the eyes, ears, face, hands, feet, or perineum.

WHAT TO LOOK FOR
Clinical findings vary with the type, degree, and depth of the burn. With a *superficial partial-thickness* burn, findings may include:
- reddened skin that blanches
- pain at the injury site
- mild swelling
- absence of blisters.

GAUGING THE SEVERITY OF A BURN

A burn may injure only the top layer of the skin—or it may extend down to the deepest layer. A first-degree burn involves the top layers of the epidermis of the skin. A second-degree burn involves both the epidermis and the dermis. A third-degree burn destroys the epidermis and dermis and may involve subcutaneous fat. A fourth-degree burn may extend through subcutaneous structures, including fat, fascia, tendon, and bone. This illustration correlates the skin layers with the major categories of burns.

A *deep partial-thickness* burn typically causes:
- mottled skin with dull white, tan, pink, or red areas
- blisters or a dry appearance
- pain at the injury site.

With a *full-thickness* burn, signs and symptoms may include:
- waxy white, charred red, or brown and leathery skin
- no blanching with pressure
- absence of pain at the injury site.

Depending on the causative agent, a *chemical burn* is likely to cause:
- blisters
- eschar formation.

With an *electrical burn*, the patient may have:
- intact skin, except at the entrance and exit sites
- a well-defined black entrance wound surrounded by grayish tissue
- underlying tissue necrosis
- cardiac arrhythmias
- respiratory arrest, cardiac arrest, or both.

With an *inhalation burn*, clinical findings may include:
- carbonaceous sputum
- coughing
- hoarseness
- dyspnea

- apnea
- airway edema
- pulmonary edema (after 24 hours).

WHAT TO DO IMMEDIATELY

For a life-threatening burn, interventions must begin as soon as possible to avoid or minimize life-threatening injuries. Specific interventions may vary with the type of burn. Immediate priorities for any burn victim are to:
- stop the burning process
- maintain a patent airway
- ensure ventilation
- restore adequate circulation.

For a thermal burn

If your patient has a serious thermal burn, follow these measures:
- Establish and maintain a patent airway. Assess the patient's respiratory status.
- If the patient isn't breathing, begin artificial respirations. Call for help. Prepare to initiate cardiopulmonary resuscitation (CPR) if respiratory arrest progresses to cardiac arrest.
- Assess for the presence of a pulse. If there is no pulse, begin CPR.
- Once pulse and respiratory rates have been assessed, rapidly assess the patient's circulatory status, including blood pressure. If all extremities have been burned, place a sterile dressing under the blood pressure cuff to prevent contamination of burned areas. A Doppler stethoscope device may be helpful. If the patient has severe burns, expect to insert an arterial line to allow continuous blood pressure monitoring.
- If the patient is in hypovolemic shock (indicated by hypotension, rapid thready pulse, restlessness, and mental status changes), immediately insert at least two large-bore I.V. lines in an unburned area, if possible. Then begin fluid resuscitation therapy, as prescribed. If peripheral access isn't possible, anticipate insertion of a central line.
- Be aware that the physician may use one of several formulas to determine the patient's fluid resuscitation needs during the first 24 hours. With any of these formulas, you'll first need to assess the amount of BSA burned. (See *Estimating burn surfaces,* page 55.)
- Once the patient's cardiopulmonary needs have been addressed, check for additional injuries. Also remove all of the patient's clothing and jewelry. Any metal (such as jewelry or buttons) that remains will retain heat and cause further burns. Clothing and jewelry can also cause constriction as edema develops in the burned areas.
- Provide emergency care for burned areas by washing them with cool water. If possible, cool burned areas by immersing them in cold but not iced water (34° to 41° F [1° to 5° C]) or by applying cold towels. Cooling that takes place within 30 minutes after the burn decreases edema and tissue damage and provides some pain relief.

B

- Then cover the burned areas with a sterile dressing. Don't apply ointment or salves at this time.
- ➡ **NurseALERT** Be sure to use aseptic technique during all care procedures, and wear a gown, mask, and cap. When giving direct care to the burned area, also wear sterile gloves.
- Cover the patient with a sheet or blanket; use bed cradles to keep linens off burned areas.
- Encourage the patient to cough to help remove secretions from the respiratory tract.

For a chemical burn

If your patient has suffered a chemical burn, expect to carry out these measures:

- Immediately remove contaminated clothing, taking care to protect yourself from direct contact with the caustic substance.
- ➡ **NurseALERT** Don't apply water to a burn caused by a dry chemical substance; water may activate the substance. Instead, gently but thoroughly brush the dry powder from the patient's skin.
- Rapidly wipe the exposed area with litmus paper to determine whether the caustic substance was acidic or alkaline. Then rapidly flush the injury site with normal saline solution or water (if normal saline solution isn't available) for 30 to 60 minutes, or until skin pH is within normal limits.
- While flushing, try to find out the name and concentration of the chemical substance. Ask a family member or a police officer to bring the substance to the hospital, if possible. If needed, call the poison control central for interventions specific to that chemical.

For an electrical burn

Take these actions for a patient with an electrical burn:

- Quickly assess the patient's cardiopulmonary status; electrical burn injuries commonly cause atrial or ventricular fibrillation or asystole.
- ➡ **NurseALERT** Never touch a patient who has sustained an electrical burn until you are certain that the patient is no longer in contact with the electrical source.
- If your patient is unresponsive, is not breathing, and has no pulse, initiate CPR and follow the advanced cardiac life support protocol for the identified arrhythmia.
- ➡ **NurseALERT** Be aware that respiratory arrest may persist even after successful cardiac resuscitation. Make sure the patient remains adequately ventilated, and provide continuous respiratory assessment after resuscitation.
- Until the extent of the patient's injuries are known, assume that she has a cervical spine injury and provide related care. She may have fallen or been thrown when the electrical burn injury occurred.
- Rapidly insert two large-bore I.V. lines for fluid resuscitation therapy.

TIPS AND TECHNIQUES

ESTIMATING BURN SURFACES

To determine the fluid resuscitation needs of a patient with a serious thermal burn, you'll need to estimate how much body surface area (BSA) is burned. You can use a visual tool such as the rule of nines, or you may refer to the modified Lund and Browder (also known as Berkow) chart.

RULE OF NINES

The rule of nines expresses BSA in multiples or fractions of nine. To use this method, visually evaluate your patient's burns by referring to the illustration. Add the corresponding percentages for each body section burned to estimate the patient's total BSA burned.

To gauge the extent of irregular burns, think of the patient's palm as being equal to 1% of total BSA, and then estimate the percentage burned accordingly.

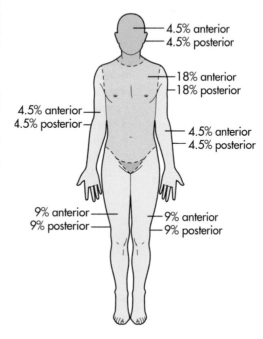

Adult	Child
9%	18%
18% front	18% front
18% back	18% back
9%	9%
9%	9%
1%	14%
18%	14%
18%	

MODIFIED LUND AND BROWDER METHOD

The modified Lund and Browder method allows more accurate calculation of burn injuries. It's especially useful for children, whose body proportions differ from those of adults.

	Under age 1	Ages 1 to 4	Ages 5 to 9	Ages 10 to 14	Age 15	Adult
Head	19%	17%	13%	11%	9%	7%
Neck	2%	2%	2%	2%	2%	3%
Anterior trunk	13%	13%	13%	13%	13%	13%
Posterior trunk	13%	13%	13%	13%	13%	13%
Right buttock	2.5%	2.5%	2.5%	2.5%	2.5%	2.5%
Left buttock	2.5%	2.5%	2.5%	2.5%	2.5%	2.5%
Genitalia	1%	1%	1%	1%	1%	1%
Right upper arm	4%	4%	4%	4%	4%	4%
Left upper arm	4%	4%	4%	4%	4%	4%
Right lower arm	3%	3%	3%	3%	3%	3%
Left lower arm	3%	3%	3%	3%	3%	3%
Right hand	2.5%	2.5%	2.5%	2.5%	2.5%	2.5%
Left hand	2.5%	2.5%	2.5%	2.5%	2.5%	2.5%
Right thigh	5.5%	6.5%	8%	8.5%	9%	9.5%
Left thigh	5.5%	6.5%	8%	8.5%	9%	9.5%
Right leg	5%	5%	5.5%	6%	6.5%	7%
Left leg	5%	5%	5.5%	6%	6.5%	7%
Right foot	3.5%	3.5%	3.5%	3.5%	3.5%	3.5%
Left foot	3.5%	3.5%	3.5%	3.5%	3.5%	3.5%

➡ **NurseALERT** For a patient with an electrical burn, base fluid resuscitation volumes on the patient's blood pressure, not on the percentage of BSA burned. If hypotension occurs, be prepared to give a bolus of normal saline solution, 20 ml/kg. As ordered, give subsequent fluid volumes based on vital signs and urine output.

- Provide emergency care for burns at the entry and exit points as you would for a thermal burn.
- Splint affected limbs in functional positions to minimize edema and contracture formation.
- Assess the neurovascular status of affected limbs at least hourly.

For an inhalation burn

If your patient has sustained an inhalation burn, take these actions:

- Rapidly evaluate the patient's level of consciousness and respiratory status. Check for burns and soot on her face and neck, for singed nasal or facial hair, and for carbonaceous sputum.
- Administer humidified oxygen with a nonrebreathing reservoir mask at a rate of 10 to 12 L/minute, as prescribed. If the patient isn't breathing, prepare for endotracheal intubation and help initiate mechanical ventilation.
- If you detect signs and symptoms of respiratory distress (stridor, wheezing, hoarseness, or dyspnea), give bronchodilators, as prescribed.
- Prepare the patient for emergency fiber-optic bronchoscopy to assess the extent of inhalation burns and help determine appropriate treatment.
- Monitor the patient's oxygen saturation values by way of pulse oximetry, and obtain and monitor arterial blood gas (ABG) values, as indicated.
- Monitor closely for signs and symptoms of acute respiratory distress syndrome and report them immediately.

WHAT TO DO NEXT

When the patient is stabilized, be prepared to take these actions:

- Insert an indwelling urinary catheter to monitor hourly urine output.
- Anticipate adjusting fluid intake to achieve a urine output of 30 to 50 ml/hour for an adult and 1 ml/kg/hour for a child.
- Monitor vital signs every hour. Tachycardia that persists after initial resuscitation usually indicates inadequate fluid replacement and ineffective pain management. Discuss your findings with the physician and anticipate changes in fluid and analgesic orders.
- Obtain the patient's baseline weight, and then take daily weights to help evaluate fluid and nutritional status.
- Take a history of the burn injury.
- Review the patient's past medical history, including tetanus immunization status. If necessary, prepare to give the immunization.

- If indicated, withhold oral foods and fluids. Prepare to insert a nasogastric tube for gastric decompression if burns are serious or the patient risks aspiration.
- Administer I.V. pain medications, such as morphine and meperidine (Demerol), as prescribed and as the patient's status permits.
- ➡ **Nurse**ALERT Don't give any intramuscular (I.M.) injections except the tetanus immunization. Drugs administered I.M. are sequestered in the interstitial edema, causing uneven distribution and impairing effective pain relief.
- Obtain baseline laboratory and radiologic studies, including complete blood count, hemoglobin and hematocrit values, coagulation studies, serum electrolytes, serum glucose, blood urea nitrogen, ABG and carboxyhemoglobin levels (for a patient with smoke inhalation), urinalysis, and a chest X-ray to serve as a baseline for comparison during recovery.

Additional measures for thermal burns
For the patient with a thermal burn, also take these steps:
- Maintaining asepsis, clean burned areas gently every day, using open or closed technique as prescribed. Afterward, apply the prescribed antibiotic ointment. If the physician orders a closed technique, dress burned areas with sterile dressings, as ordered.
- ➡ **Nurse**ALERT Don't put any creams, ointments, or topical medications on a burn wound until you know whether the patient will be transported to a burn center. If she will, these preparations must be scrubbed off (a painful procedure) so that the new burn team can assess the extent of the patient's injuries.
- When possible, elevate the burned area above the level of the patient's heart to limit edema at the injury site.
- If the patient has a full-thickness burn, prepare her for escharotomy. (See *Understanding escharotomy*, page 58.)

FOLLOW-UP CARE
- If burns are extensive or severe, prepare the patient for transport to a burn center.
- Continue to monitor all physiologic parameters.
- Maintain aseptic technique and assess burn wound healing during dressing changes and invasive procedures.
- Obtain repeat laboratory studies, as indicated, and evaluate results.
- Provide emotional support for the patient and family. Explain all treatments and procedures.
- Take steps to relieve impaired circulation if the patient has circumferential burns. Monitor closely for signs and symptoms of compartment syndrome. To help detect compartment syndrome, take circumferential measurements of extremities at least every 4 hours and use a

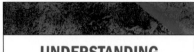

UNDERSTANDING ESCHAROTOMY

In escharotomy, the physician makes an incision into the eschar (dead tissue) down to the subcutaneous fat layer, extending the entire length of the eschar in the lateral or medial line of the limb or through circumferential eschar around the thorax.

Escharotomy helps to relieve constriction that has compromised distal blood flow in the extremities or limited respiratory movements of the chest.

FASCIOTOMY

For deep burns, fasciotomy—a deeper incision made into the muscle—may be necessary if escharotomy doesn't relieve constriction and restore distal tissue perfusion.

Doppler device to assess distal pulses. Perform neurovascular checks every 4 hours, or more frequently, if indicated, and report any pain, paresthesias, pallor, pulselessness, or paralysis.

SPECIAL CONSIDERATIONS

- During early phases of burn care, incorporate measures to limit or prevent long-term complications, such as contractures or infections that would delay healing. To prevent contractures, for example, apply splints to the extremities as ordered and institute active and passive range-of-motion exercises. To prevent infection, use strict aseptic technique when performing wound care and provide optimal nutrition.
- Anticipate the need for extensive rehabilitation after a major burn.
- Keep in mind that a patient with extensive or full-thickness burns may need to undergo skin grafting.
- A serious or an extensive burn can permanently alter a patient's appearance and body functions. Expect the patient and family to exhibit signs of grieving or loss, such as denial, anger, and withdrawal. Provide emotional support and make appropriate referrals as indicated.

CARDIAC ARREST

In cardiac arrest, the victim becomes pulseless and stops breathing as electrical activity in the ventricles becomes disrupted (as in ventricular fibrillation) or stops (as in asystole). Ventricular contractions then become inadequate or cease altogether.

The most common cause of cardiac arrest is ventricular fibrillation, which usually results from underlying coronary artery disease. Less common causes include heart failure, hypoxia, metabolic acidosis, hyperkalemia, pulmonary embolism, and use of such drugs as cocaine.

Cardiac arrest carries a high mortality, even in hospitalized patients. Without immediate treatment, the victim stands virtually no chance of surviving. What's more, a person who survives cardiac arrest may suffer permanent functional or cognitive impairment.

Rapid interventions—including arrhythmia recognition, defibrillation, cardiac pacing, and administering emergency medications—can make the difference between life and death.

WHAT TO LOOK FOR

Some victims of cardiac arrest have no known history of heart disease. Many experience no warning signs, although a few have palpitations.

During cardiac arrest, signs and symptoms include:

- unresponsiveness
- pulselessness

- apnea
- an arrhythmia, such as ventricular fibrillation, ventricular tachycardia, bradycardia, or asystole, on the ECG.

WHAT TO DO IMMEDIATELY

To help your patient survive cardiac arrest, take these actions:

- Verify that your patient is unresponsive by calling his name and shaking his shoulder. If he doesn't respond, call for help immediately.
- Position the patient flat, with a board or other firm surface under his upper back.
- Assess the patient's breathing. Open his airway using the head-tilt, chin-lift or head-tilt, neck-lift method. Then look, listen, and feel for respirations.
- If the patient is not breathing, administer two slow artificial breaths.
- Check for a pulse. If it's absent, begin cardiopulmonary resuscitation (CPR).
- As appropriate, assign one staff member to call for the emergency resuscitation (code) team and another to get the emergency (code) cart. Have another nurse attach the patient to the monitor-defibrillator to determine his heart rhythm.
- ➡ **NurseALERT** If the ECG shows ventricular fibrillation and you're qualified to perform defibrillation, do so immediately. Defibrillation is the single most important factor in survival—even more important than emergency drug administration.

WHAT TO DO NEXT

Your next actions depend on your patient's cardiac rhythm.

For ventricular tachycardia or ventricular fibrillation

- If your patient is in ventricular tachycardia or ventricular fibrillation, defibrillate immediately—up to three times—delivering increasing energy levels of 200 joules, 200 to 300 joules, and 360 joules. Before defibrillating, make sure everyone is clear of the patient's bed.
- If defibrillation fails to terminate ventricular tachycardia or ventricular fibrillation, continue giving CPR while other team members intubate the patient and establish I.V. access.
- As prescribed, administer epinephrine and then defibrillate within 30 to 60 seconds. Next, give lidocaine, as prescribed, again followed by defibrillation. The physician also may order bretylium (Bretylol), magnesium sulfate, and procainamide (Pronestyl), alternating drug administration with defibrillation.
- Continue to assess the patient's airway and respiratory and pulse rates. Continue CPR until the patient regains adequate cardiac and respiratory function.

For asystole

If the cardiac monitor shows no electrical activity, assume that your patient is in asystole. Always verify asystole in more than one ECG lead.

Make sure that no leads are loose and that the monitor is securely connected to the patient.

After verifying asystole, take the following actions:

- Continue CPR. Assist with endotracheal intubation and start an I.V. line if one's not already in place.
- Prepare for immediate transcutaneous pacing. Be aware that this intervention is most effective when done as soon as possible and performed simultaneously with emergency drug administration. (See *Performing transcutaneous pacing*.)
- Administer epinephrine and atropine by I.V. push, as prescribed.
- Be aware that if no reversible cause of asystole can be found and your patient fails to respond to treatment, a physician may call a halt to resuscitative efforts.

For pulseless electrical activity

Previously called electromechanical dissociation (EMD), pulseless electrical activity (PEA) occurs when electrical activity other than ventricular fibrillation or ventricular tachycardia appears on the cardiac monitor of a pulseless patient. (*Note:* In pseudo-EMD, a related condition, heart contractions are too weak to detect a palpable pulse.) If your patient has PEA, follow these steps:

- Continue CPR.
- Assist with endotracheal intubation, and start an I.V. line.
- Confirm lack of a pulse and blood flow with Doppler ultrasound.
- Begin appropriate interventions, as ordered, to correct an identified cause of PEA, such as hypovolemia.
- Administer epinephrine by I.V. push, as prescribed.
- If the patient has bradycardia (a heart rate slower than 60 beats/minute) or relative bradycardia, give atropine I.V., as prescribed.

FOLLOW-UP CARE

- Prepare the patient for transfer to an intensive care unit if he's not already in one.
- Continuously monitor his ECG.
- Regularly check vital signs, heart and breath sounds, neurologic status, arterial blood gas values, and serum electrolyte levels.
- Administer antiarrhythmics, as prescribed.
- Assess the sensing, pacing, and capture functions of the temporary pacemaker, if present.
- Provide care as needed if the patient requires mechanical ventilation.
- Administer ordered treatments to correct the underlying cause of cardiac arrest, such as hypoxia or hyperkalemia.
- Provide emotional support to the patient and family. Prepare family members for the patient's condition, and explain any new equipment.
- Document the events of the cardiac arrest.

TIPS AND TECHNIQUES

PERFORMING TRANSCUTANEOUS PACING

Transcutaneous pacing is a quick, noninvasive way to pace your patient's heart until a transvenous pacemaker can be inserted or definitive therapy can begin. In this technique, two large electrode pads are applied to the patient's chest and back (see illustration below). The electrodes depolarize the patient's heart through the chest wall.

An external pulse generator has controls for rate and voltage, and an ECG lead allows demand pacing. In demand pacing, the pacemaker takes over if the patient's heart fails to maintain a predetermined rate.

STEPS TO FOLLOW
If your patient needs transcutaneous pacing, follow these steps:
- Begin continuous ECG monitoring.
- Explain to the patient what a pacemaker does and why he needs a transcutaneous one. Emphasize that this type of pacemaker is only temporary.
- Forewarn the patient that he'll feel muscle twitches and contractions when the pacemaker produces electric current. Reassure him that he'll receive analgesics, if needed, to make him feel more comfortable.
- Trim the patient's chest hair, if necessary. Don't shave his chest because the resulting nicks can make the electrical charge more uncomfortable and increase his risk for infection.
- Attach monitoring electrodes to the patient's chest in the lead I, II, or III position. These electrodes will

be connected to the pacemaker. (Even with continuous cardiac monitoring, the patient still needs these electrodes.)
- Turn the monitor on and check for an ECG waveform.
- Turn the alarm on and set high and low parameters.
- Make sure your patient's skin is clean and dry, and then place a pacing electrode pad on his chest (between leads V_2 and V_5).
- Place the other pad on your patient's back, between the spine and left scapula, over his heart.
- Attach the external pulse generator.
- Set the pacer rate at 10 to 20 beats higher than the patient's own rhythm and watch for the pacer spike. If the patient doesn't have a rhythm, set the rate at 60.
- Adjust the milliamperes (mA, the amount of energy delivered) until you see a pacer spike followed by a QRS complex. This is called the *threshold* (usually between 40 and 80 mA). To ensure capture, increase it by 10%.

Troubleshooting
- If the pacemaker fails to capture, check the connectors and electrode placement. If you don't find any problems, turn up the voltage until capture occurs. The patient's paced heart rate should be the same as the set rate on the pacemaker.
- If the pacemaker isn't pacing, check that the electrode pads are securely attached to the skin.
- Remember that if an ECG electrode becomes detached, the pacemaker will interpret the result as asystole and produce an electric current.

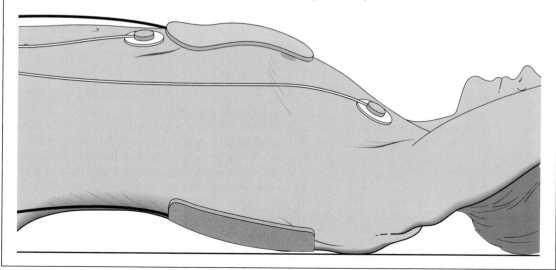

SPECIAL CONSIDERATIONS

➡ **NurseALERT** If a peripheral I.V. line isn't already in place when resuscitation begins, give epinephrine, lidocaine, and atropine through your patient's endotracheal tube, as prescribed, in doses 2 to 2½ times the recommended I.V. dose. Dilute medications in normal saline solution or distilled water. Using a plastic catheter, not a needle, inject the medication into the distal end of the endotracheal tube. Before drug administration begins, chest compressions should stop. After administering the medication rapidly, hyperventilate the patient several times and resume chest compressions and mechanical ventilation.

• If the patient doesn't survive despite resuscitative efforts, provide emotional support to family members. Ask if they would like to see the patient. Offer to accompany them to his room; if they prefer to be alone, respect their wishes and remain nearby. Also ask if they would like to see the hospital clergyperson or their own clergyperson.

CARDIAC TAMPONADE

A perilous development, cardiac tamponade occurs when pressure from fluid in the pericardial sac prevents the heart from filling during diastole, causing a dangerous drop in cardiac output. If your patient is at risk for cardiac tamponade, you'll need to know how to identify signs and symptoms and intervene promptly. Quick action on your part may be her only hope for avoiding progression to cardiogenic shock and almost certain death.

Normally, the pericardial space houses just a small amount of fluid. This fluid lubricates the pericardial space, aiding movement of the ventricles during contractions. (See *Inside view of the pericardial sac*.)

When fluid volume rises too quickly

If pericardial fluid volume rises slowly, such as from a slow leak into the pericardial sac, cardiac tamponade develops gradually. To accommodate the increased volume, the pericardial fibers stretch little by little. With such a gradual rise, the pericardial space can expand to hold up to 2 L of fluid before symptoms develop.

A rapid fluid increase, on the other hand, jeopardizes the patient's life immediately. Pushed to the limit, pericardial fibers can't stretch quickly or effectively enough to make room for the excess fluid. Increased pressure from pericardial fluid restricts heart movement, preventing full ventricular contraction and expansion, limiting ventricular filling during diastole, and leading to reductions in stroke volume and cardiac output.

Understanding the causes

Cardiac tamponade usually results from acute pericarditis. Other causes include:

• bleeding into the pericardial space (hemopericardium, typically

INSIDE VIEW OF THE PERICARDIAL SAC

The heart is suspended within the pericardial sac. The sac has two portions. The *fibrous pericardium,* the outer portion, is composed of tough, fibrous tissue and protects the heart and serous membrane. The inner portion, the *serous pericardium*, consists of two layers: the *parietal layer*, which lines the inside of the fibrous pericardium; and the *visceral layer* (also called epicardium), which adheres to the heart's outer surface.

Separating the parietal and visceral layers is the *pericardial cavity*, or space. Usually, the pericardial cavity contains a minute amount of serous fluid, which lubricates the surfaces of the cavity and aids heart contractions. Abnormal fluid accumulation—for example, from pericarditis—can restrict heart movement, eventually causing cardiac tamponade, cardiogenic shock, and, possibly, death.

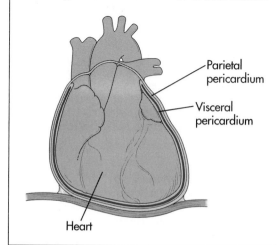

Parietal pericardium

Visceral pericardium

Heart

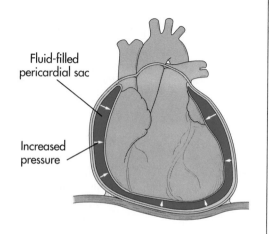

Fluid-filled pericardial sac

Increased pressure

brought on by chest trauma, cardiac surgery, myocardial rupture, aortic dissection, or anticoagulant therapy)
* malignant or uremic pericardial effusions.

WHAT TO LOOK FOR
Cardiac tamponade may cause the following signs and symptoms:
* distant, muffled, or absent heart sounds
* reduced cardiac output, leading to profound hypotension
* jugular vein distention on inspiration
* pulsus paradoxus—a systolic blood pressure decrease of more than 15 mm Hg during inspiration (see *Understanding pulsus paradoxus,* page 64)
* apprehension, anxiety, or fear progressing to panic
* pale, cool skin
* diaphoresis
* tachypnea and dyspnea progressing to marked respiratory distress
* tachycardia
* substernal chest pain
* decreased or absent peripheral pulses

UNDERSTANDING PULSUS PARADOXUS

Always stay alert for pulsus paradoxus (also called paradoxical pulse) if your patient has suspected cardiac tamponade or is at risk for developing this potentially fatal condition. A classic sign of cardiac tamponade, pulsus paradoxus refers to an abnormally large decrease in systolic blood pressure during inspiration. Normally, systolic pressure drops less than 10 mm Hg with inspiration; with cardiac tamponade, it typically drops more than 15 mm Hg.

Pulsus paradoxus reflects the exaggerated changes in left ventricular stroke volume that accompany inspiration and expiration. Stroke volume (the amount of blood ejected from the left ventricle with each heartbeat) is closely linked to cardiac output (the amount of blood ejected in 1 minute). Normally, a slight drop in stroke volume accompanies inspiration, as blood pools in the pulmonary vasculature and intrathoracic pressure rises. Because cardiac output is a component of blood pressure, any decline in cardiac output affects blood pressure.

WHAT CAUSES SYSTOLIC PRESSURE TO DECREASE?

In cardiac tamponade, fluid or air in the pericardial space causes mechanical compression of the myocardium, which prevents complete filling of the ventricles. As a result, the ventricles eject less blood during systole. During inspiration, incomplete myocardial contraction and expansion intensifies the normal decline in systolic pressure.

ASSESSING FOR PULSUS PARADOXUS

The most accurate way to detect pulsus paradoxus is through direct intra-arterial measurement. If your patient doesn't have an arterial line, you'll need to use a blood pressure cuff, manometer, and stethoscope. Follow these steps:
- Wrap a cuff around the arm you've been using to measure the patient's blood pressure.
- Inflate the cuff 20 mm Hg above the patient's most recent blood pressure reading. Then instruct him to breathe normally.
- Slowly deflate the cuff, and note the point at which you first hear Korotkoff's (blood pressure) sounds. Normally, you can hear these sounds during expiration but not during inspiration.
- As you continue to deflate the cuff, note the point at which Korotkoff's sounds are heard throughout the respiratory cycle. With pulsus paradoxus, the difference between the pressure reading at which you first heard Korotkoff's sounds and the reading at which you heard them consistently during expiration and inspiration will exceed 15 mm Hg.
- *Important:* Because intra-arterial blood pressure monitoring is more sensitive than that obtained by a blood pressure cuff, expect to see more dramatic blood pressure changes with an intra-arterial monitor. A difference of 10 mmg Hg recorded by cuff is equivalent to a difference of about 15 mm Hg recorded by an intra-arterial monitor.

- equalization of right- and left-sided heart pressures
- elevations in right atrial pressure, right ventricular end-diastolic pressure, and pulmonary artery wedge pressure.

WHAT TO DO IMMEDIATELY

If you suspect cardiac tamponade, notify the physician and take the following actions:
- If the patient's cardiac tamponade is a result of acute pericarditis, prepare to assist with emergency pericardiocentesis to remove excess pericardial fluid and relieve intrapericardial pressure. Performed on an emergency basis when the patient has profound hypotension or other acute, life-threatening symptoms, this procedure improves myocardial pumping action and restores hemodynamic stability. If a large amount of fluid is drained, a flexible catheter may be left in the pericardial space and attached to a drainage bag.
- Alternatively, prepare the patient for surgery, such as pericardiectomy, if indicated. In this procedure, the surgeon removes the pari-

etal and visceral layers of the pericardium, creating an opening in the pericardial sac that allows constant fluid drainage into the pleural space for reabsorption.

- If the patient's cardiac tamponade results from surgery or trauma, prepare to assist the physician with opening the chest immediately or inserting a large-bore chest tube.
- Give colloid or crystalloid infusions, as prescribed. These agents increase ventricular pressure, improving stroke volume and cardiac output.
- Administer inotropic and vasoactive medications, as prescribed, to improve cardiac output and raise blood pressure. Keep in mind that these medications may not be necessary if excess pericardial fluids can be removed immediately.
- Check the patient's blood pressure and pulse and respiratory rates every 5 to 15 minutes.
- To evaluate for ventricular impairment, monitor pulse pressure, pulmonary artery pressures, stroke volume, and level of consciousness every 5 to 15 minutes.
- ➡ **NurseALERT** Assess heart sounds and neck veins hourly. Notify the physician if heart sounds become muffled or if you detect a third or fourth heart sound (S_3 or S_4), summation gallop, new murmur, irregular heart rhythm, pulsus paradoxus, or jugular vein distention—all signs of worsening cardiovascular function.
- As indicated, place the patient on continuous cardiac monitoring and watch for such changes as low voltage of the P wave, QRS complex, and T wave and for electrical alternans of the P wave and QRS complex (alternating amplitude variations from one heartbeat to the next).
- As indicated and ordered, administer oxygen and prepare for endotracheal intubation and mechanical ventilation if the patient experiences respiratory distress.
- To reduce myocardial oxygen demands and improve cardiac output, enforce bed rest until the patient is hemodynamically stable.
- Elevate the head of the bed 45 degrees to promote optimal respirations and comfort.

WHAT TO DO NEXT
Once your patient has stabilized, take the following measures:
- Continue to monitor his vital signs and other hemodynamic values, such as pulmonary artery pressures, if appropriate.
- Check his peripheral pulses, skin temperature, and capillary refill at least every hour.
- Monitor his fluid intake and output hourly. Notify the physician of an increase or a decrease. Be aware that urine output may decrease from impaired kidney perfusion and ischemia resulting from poor cardiac output. Conversely, urine output may increase with hemorrhage and subsequent hypovolemia.
- Withhold oral intake in preparation for surgical interventions, such as pericardiocentesis or pericardial window. Pericardial window, a

form of pericardiectomy, involves creation of a small window and removal of a portion of pericardial tissue. Pericardiectomy may be done once the patient has been stabilized and evaluated more fully, such as with echocardiography or cardiac catheterization.

- Maintain parenteral therapy with colloids and crystalloids, as indicated and prescribed, to improve cardiac output and raise blood pressure.

FOLLOW-UP CARE

- Monitor blood test results for abnormalities. Elevated leukocyte counts or an increased sedimentation rate may signal pericardial infection or inflammation; sharp drops in hemoglobin and hematocrit could indicate hemorrhage.
- Auscultate the patient's heart sounds for a pericardial friction rub, a sign of pericarditis.
- If cardiac tamponade resulted from hemorrhage caused by anticoagulant therapy, expect to discontinue anticoagulants or reduce the dose. Monitor the patient's prothrombin time and activated partial thromboplastin time, and report prolongation.
- Assess your patient's pain level. If the patient has acute pericarditis, administer analgesic and anti-inflammatory medications, such as nonsteroidal anti-inflammatory drugs, as indicated and prescribed. To reduce chest pain, instruct the patient to sit up and lean forward.

SPECIAL CONSIDERATIONS

- As indicated, keep necessary equipment available for emergency procedures, such as pulmonary artery catheter or central venous catheter insertion for pericardiocentesis, endotracheal intubation, or thoracotomy. Also keep a defibrillator and an emergency cart on hand.
- If your patient goes into cardiac arrest, check for a pulse to confirm the return of a cardiac rhythm. In cardiac tamponade, mechanical compression of the heart muscle by fluid or air may lead to pulseless electrical activity—the presence of a cardiac rhythm (even a normal sinus rhythm) despite an absence of myocardial contraction and relaxation. Be aware that peripheral pulses may be absent even in the presence of a cardiac rhythm. If this situation arises, inform the physician immediately; expect to prepare the patient for pericardiocentesis and to administer epinephrine, 1 mg I.V., repeated every 3 to 5 minutes, as prescribed.
- Maintain aseptic technique when changing a precordial dressing or when handling a pericardial drainage tube or collection device after pericardiocentesis.
- ➡ **NurseALERT** Never inject anything—including medication—into a pericardial drainage tube. Doing so may worsen cardiac tamponade, cause tissue destruction, or lead to infection. If you suspect that the tube has become obstructed, don't attempt to clear it yourself. Instead, notify the physician immediately; pericardial fluid trapped be-

hind the obstruction may trigger or worsen cardiac tamponade.
- Teach the patient about his condition and the treatments he's receiving.

CARDIOGENIC SHOCK

In cardiogenic shock, sometimes called pump failure, the heart can't maintain an output sufficient to perfuse the body's tissues. (See *What happens in cardiogenic shock*, page 68.) In most cases, the condition results from extensive myocardial infarction (MI). Cardiogenic shock also may stem from cardiomyopathy, myocarditis, ventricular septal defect, papillary muscle rupture, cardiac tamponade, or trauma.

Even in the hospital, the mortality rate for cardiogenic shock may exceed 70%. Once compensatory mechanisms fail and shock reaches the refractory or irreversible stage, organs begin to fail and death is imminent. If you can recognize and respond to cardiogenic shock in its early stages, you can give your patient a better chance for survival.

WHAT TO LOOK FOR
The earliest evidence of cardiogenic shock stems from reduced cardiac output. Clinical findings may include:
- hypotension
- cool, clammy skin
- restlessness
- slight reduction in urine output.

As the body attempts to compensate, clinical findings may include:
- tachycardia
- weak, thready pulses
- tachypnea
- respiratory alkalosis
- crackles
- increasing anxiety, restlessness
- reduced urine output
- pale skin
- slow capillary refill
- elevated left ventricular end-diastolic pressure, reflected as an increase in pulmonary artery wedge pressure (PAWP)
- S_3 and S_4 heart sounds
- jugular vein distention.

As shock progresses and compensatory mechanisms begin to fail, clinical findings may also include:
- arrhythmias
- chest pain
- respiratory distress

WHAT HAPPENS IN CARDIOGENIC SHOCK

Early in cardiogenic shock, falling blood pressure (the result of decreased cardiac output) stimulates the sympathetic nervous system to compensate by increasing the patient's heart rate in an attempt to correct hypotension and improve cardiac output. Unfortunately, however, the increased heart rate also increases the heart's workload and oxygen consumption. If the patient had myocardial ischemia to begin with, this increased demand may further impair the heart's pumping ability. As a result, blood backs up into the heart and pulmonary vasculature, leading to pulmonary edema, carbon dioxide accumulation, and eventual metabolic acidosis—which has a depressive effect on cardiac function.

Sympathetic stimulation also causes vasoconstriction, which shunts blood to the heart and brain, where it's most needed. That action deprives other organs of blood, such as the kidneys and skin. Decreased blood flow to the kidneys results in decreased urine production; pallor reflects decreased skin perfusion. Deprived of oxygen from reduced blood flow, cells turn to aerobic metabolism for energy. Production of lactic acid contributes to the development of metabolic acidosis as well.

Eventually, compensatory mechanisms fail. Indeed, a vicious cycle is established as compensatory mechanisms aggravate the underlying myocardial ischemia and actually exacerbate cardiogenic shock.

- metabolic acidosis
- oliguria
- agitation, disorientation
- decreasing level of consciousness
- elevated PAWP.

As shock progresses to the irreversible or refractory stage, clinical findings may include:
- unresponsiveness, coma
- no peripheral pulses
- slow, irregular respiratory rate
- anuria
- cyanotic skin
- absent bowel sounds
- falling systolic blood pressure, profound hypotension
- diastolic pressure as low as 0 mm Hg.

WHAT TO DO IMMEDIATELY
If you suspect cardiogenic shock, notify the physician and follow these measures:
- Establish two I.V. access lines, if not already in place. A patient in cardiogenic shock will require I.V. medications, many of which are incompatible with one another or must be administered by infusion pump to ensure dose accuracy. The patient may benefit from a central line because some of the drugs he'll receive, such as dopamine, can cause tissue necrosis if they extravasate.
- Begin continuous ECG monitoring. Report arrhythmias, ischemic ST-segment or T-wave changes, or a heart rate above 140 beats/minute.
- Monitor the patient's intake and output hourly. Insert an indwelling

urinary catheter, as ordered, to monitor urine output.
- Assist with insertion of a pulmonary artery catheter, and begin hemodynamic monitoring to evaluate your patient's response to therapy. Monitor central venous pressure (CVP), pulmonary artery diastolic (PAD) pressure, PAWP, and mean arterial pressure (MAP).
- ➡ **NurseALERT** Keep in mind that MAP shows tissue perfusion throughout the cardiac cycle. Cerebral and renal perfusion are seriously decreased when MAP drops below 60 mm Hg. If you need to calculate it, use this formula:

$$\text{MAP} = \frac{\text{systolic blood pressure} + 2(\text{diastolic blood pressure})}{3}$$

- Assess the patient's oxygen saturation levels with pulse oximetry or arterial blood gas (ABG) measurements, as ordered, and give supplemental oxygen.
- Administer morphine sulfate, as prescribed, to enhance venous pooling. Morphine also reduces dyspnea, anxiety, and pain.
- ➡ **NurseALERT** Monitor your patient's respiratory rate carefully because morphine can depress respirations. Keep naloxone (Narcan) at hand for treating overdose.
- Administer inotropic agents, such as dobutamine (Dobutrex), dopamine (Intropin), and amrinone (Inocor), as prescribed, to increase contractility, stroke volume, and, ultimately, cardiac output.
- Give vasodilators, such as nitroglycerin and nitroprusside (Nitropress), as prescribed, to reduce preload and afterload. Vasodilators also promote peripheral blood pooling and reduce myocardial oxygen consumption.
- ➡ **NurseALERT** Monitor your patient's blood pressure carefully when giving these drugs because they can cause hypotension.
- Give vasopressors, such as norepinephrine (Levophed), epinephrine, and phenylephrine, as prescribed, to promote vasoconstriction and improve ventricular contractility.
- Monitor for fluid volume overload by checking for pulmonary congestion, jugular vein distention, ascites, peripheral edema, and a positive hepatojugular reflux. Also look for increasing CVP and PAWP. In pulmonary edema, PAWP exceeds 25 mm Hg.
- Administer diuretics, such as furosemide (Lasix) and bumetanide (Bumex), as prescribed, to reduce volume overload.
- Assess for hypovolemia, as evidenced by a CVP less than 6 mm Hg or a PAWP less than 18 mm Hg. Make sure you monitor CVP and PAWP during infusion.
- Anticipate intra-aortic balloon counterpulsation therapy to reduce afterload, increase perfusion of coronary arteries, and improve cardiac output.

WHAT TO DO NEXT

Once your patient has stabilized, take these actions:

- Because many of the drugs your patient needs are prescribed in micrograms per kilogram per minute, you'll need to weigh him at about the same time each day, using the same scale and with the patient wearing the same amount of clothing. Because these drugs are potent, don't estimate your patient's weight or use his preillness weight.
- Titrate all drugs to the desired heart rate, blood pressure, MAP, CVP, PAD, and PAWP.
- Assess for signs of renal failure, including increasing blood urea nitrogen (BUN) and serum creatinine levels, electrolyte imbalances, and reduced or absent urine output.
- Monitor the patient's vital signs, heart and breath sounds, skin temperature and color, capillary refill, and peripheral pulses.
- Check his ABG values for signs of hypoxemia, including a partial pressure of arterial oxygen less than 60 mm Hg and oxygen saturation less than 90%. Also assess for increased restlessness, worsening dyspnea, and reduced level of consciousness.
- Keep in mind that cyanosis is a late sign.
- Keep watch for respiratory alkalosis (pH above 7.45 and partial pressure of arterial carbon disoxide ($PaCO_2$) less than 35 mm Hg), which can develop if your patient hyperventilates. Also watch for metabolic acidosis, which may develop later from poor tissue perfusion and lactic acid buildup (pH below 7.35, $PaCO_2$ normal or less than 35 mm Hg with compensation, and HCO_3^- less than 22 mEq/L).
- ➡ **NurseALERT** Acidosis and hypoxemia require immediate treatment because they can further reduce myocardial contractility and induce arrhythmias, perpetuating the shock cycle. Moreover, an acidotic state reduces your patient's response to drug therapy. Monitor your patient's lactate levels to detect anaerobic metabolism.
- Continue to monitor the patient's ECG for evidence of ischemia and infarction. If cardiogenic shock causes an extension of his MI, he'll report chest pain and you'll see ST-segment and T-wave changes on his ECG.
- Treat arrhythmias, such as ventricular tachycardia and ventricular fibrillation, according to your facility's policy and advanced cardiac life support algorithms.
- Anticipate coronary artery bypass grafting or percutaneous transluminal coronary angioplasty to improve the patient's myocardial perfusion and limit myocardial necrosis. He may need corrective surgery if the cardiogenic shock stems from papillary muscle rupture or ventricular septal defect.
- Assess your patient's pulmonary status. Observe whether he's using accessory muscles for breathing, auscultate his lungs for increasing crackles, and monitor his respiratory rate and ABG results.

➡ Nurse**ALERT** A respiratory rate above 30 breaths/minute is a sign of declining respiratory status. Anticipate endotracheal intubation and mechanical ventilation.

• Watch for signs of pulmonary edema, including dyspnea, cough, frothy sputum, and cyanosis. The patient may have an increasing respiratory rate and falling blood pressure. PAWP exceeds 25 mm Hg.

➡ Nurse**ALERT** If your patient complains of chest pain, administer nitroglycerin promptly, as prescribed, to prevent further ischemia and infarction and to preserve as much myocardium as possible.

• Anticipate insertion of a ventricular assist device if your patient doesn't respond to other therapies. (See *Understanding ventricular assist devices*, page 72).

FOLLOW-UP CARE

• Monitor the patient's response to medications, and assess vital signs, heart and breath sounds, skin temperature and color, and capillary refill.

• Encourage your patient to cough and deep breathe every 2 hours once he is hemodynamically stable.

• Keep him on bed rest to reduce metabolic demands until he is hemodynamically stable, and then help him increase his activity, as tolerated. Help him change positions every 2 hours.

• Monitor laboratory results and report abnormal values, including elevated white blood cell (WBC) count and BUN, creatinine, carbon dioxide, and lactate levels. You also may see electrolyte abnormalities and, if your patient has had an MI, a characteristic rise and fall of cardiac enzyme levels.

• Check the insertion site for your patient's pulmonary artery catheter, and report any redness, swelling, warmth, tenderness, or drainage around the site. Also report fever and increased WBC count.

• Minimize noise, and plan your nursing care to give your patient uninterrupted sleep and rest periods, if possible.

SPECIAL CONSIDERATIONS

• Cardiogenic shock is a life-threatening condition and frightening for both the patient and his family. Fear and anxiety can place further demands on the patient's already compromised heart through stimulation of the sympathetic nervous system. Whenever possible, include the patient and his family in care, and take time to explain treatments and procedures. Allow the patient to verbalize his fears and concerns. Clarify misconceptions, and reassure him that his condition is being monitored closely.

UNDERSTANDING VENTRICULAR ASSIST DEVICES

A ventricular assist device (VAD) takes over the work of your patient's failing heart so that his body can continue to be supplied with blood and oxygen while his heart rests and recovers or until a donor heart becomes available for transplantation.

Several types of VADs are available, but all divert blood around the failing ventricle by directing it through an inflow cannula to the assist device, which pumps it back into the great vessels (aorta or pulmonary artery, depending on which ventricle is being assisted). The pump (which may be electrically, pneumatically, or centrifugally driven) is either implanted in the abdomen or positioned outside the body. Although a left VAD is more common, as shown in the illustration, you'll also see patients with right VADs, or even both.

NURSING CARE

- Check the VAD, its tubing, and blood flow every 15 minutes until your patient is stable. Then check them every hour. Avoid pulling or kinking the tubes.
- Assess the patient's cardiovascular status frequently, including vital signs, heart rhythm, peripheral pulses, central venous pressure, pulmonary artery pressures, cardiac output, urine output, and heart and breath sounds.
- Inspect all incisions, and report any redness, warmth, swelling, or drainage. Also report fever and increased white blood cell count. Administer antibiotics, as ordered.
- Give a continuous infusion of heparin, if ordered, and give an aspirin tablet, as prescribed, to prevent clot formation. Monitor for signs and symptoms of bleeding.
- If your patient has biventricular failure but only has a VAD for the left side, assess for evidence of right ventricular failure, such as jugular vein distention, ascites, hepatomegaly, and edema.
- Observe the mediastinal chest tube drainage and report excessive bleeding (output greater than 150 ml/hour for more than 2 hours). If chest tube drainage abruptly stops, check for clots in the tubing.
- Monitor the patient's prothrombin time, activated partial thromboplastin time, platelet count, and fibrinogen levels. Report abnormal results, and prepare to give fresh frozen plasma, platelets, or clotting factors.
- Assess for evidence of an air embolus or a thrombus, including changes in level of consciousness, reduced urine output, pulselessness, pallor, pain,

paresthesias, and paralysis of an extremity.
- Wean your patient from the VAD by gradually reducing the flow rate, as ordered, so that the ventricle can gradually increase functioning. Assess the patient's cardiovascular status frequently during the weaning process.

Special considerations

- The thermodilution method commonly used to determine cardiac output can only be used for a patient with a left VAD, not a right VAD.
- If cardiac arrest occurs, follow advanced cardiac life support guidelines and anticipate internal cardiac massage and defibrillation rather than external compressions and defibrillation.
- A patient who needs a VAD is seriously ill. Try to include his family in your nursing care as much as possible, and urge them to verbalize concerns and fears.

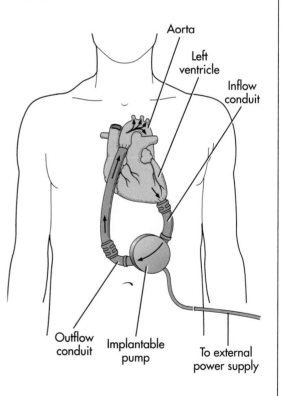

CENTRAL VENOUS CATHETER OCCLUSION

Invaluable in treating critically ill patients, a central venous catheter (CVC) delivers medications, I.V. fluids, and blood and blood products. It also allows continuous monitoring of right atrial (central venous) pressure.

Like any medical device, a CVC must be set up and maintained properly, and it must be inspected often during use to prevent and detect malfunctions that could endanger the patient. For example, if it becomes partially or totally occluded, it won't deliver the proper amount of medications or fluids, and you'll lose venous access. Even worse, if air enters the patient's heart, as from a disconnected or damaged CVC, a lethal air embolism may occur.

By understanding the causes of CVC occlusion and staying alert for signs of partial occlusion, you can take swift action to avert complete occlusion. To ensure your patient's well-being, you also must know how to deal with CVC occlusion or air embolism promptly once it occurs.

Causes of CVC occlusion
Most commonly, a CVC becomes occluded when blood residue accumulates within its lumen. One cause of such accumulation is delayed flushing after infusing a medication or solution; the delay allows blood to reflux into the catheter, where it begins to clot. Other causes of occlusion include:
- formation of drug precipitates when incompatible substances contact each other in the catheter lumen; the resulting insoluble salts or solids may fill the lumen
- kinking of the external or internal catheter track
- a closed clamp or clip in the catheter track.

Causes of an air embolism
The most dangerous complication of CVC occlusion is an air embolism, which can occur if the CVC becomes disconnected or damaged or if the I.V. infusion runs dry. Air then may enter your patient's right ventricle.

A large bolus of air in the right ventricle may prevent blood from entering the pulmonary circulation, leading to cardiopulmonary arrest.

WHAT TO LOOK FOR
If your patient has a CVC, watch for the following signs of partial or complete *occlusion*:
- sluggish infusion when administering a solution by gravity or an I.V. infusion device
- bulging of the catheter material above the hub during attempted irrigation
- resistance to instillation of a flush solution
- resistance to instillation of any fluid by gravity, manual pressure, or an infusion device

- deterioration in the patient's clinical condition despite seemingly proper treatment.

With an *air embolism*, clinical findings typically include:
- dyspnea or tachypnea
- chest pain
- tachycardia
- cyanosis
- hypotension
- anxiety or a sudden feeling of doom
- confusion
- loss of consciousness followed by shock and cardiac arrest (with a massive embolism).

WHAT TO DO IMMEDIATELY

If you suspect that your patient's CVC is occluded, stop the infusion and take the following actions:
- Inspect for a closed clamp or slide clip, checking from the external hub to the CVC insertion point.
- Check the CVC insertion site for "pinch-off" kinks in the catheter.
- Look for blood residue in the hub or lumen. Be aware that in the lumen of a Silastic or polyurethane catheter, blood residue appears pink or red.
- Review the medications and solutions your patient is receiving through the CVC for possible incompatibilities. To help prevent incompatibilities, use the saline-admixture-saline-heparin (SASH) technique to clear the line. First administer a normal saline solution flush, then administer the prescribed admixture or medication, and follow with another saline flush. Finally, flush with heparin. By flushing the I.V. line with normal saline (which is compatible with most I.V. solutions and medications), you'll prevent two incompatible solutions or medications from coming in contact with each other, which can cause a precipitate to form in the I.V. line or catheter.
- ➡ **NurseALERT** To avoid excessively high pressure, which could rupture the catheter lumen, always use a 5-ml or larger barrel syringe when irrigating a CVC. Also, never attempt to forcibly clear an obstruction by irrigation. You could inadvertently dislodge a clot, causing an embolism.

Dealing with an air embolism

If you suspect an air embolism, ask someone to notify the physician while you take the following measures:
- Stop any ongoing I.V. infusion and clamp the CVC. Place the patient on her left side in the Trendelenburg position. This position aids the flow of air bubbles toward the right atrium and away from the pulmonary artery, allowing blood to enter the lungs.
- If appropriate, try to aspirate the air from the CVC, using a syringe.
- Check the integrity of the I.V. solution and line, and replace them if

DECLOTTING A CENTRAL VENOUS CATHETER

If you're unable to aspirate more than 1 ml of blood from your patient's central venous catheter (CVC), a blood clot may be obstructing it. If so, you'll need to assess the situation and intervene swiftly.

First obtain an order to instill urokinase (Abbokinase) or another thrombolytic agent to dissolve the clot, and then follow the procedure below, using standard precautions.

KEY STEPS TO FOLLOW

- Gather one vial (5,000 IU) of urokinase, sterile gloves, a three-way stopcock, two 10-ml syringes, two packages of sterile 4" x 4" gauze squares, and one male adapter cap.
- Locate the hub of the catheter lumen.
- Because urokinase is available in a two-compartment glass vial, you'll need to mix the contents of the two compartments. To do this, push down the rubber stopper on top of the vial. This action forces the rubber stopper separating the diluent from the powdered medication to move into the lower vial, thus allowing the diluent to mix with the powdered medication and prepare it for use.
- Draw up the activated urokinase into one of the 10-ml syringes.

- Using sterile technique, attach the three-way stopcock to the catheter hub. Then attach the second (empty) 10-ml syringe to the opposite end of the stopcock.
- Attach the syringe of urokinase to the side port of the stopcock.
- Using the empty 10-ml syringe, draw all air and blood from the catheter lumen. Then close off the lumen with the stopcock lever.
- Once a vacuum forms, let it pull the urokinase into the lumen. Allow the urokinase to remain there for 15 to 45 minutes, to give it time to dissolve the clot.
- After the designated amount of time, try to aspirate the dissolved clot through the stopcock, using the empty 10-ml syringe.
- If you can aspirate the clot or if the urokinase successfully dissolves the clot, flush the CVC according to your facility's policy, such as with normal saline solution followed by heparin. Then reconnect the infusion tubing to the catheter.
- If your first aspiration attempt fails, try again—this time letting the urokinase remain in the lumen for up to 12 hours.
- If this second attempt fails, expect the physician to replace the occluded CVC with a new one.

C

---

indicated. Also check all connections to make sure that none are loose or dislodged.

- Administer supplemental oxygen, as prescribed.
- Before reconnecting the I.V. line to the CVC, flush the system to remove any air. If there is a possibility that the I.V. tubing was contaminated by disconnection, replace it and the I.V. solution.

WHAT TO DO NEXT

Once you've determined the most likely cause of the occlusion, follow these steps:

- Remove or release any clamps or clips that were closed.
- Attempt to straighten any kinks in the CVC. Using sterile technique, remove the dressing over the insertion site, and then reposition and secure the kinked catheter. You may use stabilizing sterile tape strips to hold the catheter straight if it's badly kinked or made of a stiff, Teflon-type material. After straightening the CVC, clean and redress the insertion site according to your facility's policy, and gently repeat your attempt to irrigate the catheter.
- Obtain an order to declot the catheter, according to your facility's policy, such as by instilling a thrombolytic agent into the lumen. (See *Declotting a central venous catheter*.)

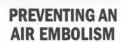

PREVENTING AN AIR EMBOLISM

You can help prevent an air embolism in a patient with a central venous catheter by taking these measures:
- Use luer-lock connections to help prevent tubing disconnections.
- Use an air-eliminating filter on the terminal end of the I.V. tubing to remove any air that inadvertently enters the I.V. line.
- Change all I.V. solution containers before they run completely dry so that air won't enter the tubing.
- Teach the patient how to perform Valsalva's maneuver (unless contraindicated). Instruct her to perform it during catheter insertion and tubing changes to minimize the chance of air entry during these procedures.

- If you suspect that drug incompatibility contributed to the CVC occlusion, ask the pharmacist which agent to instill into the lumen to help eliminate precipitates. For instance, solids may be dissolved by instilling hydrochloric acid or sodium bicarbonate solution, as prescribed.
- After removing the occluding substance, flush the catheter lumen with 10 to 20 ml of sterile normal saline solution for injection. Preferably, use a pulsing flush technique to remove all residue of blood, drugs, and solutions from the internal lumen. To help maintain catheter patency, follow by instilling a heparin solution.

For an air embolism
- Monitor arterial blood gas (ABG) values if ordered.
- Assess the patient's vital signs every 5 to 15 minutes.
- Monitor the patient's oxygen saturation, using pulse oximetry or ABG values.

FOLLOW-UP CARE
- Always flush a CVC with a turbulent-style flush: First infuse 1 ml of normal saline solution, then pause, infuse another 1 ml, and pause again until the flush is completed. The pause at the end of each 1-ml increment of normal saline causes a slight backswirl of saline in the catheter. This backswirl removes more residue from the internal catheter lumen.
- Be sure to use the proper volume of saline solution when flushing the CVC. As a general rule, use an amount that's twice the internal volume of the lumen. With the CVCs most commonly used today, this means flushing with 5 to 8 ml of saline solution.
- Learn about all ordered infusates before administering them to help prevent incompatibilities.
- Use the SASH technique to maintain your patient's CVC.
- Routinely monitor her vital signs and neurologic signs to check for an air embolism.

SPECIAL CONSIDERATIONS
- To reduce the risk of an air embolism, use the proper I.V. connections and filters. (See *Preventing an air embolism*.)
- When clearing an occluded CVC, always *aspirate*—never infuse—the agent out of the lumen. If you're unable to aspirate it, notify the physician and expect to discontinue the CVC.
- To help prevent CVC occlusion, flush the catheter with normal saline solution before and after withdrawing blood and infusing a medication or solution.
- If your patient is receiving a nutritional solution with a lipid component, the lumen may become obstructed by a waxy buildup. To restore proper flow, ethyl alcohol, a solvent, may be instilled and removed by aspiration, unless the catheter is made of polyurethane.

➡ **NurseALERT** Using ethyl alcohol on a polyurethane catheter may damage the catheter material.

CEREBRAL ANEURYSM, RUPTURED

A cerebral aneurysm is a weakened, bulging area on an intracranial blood vessel. The exact cause of these vascular defects is unknown, although their development has been linked to atherosclerosis, congenital abnormalities, inflammation, trauma, and infection.

About 4% of Americans experience cerebral aneurysms and remain asymptomatic. But each year, about 26,000 face the potentially life-threatening consequences of aneurysm rupture.

When a rupture occurs, blood flows from the torn vessel into the subarachnoid space between the arachnoid and pia layers of the meninges, the protective covering of the brain and spinal cord. Intracranial pressure (ICP) rises in response to bleeding and, along with pressure from local tissues, may be sufficient to stop the bleeding. However, the escaped blood circulating in cerebrospinal fluid around the brain and basal cisterns acts as an irritant. The resulting vasospasm impairs cerebral blood flow and may induce cerebral ischemia and infarction. If the bleeding from the aneurysm is great, ICP can increase profoundly, leading to brain herniation and sudden death.

A ruptured cerebral aneurysm can quickly turn deadly. A rapid and accurate response to this emergency can help improve your patient's outcome.

WHAT TO LOOK FOR
Before a cerebral aneurysm ruptures, the patient may have vague signs and symptoms that are easy to overlook or attribute to other causes. Clinical findings may include:
- complaints of hearing "noise" in the head (caused by a bruit)
- headache (localized or general)
- visual disturbances (blurred vision, diplopia, eye movement disorders)
- focal neurologic deficits.

If the aneurysm ruptures, clinical findings may include:
- a sudden, explosive headache (the classic sign of ruptured cerebral aneurysm)
- sudden, transient loss of consciousness or change in level of consciousness (restlessness, irritability)
- stiff neck (meningeal irritation)
- Kernig's and Brudzinski's signs (meningeal irritation)
- photophobia
- nausea and vomiting
- neurologic deficits involving cranial nerves III, IV, and VI, such as diplopia, ptosis, dilated pupils, and deviated eye movements

- focal deficits, such as weakness or paralysis of an arm or a leg
- seizures
- coma.

WHAT TO DO IMMEDIATELY

If you think your patient has suffered a ruptured cerebral aneurysm, notify the physician. Then take these steps:

- Secure and maintain the patient's airway. A person who survives initial rupture of a cerebral aneurysm typically has an altered level of consciousness and therefore cannot maintain an adequate airway.
- Assist with endotracheal intubation and mechanical ventilation, as needed.
- Maintain supplemental oxygen, as prescribed. Monitor oxygen saturation levels with pulse oximetry and arterial blood gas analyses. If the patient needs suctioning, preoxygenate him to avoid hypoxia.
- Assess and document the patient's level of consciousness, including the type and amount of stimulation required for a response; pupil size, shape, and response to light; extraocular eye movements; strength and movement of extremities; and presence or absence of protective reflexes.
- Carefully document any focal neurologic deficits. Then continue to monitor the patient's neurologic status. Remember that once an aneurysm ruptures, disability and death most commonly result from rebleeding, vasospasm, or both.
- Assist with measures to regulate the patient's blood pressure to promote adequate cerebral perfusion.
- ➡ **NurseALERT** Be aware that careful management of blood pressure can help prevent rebleeding and vasospasm. Your goal is to keep systolic pressure between 140 and 150 mm Hg. Higher pressures can contribute to rebleeding. Lower pressures can compromise cerebral blood flow. Anticipate giving labetalol because it doesn't cause abrupt pressure changes.
- Monitor your patient's blood pressure and pulse and respiratory rates every 15 minutes until he is stable. Take his temperature every 4 hours (the body's inflammatory response to blood in the subarachnoid space raises body temperature). Be prepared to treat hyperthermia promptly.

WHAT TO DO NEXT

Once your patient is stable, take the following actions:

- Begin aneurysm precautions designed to prevent increased ICP and, possibly, rebleeding. For example, place the patient on bed rest with the head of the bed elevated 15 to 30 degrees. Maintain a quiet environment and assess carefully for agitation. If necessary, obtain orders for a mild sedative, such as phenobarbital, to help the patient rest. Keep the room dark to decrease photophobia. Follow a bowel management program that includes a stool softener to help the patient avoid straining.

DIAGNOSTIC TESTS

CONFIRMING A CEREBRAL ANEURYSM BY ANGIOGRAPHY

Cerebral angiography can pinpoint the location of your patient's cerebral aneurysm and help in planning a surgical approach. An angiogram also reveals vessel size and shape, blood flow through the aneurysm, and the condition of surrounding vessels.

PERFORMING THE TEST

To perform cerebral angiography, the radiologist threads a catheter through a puncture site, usually in the groin, up to the cerebral vessels. Typically, the catheter travels in the femoral artery, although the radiologist sometimes uses the brachial or carotid artery instead.

After confirming catheter placement by fluoroscopy or X-ray, the radiologist injects a contrast dye into the cerebral vasculature. During the injection, the patient may feel warmth, flushing, and a burning sensation that lasts about 5 seconds. As the dye moves through cerebral vessels, serial X-rays allow evaluation of these vessels.

EXPECTED RESULTS

With a cerebral aneurysm, the angiogram reveals alterations in cerebral circulation and vessel lumen size as well as differences in arterial filling. Because about one patient in every five has multiple aneurysms, the radiologist looks carefully at all vessels feeding into the intracranial circulation.

ALTERNATIVE STUDIES

Another diagnostic test, magnetic resonance imaging (MRI) is sensitive to soft-tissue changes and reveals intracranial blood vessels, the extent of hemorrhage, and the location of an aneurysm. Unlike cerebral angiography, an MRI seldom produces the level of detail about the vasculature itself that is necessary for a surgeon to determine how to treat the aneurysm.

- Continue to monitor vital signs and neurologic status hourly. Report a decline in neurologic status immediately.
- Prepare the patient for cerebral angiography to outline the aneurysm and identify multiple aneurysms. Provide information to help plan surgery. Be sure to check the patient's prothrombin time, activated partial thromboplastin time, and blood urea nitrogen and creatinine levels before the procedure. (See *Confirming a cerebral aneurysm by angiography*.)
- Provide the patient and family with an explanation of his condition, and offer support and encouragement.
- Monitor fluid intake and output. Careful fluid management can help reduce the risk of increased ICP and elevated blood pressure.
- Administer prophylactic anticonvulsants, as prescribed, and assess for signs of seizures.
- Provide analgesics to control headache, as prescribed, and assess their effectiveness.
- Prepare the patient for surgery, if indicated. If the patient's condition and the aneurysm's location allow, surgical clipping or wrapping of the aneurysm is the treatment of choice. If his neurologic status is good, expect him to undergo surgery within 72 hours after the rupture.
- If appropriate, prepare the patient for other types of treatment, such as coiling and balloon occlusion, which are typically performed with angiography.
- Continue giving nimodipine for 21 days after the rupture, as ordered, to improve collateral blood flow and decrease the risk of vasospasm.

FOLLOW-UP CARE

- After surgery, monitor your patient's neurologic status closely. Be aware that he is at increased risk for vasospasm (which typically occurs after the second postoperative day up to 8 days postoperative) and hydrocephalus. Stay alert for changes in mental status, which suggest hydrocephalus.
- Because headache is an ongoing problem, assess your patient's need for analgesics repeatedly and monitor his response.
- Maintain fluid therapy, as prescribed, to minimize the risk of vasospasm.
- Monitor serum electrolyte levels carefully, especially sodium and potassium. Common abnormalities include hyponatremia and hypokalemia.

SPECIAL CONSIDERATIONS

- If the patient isn't a surgical candidate, medical therapy will continue for about 4 weeks. Maintain aneurysm precautions throughout that period.
- Provide plenty of support and encouragement to the patient and family.
- Teach the patient ways to prevent increased ICP, such as not straining or coughing excessively.
- If the patient has permanent neurologic deficits, seek appropriate referrals for rehabilitation services or home health follow-up.

CEREBROVASCULAR ACCIDENT

In a cerebrovascular accident (CVA)—commonly called a stroke—a cerebral vessel ruptures (hemorrhagic CVA) or becomes occluded by a thrombus or an embolism (thrombotic CVA). As a result, blood flow to the part of the brain served by the affected vessel is interrupted. Without adequate blood flow, cerebral oxygenation diminishes.

Within 4 to 5 minutes, pathophysiologic changes begin at the cellular level. Stores of glucose, glycogen, and adenosine triphosphate become depleted, metabolism ceases, and the sodium-potassium pump fails. Sodium then draws water into cells, causing them to swell. Cerebral edema compresses cerebral vasculature and further decreases blood flow.

When severe or prolonged, ischemia leads to cellular death and permanent neurologic deficits. Consequently, your patient's prognosis depends largely on how quickly blood flow is restored to affected brain tissue. Swift action on your part may improve your patient's chance for recovery, especially if he is a candidate for thrombolytic therapy and other new treatments that offer the hope of nearly complete recovery.

WHAT TO LOOK FOR

Expect to detect neurologic, sensory, and motor problems contralaterally—on the side of the body opposite the affected brain region. In addition, general clinical findings in a patient with a CVA may include:

UNDERSTANDING TRANSIENT ISCHEMIC ATTACKS

A transient ischemic attack (TIA) is a brief episode of cerebral ischemia that causes temporary neurologic dysfunction. Sometimes called a "ministroke," a TIA typically results from the same conditions that produce cerebrovascular accidents (CVAs): thrombosis (the most common) or embolism.

In fact, a TIA is a warning sign that a CVA may be imminent. At least half the patients who experience a TIA suffer a CVA within 2 to 5 years.

NEUROLOGIC MARKERS

Signs and symptoms of TIA range from transient focal deficits that involve some degree of motor or sensory dysfunction to loss of consciousness and loss of motor and sensory function for a brief time. Most commonly, the patient experiences weakness of the lower part of the face and of the arms, hands, fingers, and legs on the side opposite the affected brain region. Other typical findings include transient dysphagia and sensory dysfunction, such as numbness and tingling of the face or lips or an extremity. Neurologic deficits resolve within 24 hours.

TIAs may recur intermittently over days, weeks, months, or years. Between episodes, the patient's neurologic status is normal.

RESPONDING TO A TIA

If you suspect that your patient is experiencing a TIA, notify the physician immediately. Evaluate the patient's neurologic status closely. When the episode resolves, prepare him for diagnostic tests, such as carotid Doppler ultrasound, to evaluate his condition.

Once the patient's condition stabilizes, teach him and his family ways to reduce his risk factors for CVA. Provide instruction on prescribed medications, such as vasodilators, anticoagulants, and antiplatelet agents.

- unilateral limb weakness
- speech difficulties
- unilateral numbness
- blurred vision
- headache
- dizziness
- anxiety
- altered level of consciousness
- previous diagnosed or suspected transient ischemic attack (TIA). (See *Understanding transient ischemic attacks*.)

How findings vary with the affected vessel

Additional clinical findings vary with the particular cerebral vessel affected. For instance, if the CVA involved the *middle cerebral artery* (most common), signs and symptoms may include:

- contralateral paralysis or motor loss (more pronounced in the face and arm than in the leg)
- contralateral sensory losses
- blindness or visual defects in the left or right halves of the visual fields of both eyes (homonymous hemianopia)
- aphasia, if the dominant brain hemisphere was involved
- apraxia, agnosia, and neglect, if the nondominant hemisphere was involved.

If the CVA affected the *anterior cerebral artery*, the patient may experience:
- contralateral paralysis of the leg and foot

- gait impairment
- inability to make decisions
- personality changes, including flat affect, inappropriate emotional responses, and distractibility
- urinary incontinence.

With involvement of the *posterior cerebral artery,* expect the following findings:
- homonymous hemianopia
- cortical blindness
- memory dysfunction
- perseveration (abnormal persistence of a response).

With involvement of the *vertebral* or *basilar artery,* signs and symptoms may include:
- weakness of the tongue
- facial numbness and weakness on the same side as the brain injury
- dizziness
- nystagmus
- dysphagia
- dysarthria
- gait dysfunction and ataxia
- "locked-in" syndrome (quadriplegia and mutism with intact consciousness).

WHAT TO DO IMMEDIATELY
If you suspect your patient has suffered a CVA, check his airway, breathing, and circulation. Notify the physician. Then take these actions:
- Establish and maintain a patent airway. Remember that a patient with an altered level of consciousness may have difficulty breathing, particularly if the CVA has affected the posterior cerebral circulation or the vertebral or basilar artery.
- Ensure adequate oxygenation by providing supplemental oxygen, as prescribed. Maintain oxygen saturation above 93%.
- Perform a baseline neurologic assessment, and then reassess the patient's neurologic status every 15 to 30 minutes. Be sure to evaluate level of consciousness, motor and sensory functions, speech difficulty, and protective reflexes.
- Assess the patient's vital signs every 15 minutes until he is stable.
- ➡ **NurseALERT** If the physician prescribes an antihypertensive, such as nitroprusside (Nitropress), to reduce a severely elevated blood pressure, be sure to monitor your patient's intra-arterial blood pressure closely. The goal of antihypertensive treatment is to keep the patient mildly hypertensive, not to lower the blood pressure to the normal range. By keeping the patient mildly hypertensive, adequate cerebral perfusion will be maintained in the face of increased intracranial pressure (ICP) from edema surrounding the cerebral infarction. Lowering

the patient's blood pressure too much can increase cerebral ischemia.

- Try to pinpoint the time of symptom onset. A patient who receives medical attention within 3 hours of the onset of neurologic dysfunction and whose CVA is thrombotic in origin may be eligible for thrombolytic therapy. If your patient is a candidate for this therapy, assess for possible contraindications, such as evidence of intracranial hemorrhage; recent intracranial surgery, serious head trauma, or CVA; active internal bleeding; and uncontrolled hypertension.
- Establish I.V. access, and administer fluids and electrolytes, as prescribed.
- Begin anticoagulation therapy, as prescribed. Heparin is the most common anticoagulant used to treat thrombotic CVA; it's usually administered 1 to 2 hours after thrombolytic therapy.
- Prepare the patient for ordered diagnostic tests, such as computed tomography to rule out hemorrhage and carotid Doppler studies or two-dimensional echocardiography to identify the cause of the CVA.

WHAT TO DO NEXT
Once your patient's condition stabilizes, carry out the following interventions:

- Continue to monitor his neurologic status, and immediately report any change. Keep in mind that neurologic deterioration may signal a new hemorrhage caused by reperfusion or extension of the CVA.
- Maintain the patient's blood pressure within desired parameters.
- Continue anticoagulation therapy, as prescribed. Assess the patient's coagulation values, including activated partial thromboplastin time. Adjust anticoagulant doses, as prescribed and indicated.
- If your patient has dysphagia, watch closely for signs of aspiration of food or fluids. Institute appropriate safety measures, such as encouraging the patient to take small mouthfuls of food, placing the food in the unaffected side of the mouth, and checking his mouth for residue at the end of the meal. Anticipate feeding him by way of a gastric tube. Also anticipate that the patient will undergo an evaluation of his swallowing, possibly with video fluoroscopy.
- As appropriate, arrange for the patient to start rehabilitation therapies, including speech therapy, physical therapy, and occupational therapy, within 24 hours of admission (unless contraindicated).
- Manage GI problems as needed. Assess for adequate elimination, provide sufficient fluids, and, if necessary, administer stool softeners or laxatives to promote elimination.
- Evaluate for urinary incontinence. If indicated, begin a bladder retraining program.
- If the patient has trouble speaking, establish an alternative communication method.
- Explain all diagnostic tests and treatments to the patient and family, using simple terms.

CEREBRAL EDEMA: PERILOUS AFTERMATH OF C.V.A.

By decreasing blood flow to brain cells, a cerebrovascular accident (CVA) may lead to cerebral edema through cellular changes that impair the sodium-potassium pump.

The leading cause of death after a CVA, cerebral edema peaks 24 to 72 hours after a CVA and is most common in elderly people and when the CVA involves a large portion of the brain.

RECOGNIZING CEREBRAL EDEMA

Signs and symptoms of increased intracranial pressure (ICP) are the hallmark of cerebral edema and include:
- decreasing level of consciousness
- restlessness and irritability
- increasing systolic blood pressure
- widening pulse pressure
- papilledema
- projectile vomiting
- unequal pupils, change in pupil reaction to light
- changes in respiratory pattern
- decorticate or decerebrate posturing, both of which warn of the patient's grave condition (see accompanying illustrations).

TAKING ACTION

If you suspect your patient has cerebral edema, take the following measures:
- Closely monitor vital signs and neurologic status. Be especially alert to changes in level of consciousness. Restlessness and irritability are often the earliest clues to decreasing level of consciousness.
- Maintain a patent airway and adequate oxygenation. If necessary, suction nasotracheally to remove secretions (which can impair gas exchange, increasing cerebral ischemia and edema), but limit suction-ing time to a minimum. Don't suction routinely.
- Position the patient with the head of the bed elevated at least 30 degrees and his head and neck in neutral body alignment, which promotes venous outflow from the head.
- Avoid hip flexion, which increases intra-abdominal and intrathoracic pressure and can ultimately increase ICP.
- Administer osmotic diuretic agents, as prescribed. Take care to prevent hypovolemia because this will lower blood pressure and decrease cerebral perfusion.
- Monitor serum electrolyte levels carefully if the patient is receiving osmotic diuretics. Keep a meticulous record of fluid intake and output.
- Maintain adequate blood pressure to support cerebral perfusion. If administering antihypertensive drugs, make sure that the patient's blood pressure doesn't fall below the prescribed level. The goal is to keep the patient mildly hypertensive (systolic, 140 to 150 mm Hg) to maintain cerebral perfusion.
- Space treatments and physical care to allow the patient time to rest. These activities can cause transient increases in ICP, which can have a cumulative effect.
- Teach the patient to avoid the Valsalva maneuver. Turn and reposition him passively—he shouldn't pull on the side rails or use an overhead trapeze. Give stool softeners, as prescribed.
- Talk to the patient as you care for him, even if he is unresponsive or comatose. Allow the family to remain at the bedside when possible. These actions have been shown to lower ICP.

FOLLOW-UP CARE

- Monitor the patient's vital signs and neurologic status as his activity level increases.
- → Nurse**ALERT** Watch closely for signs of increasing ICP and other signs of cerebral edema, which tends to peak 24 to 72 hours after an ischemic CVA. Suspect increasing ICP if you note a change in the patient's level of consciousness. Stay especially alert for signs of cerebral edema if your patient's CVA involved a large portion of one brain hemisphere, as indicated by the degree of neurologic dysfunction. (See *Cerebral edema: Perilous aftermath of CVA.*)
- Administer prescribed medications, such as anticoagulants, antiplatelet agents, and anticonvulsants, and assess for adverse effects.
- Perform meticulous skin care, especially on the affected side.

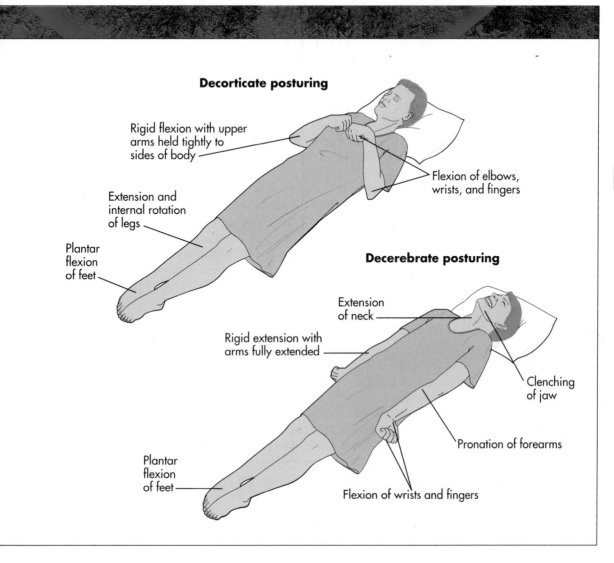

Decorticate posturing

Rigid flexion with upper arms held tightly to sides of body

Flexion of elbows, wrists, and fingers

Extension and internal rotation of legs

Plantar flexion of feet

Decerebrate posturing

Extension of neck

Rigid extension with arms fully extended

Clenching of jaw

Pronation of forearms

Plantar flexion of feet

Flexion of wrists and fingers

C

- Check regularly for signs and symptoms of pulmonary embolism, such as sudden onset of acute dyspnea, restlessness, or decreased oxygen saturation, especially if your patient isn't receiving anticoagulants.
- Teach the patient how to modify his activities of daily living, given his disability. Encourage him to participate in self-care to the extent possible. Also urge family members to participate in his care, especially if he'll be discharged to his home.
- Initiate a referral to an acute or a subacute rehabilitation facility as necessary.
- Teach the patient and his family about prescribed drugs and related precautions and about CVA risk factors and how to reduce them.

- Inform the patient and his family which signs and symptoms of CVA recurrence to report immediately.
- Refer the patient and his family for home care services to aid rehabilitation, if necessary. Help them obtain any medical equipment the patient may need to remain independent at home.

SPECIAL CONSIDERATIONS

- If your patient receives thrombolytic therapy, expect him to be monitored in the intensive care unit for at least 24 hours after therapy. Watch for and report signs of neurologic deterioration, which may indicate hemorrhage.
- After thrombolytic therapy, maintain systolic blood pressure below 185 mm Hg and diastolic pressure below 110 mm Hg. Carefully monitor for signs and symptoms of bleeding (the most common adverse effect of thrombolytics).
- ➡ **NurseALERT** Don't give warfarin (Coumadin) or aspirin for at least 24 hours after thrombolytic therapy. These agents could increase the patient's risk for hemorrhage.

CONSCIOUSNESS, ALTERED LEVEL OF

The state of being aware of oneself and oriented to the environment, level of consciousness (LOC) results from smooth functioning of the brain's reticular activating system and its connections with the cerebral cortex. The aspect of consciousness known as cognition relies largely on the cerebral cortex. The aspect known as arousal, or wakefulness, depends largely on the reticular activating system.

Changes in LOC can vary from slight to severe and can develop suddenly or gradually, depending on the cause. Some causes of altered LOC include structural brain abnormalities that result in edema; metabolic disturbances; central nervous system infections; cardiopulmonary disorders; certain drugs, such as steroids, anticonvulsants, and salicylates; and degenerative disorders.

Restlessness and irritability are some of the earliest signs of a decreasing LOC. As LOC decreases, the patient becomes confused and disoriented to time, then place, and finally people. Wakefulness also decreases, and the patient becomes lethargic, less responsive, and, finally, comatose. Therefore, any change in a patient's LOC requires a swift and certain response from you and your fellow health-care professionals.

WHAT TO LOOK FOR
Clinical findings vary, depending on which aspect of LOC is affected. Findings that suggest a change in *wakefulness and arousal mechanisms* include:
- restlessness, irritability
- sleepiness
- lethargy

- disorientation to time, place, and person
- markedly short attention span
- inability to follow simple commands
- the need for a tactile or strong stimulus to elicit a response.

Clinical findings that suggest a change in *cognitive function* may include:
- disorientation to person, place, and time
- poor memory
- poor judgment
- inability to solve problems
- inability to follow two-step or sequenced commands.

C

WHAT TO DO IMMEDIATELY
If you suspect your patient has an altered LOC, notify the physician. Then take these steps:
- Assess the patient's respiratory rate and depth; make sure she has a patent airway.
- ➡ **NurseALERT** Remember that when altered LOC stems from an acute problem, your patient quickly may progress to unconsciousness. Be sure to keep emergency equipment at hand, and anticipate the need for endotracheal intubation and mechanical ventilation. Keep in mind that inadequate oxygenation is a cause of decreased LOC.
- Reassess her frequently, using standard LOC assessment tools. If she is unstable, check her every 5 to 10 minutes. If she seems stable and her LOC decrease occurred gradually, assess her at least every 4 hours. (See *Assessing level of consciousness*, page 88.)
- Prepare the patient for diagnostic tests, such as computed tomography of the head, as indicated.
- Take steps to protect her from injury. For instance, if she is restless or agitated, supervise her closely to prevent falls and other injuries.

WHAT TO DO NEXT
Next, you'll need to take the following actions:
- Continue to monitor the patient's neurologic status carefully.
- Assess the need to protect her from aspiration if swallowing is affected or if she is lethargic.
- Implement treatments, as ordered, based on the cause of her decreased LOC.
- To help decrease the patient's confusion, limit environmental stimulation, such as by limiting visitors and keeping the room quiet. Reorient the patient often and keep all explanations simple.
- If the patient is immobile from a severely reduced LOC, apply elastic stockings or compression boots to help prevent deep vein thrombosis.
- Provide meticulous skin care; turn and reposition the patient every 2 hours, and keep her skin clean and dry.

ASSESSING LEVEL OF CONSCIOUSNESS

To assess your patient's level of consciousness accurately and objectively, start with a normal level of stimulus and increase stimulus strength, as appropriate, until she responds.

Using a normal tone of voice, start by asking questions that will reveal if the patient is disoriented. If she doesn't respond, try speaking louder or clapping your hands to get her attention, and then ask her the questions again. Note whether she responds to the louder noise. If she does respond, determine whether she answers your questions appropriately or whether she drifts back to sleep.

If auditory stimulation doesn't arouse her, try tactile stimulation by touching her gently while calling her name. If she doesn't respond to touch, gently shake her shoulder. If that doesn't elicit a response, try a stronger stimulus. Using a pen or another hard object, apply pressure to her nail bed and watch her response.

If there is no response to this peripheral stimulus, assess her response to a strong stimulus applied centrally. Pinch her trapezius or pectoralis major muscle and watch her response. Don't pinch near a nipple (the tissue bruises too easily), perform a sternal rub, or apply supraorbital pressure. Never use a pin to deliver a painful stimulus because you may cause injury and infection.

USING THE GLASGOW COMA SCALE

For an objective, standardized assessment of your patient's level of consciousness, use the Glasgow Coma Scale, shown below. With this scale, you'll add the scores in each of three categories to arrive at a total score of 3 to 15. A patient who's fully awake and alert will receive a 15. A patient who scores less than 7 is considered to be in a coma; a score of 3 indicates a deep coma.

Eye opening	Spontaneous	4
	To voice	3
	To pain	2
	No response	1
Best verbal response	Oriented	5
	Confused	4
	Inappropriate words	3
	Incomprehensible sounds	2
	No response	1
Best motor response	Obeys command	6
	Localizes pain	5
	Withdraws from pain	4
	Flexion with pain	3
	Extension with pain	2
	No response	1
Total score		3 to 15

- Place her joints in functional positions and elevate them slightly to prevent dependent edema. Perform passive range-of-motion exercises every 4 hours.
- Provide adequate nutrition and hydration. Discuss the appropriateness of tube feedings with the physician.

FOLLOW-UP CARE

- Begin ordered therapy to improve the patient's cognitive skills as soon as she can participate. Keep in mind that most patients with an altered LOC regain neurologic function over time.
- Provide emotional support to the patient's family because recovery can be slow. Help them identify needs and make discharge plans.

SPECIAL CONSIDERATIONS

- When assessing for causes of an altered LOC, evaluate the patient's history carefully for contributing factors, such as medications, traumatic injury, or a history of neurologic problems.
- Anticipate the need for follow-up home care to aid rehabilitation.

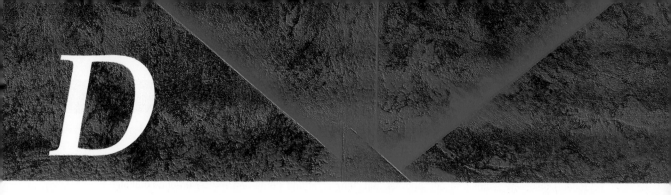

DEHYDRATION, ACUTE

Dehydration refers to a shortage of water in the body—commonly from prolonged fever, diarrhea, or vomiting. To understand the clinical significance of dehydration, you need to understand why this water shortage can have fatal effects.

The danger of dehydration lies in the shift of fluids and electrolytes that ensues—a shift that upsets the delicate balance of substances floating between the intracellular and extracellular compartments. Indeed, dehydration may be isotonic, hypertonic, or hypotonic. (See *Distinguishing among the types of dehydration*, page 90.)

Regardless of the type of dehydration your patient has, you'll need to intervene promptly to prevent a downward spiral to hypovolemic shock, multisystem organ failure, coma, and death.

WHAT TO LOOK FOR
Clinical findings in dehydration (and the underlying problem of hyponatremia or hypernatremia) may include:
- thirst
- dry skin, dry mucous membranes, decreased perspiration
- poor skin turgor
- dry, fissured tongue
- difficulty speaking
- dizziness, weakness, fatigue
- hypotension (particularly orthostatic)
- lethargy
- confusion, delirium
- fever
- tachycardia at rest
- weight loss
- oliguria or anuria
- sunken eyes
- muscle twitching
- seizures
- shock
- abnormal serum sodium and osmolality levels.

DISTINGUISHING AMONG THE TYPES OF DEHYDRATION

Normally, intracellular, interstitial, intravascular, and transcellular (such as cerebrospinal, pleural, and peritoneal) fluids are isotonic to one another. But dehydration can alter their delicate balance in several ways. For one, fluids outside the cells may contain more water than fluids inside the cells, which prompts water to enter the cells, causing them to swell and, possibly, rupture. Likewise, if fluids inside the cells contain more water than fluids outside the cells, water leaves, causing the cells to shrink and eventually, if untreated, to die.

Because of these differences, dehydration can be classified as isotonic, hypertonic, or hypotonic.

ISOTONIC DEHYDRATION

In isotonic dehydration, proportional changes in electrolytes accompany changes in total body water. Because total body water loss equals electrolyte loss, serum electrolyte levels and osmolality stay within normal limits. Common causes of isotonic dehydration include hemorrhage, excessive diaphoresis, vomiting, diarrhea, burns, and excessive wound drainage.

HYPERTONIC DEHYDRATION

In hypertonic dehydration, water loss exceeds loss of electrolytes (mainly sodium), and serum sodium levels and osmolality rise above normal. Typically, hypertonic dehydration results from impaired thirst mechanism, fever, hyperventilation, ketoacidosis, and excessive fluid or sodium bicarbonate administration.

HYPOTONIC DEHYDRATION

In hypotonic dehydration, loss of electrolytes (mainly sodium) exceeds water loss, and serum sodium levels and osmolality drop below normal. Causes of hypotonic dehydration include chronic illnesses (such as renal failure and malnutrition) and excessive ingestion of hypotonic fluids.

WHAT TO DO IMMEDIATELY

If you suspect your patient is dehydrated, notify the physician. Then take these steps:

- Assess the patient's vital signs.
- Record his baseline weight. Keep meticulous documentation of fluid intake and output.
- Prepare him for I.V. therapy, and establish a peripheral I.V. line. Stay alert for signs of infiltration.
- Obtain blood samples to measure serum electrolyte and hemoglobin levels, hematocrit, and white blood cell count.
- Place the patient on continuous cardiac monitoring, and monitor his ECG for tachycardia and other arrhythmias.
- Assist with diagnostic tests or procedures to identify the underlying cause of dehydration.
- Monitor the patient's electrolyte status carefully; the treatment you implement relates directly to the imbalance involved, as outlined below.

For isotonic dehydration

- Administer isotonic saline solution to promote rehydration, as prescribed. Expect to continue this infusion as long as the patient shows evidence of hemodynamic compromise.

For hypertonic dehydration and hypernatremia

- Give I.V. hypotonic electrolyte solution (0.2% or 0.45% sodium chloride) or a salt-free solution, such as dextrose 5% in water, as prescribed.

- Document the time I.V. therapy began to ensure a *gradual* reduction of the serum sodium level to normal—a process that should take at least 48 hours.
- ➡ **NurseALERT** Remember that if you correct hypernatremia too quickly, your patient could develop cerebral edema. Watch for such telltale signs and symptoms as lethargy, headache, nausea, vomiting, brady-cardia, and hypertension.
- Check your patient's blood pressure, pulse and respiratory rates, and level of consciousness every 5 to 15 minutes, watching especially for bradycardia and hypertension. Keep in mind that loss of conscious-ness may progress to coma and, if the underlying condition is uncor-rected, permanent neurologic damage or even death.

For hypotonic dehydration and hyponatremia

- Slowly administer normal saline solution I.V. For severe hypona-tremia (a serum sodium level less than 115 mEq/L), administer 3% to 5% sodium chloride solution I.V., as prescribed.
- ➡ **NurseALERT** Know that incorrect sodium chloride administration could cause pulmonary edema and a worsening neurologic status. Specifically, a rapid correction of hyponatremia can cause central pontine myelinolysis, which may result in quadriplegia, cranial nerve abnormalities, or changes in level of consciousness. To prevent fluid overload, use a volume-control device and monitor the infusion closely. Be particularly cautious if your patient has heart failure or re-nal failure. (Ideally, a patient receiving I.V. sodium chloride should be in the intensive care unit to ensure close monitoring.)
- Be aware that sodium chloride solution is irritating to the vein. Moni-tor the I.V. site frequently as the infusion begins and every 30 minutes thereafter.
- Report signs and symptoms of circulatory overload—such as dysp-nea, crackles on auscultation, and jugular vein distention—to the physician at once.
- Obtain blood samples for serum sodium and osmolality measure-ment and evaluate laboratory results. Remember that the sodium level must increase *slowly* to avoid complications.
- As prescribed, administer furosemide (Lasix) to promote water loss and prevent pulmonary edema. Also monitor the patient's urine out-put, and send a urine specimen to the laboratory to measure sodium and potassium levels.
- Implement seizure precautions, such as raising and padding the side rails, as needed. If the patient has a seizure, make sure he has a patent airway and that he is safe. Then notify the physician at once.

WHAT TO DO NEXT
Once the patient is stable, take the following actions:
- Continue to monitor blood test results, as indicated; report signifi-cant changes, especially in sodium levels and osmolality.

- Continue to assess your patient's vital signs and level of consciousness every hour initially during I.V. therapy and then every 4 hours. An improved level of consciousness and increased muscle strength verify the effectiveness of the therapy.
- ➡ **NurseALERT** Keep in mind that diminished urine output may lead to cerebral edema or circulatory overload.
- Monitor and document the patient's weight daily.
- Continue seizure precautions. As the imbalance resolves, the risk of seizures declines (unless the patient has another risk factor).
- Provide oral intake, as prescribed. Document the amount consumed on the patient's intake record. Track the patient's hourly fluid intake and output.
- Institute safety precautions, as indicated. Severely dehydrated patients are weak and may experience orthostatic hypotension, resulting in falls.

FOLLOW-UP CARE
- Continue to monitor the patient's vital signs, daily weight, and intake and output accurately.
- Check his serum sodium level and osmolality. If you see any fluctuation, notify the physician immediately.
- Monitor the patient's urine specific gravity to detect concentrated or dilute urine.
- Assess his level of consciousness; a sudden change could indicate electrolyte imbalances.
- Educate the patient about the importance of maintaining his fluid and electrolyte levels within normal limits.

SPECIAL CONSIDERATIONS
- Remember that elderly people and infants are particularly susceptible to dehydration.

DIABETES INSIPIDUS

In diabetes insipidus, the body produces large amounts of dilute urine from deficient antidiuretic hormone (ADH) or, less often, from the kidneys' inability to respond to ADH. Without ADH, the kidneys can't concentrate urine in relation to the body's hydration status, triggering severe polyuria. Urine output may increase to as much as 1 L/hour.

If the patient loses enough fluid, she rapidly may deteriorate to life-threatening hypovolemic shock. You'll need to take quick action to prevent circulatory collapse and death.

Diabetes insipidus most often occurs as the result of damage to the cells in the hypothalamus, which produce ADH, or the pituitary gland (where ADH is stored and secreted). Called neurogenic (or central) diabetes insipidus, this disorder can develop after a traumatic head injury or intracranial neurosurgery or as a result of cerebrovascular lesions or infectious processes. Neurogenic diabetes insipidus can be transient (if related to edema, such as from surgery) or permanent (if the cells that produce or secrete ADH are destroyed).

   If you suspect your patient has developed diabetes insipidus, you'll need to take quick action to prevent serious electrolyte disturbances, severe dehydration, and, possibly, circulatory collapse.

WHAT TO LOOK FOR
Clinical findings in diabetes insipidus include:
- sudden onset of polyuria (3 to 24 L/24 hours)
- dilute urine that looks like water
- urine specific gravity less than 1.005
- intense thirst unrelieved by fluid intake
- poor skin turgor
- dry mucous membranes
- orthostatic hypotension
- tachycardia.

WHAT TO DO IMMEDIATELY
If your patient shows signs or symptoms of diabetes insipidus, notify the physician. Then follow these guidelines:
- Quickly check your patient's vital signs. Check the specific gravity of her urine if a urinometer is available (or obtain a urine specimen to send to the laboratory, as ordered).
- Establish I.V. access, and begin fluid resuscitation therapy with a hypotonic solution, as prescribed.
- Immediately administer aqueous vasopressin (exogenous ADH) parenterally, as prescribed.
- Monitor the patient's fluid intake and output. If she doesn't already have an indwelling urinary catheter in place and develops signs and symptoms of hypovolemic shock (severe hypotension, tachycardia, and an altered level of consciousness), insert a urinary catheter to monitor output more accurately.
- Prepare to assist with insertion of a hemodynamic monitoring device, such as a central venous catheter, if indicated, to monitor the effectiveness of rehydration therapy.

WHAT TO DO NEXT
Once therapy for diabetes insipidus begins, take the following steps:
- Continue to monitor your patient's vital signs, urine specific gravity, and fluid intake and output at least hourly.
- Adjust the flow rate of the I.V. fluid infusion. As a rule of thumb, expect to give 1 ml of fluid for every 1 ml of urine excreted.
- Give subsequent vasopressin doses based on your patient's urine output, according to the physician's order. (See *Medications for diabetes insipidus*, page 94.)
- Assess the patient closely for signs and symptoms of water intoxication (severe water retention and hyponatremia), including peripheral

TREATMENT OF CHOICE

MEDICATIONS FOR DIABETES INSIPIDUS

Exogenous antidiuretic hormone (ADH) is a cornerstone of therapy for the patient with diabetes insipidus. Here's what you need to know about the ADH forms available and how to administer them. After giving any form of ADH, always monitor the patient closely for water intoxication.

VASOPRESSIN
Vasopressin controls polyuria for up to 8 hours. In an emergency, this drug most commonly is given subcutaneously (S.C.). However, it also may be given intramuscularly or nasally.

Nasal preparations may be given by spray, cotton pledget, or dropper. Usually, though, nasal forms are reserved for chronic rather than emergent cases.

DESMOPRESSIN ACETATE (DDAVP)
Desmopressin acetate controls polyuria for up to 24 hours. It's the only form of ADH that can be given I.V.; it also may be given by the S.C. or nasal route.

When giving desmopressin I.V., dilute it in 10 to 50 ml of normal saline solution and infuse it over 15 to 30 minutes. Nasal preparations, which can be administered by spray, cotton pledget, or dropper, usually are reserved for chronic cases.

---

edema, dyspnea, crackles, and altered level of consciousness during fluid resuscitation. Report these findings immediately.
- Monitor the patient's serum electrolyte levels and serum and urine osmolality, as ordered.

FOLLOW-UP CARE
- Weigh the patient daily at the same time, on the same scale, and in similar clothing. Notify the physician if she loses more than 1 kg/day.
- Check the patient's urine specific gravity and monitor her vital signs every 4 to 6 hours.
- Taper the patient from vasopressin therapy, if possible and as ordered. When doing this, assess her urine output carefully to determine whether diabetes insipidus has resolved or become permanent. With resolution, urine output returns to normal without vasopressin therapy; in permanent diabetes insipidus, urine output increases each time vasopressin therapy stops.

SPECIAL CONSIDERATIONS
- If diabetes insipidus becomes permanent, teach the patient how to self-administer vasopressin and which adverse effects to report. If desmopressin acetate (DDAVP) is prescribed (instead of vasopressin), teach the patient how to administer it intranasally.
- Instruct the patient how to measure urine specific gravity and monitor daily fluid intake and output.
- Review signs and symptoms of dehydration and water intoxication, and explain when the patient should seek medical attention.
- Stress the importance of obtaining a medical identification bracelet or necklace to wear at all times.
- Urge the patient to keep all follow-up medical appointments.

DIABETIC KETOACIDOSIS

A life-threatening metabolic disorder, diabetic ketoacidosis (DKA) most commonly affects people with insulin-dependent (type I) diabetes. DKA stems from a severe insulin deficiency that occurs when the pancreas can no longer meet minimal insulin requirements or when the patient's health or lifestyle changes enough to render his normal insulin dosage grossly insufficient.

The severe insulin shortage in DKA prevents glucose from entering cells, which causes the body to burn fat as an alternate fuel. During fat breakdown, ketone bodies are released. If fat breaks down faster than the body can excrete ketone bodies, these bodies build up in the blood. When ketone bodies accumulate in the blood, pH drops and metabolic acidosis results in a condition called ketoacidosis.

Meanwhile, glucose—unable to enter the cells because of the insulin deficiency—also builds up in the blood, producing hyperglycemia. As the body attempts to compensate by removing excess glucose through the renal system, large amounts of water and electrolytes are lost in urine. These fluid and electrolyte losses may cause severe dehydration, a hyperosmolar state, and marked electrolyte imbalances—conditions that worsen metabolic acidosis.

To prevent your patient from developing hypovolemic shock and potentially lethal cardiac arrhythmias, you'll need to take quick action if you suspect he has DKA.

WHAT TO LOOK FOR
Clinical findings in DKA may include:
- excessive urination (polyuria)
- excessive thirst (polydipsia)
- excessive hunger (polyphagia)
- ketonuria
- glycosuria
- rapid, deep respirations (Kussmaul's respirations)
- fruity breath odor
- altered level of consciousness
- weakness
- warm, dry skin
- dry mucous membranes
- poor skin turgor
- severe abdominal pain
- nausea and vomiting
- tachycardia
- hypotension
- hypothermia.

D

WHAT TO DO IMMEDIATELY

If your patient shows signs and symptoms of DKA, notify the physician. Then take these steps:

- Double-check your patient's blood glucose level. Also check his urine for ketones.
- Begin continuous cardiac monitoring.
- Obtain an arterial blood sample for arterial blood gas analysis and a venous blood sample, as ordered, to check serum electrolyte levels.
- Establish I.V. access for fluid replacement and insulin therapy.
- Expect to begin I.V. fluid replacement by giving 10 to 20 ml/kg of isotonic normal saline solution over 30 to 60 minutes. Watch closely for signs and symptoms of fluid overload, especially if the patient has heart or kidney disease.
- Start insulin therapy, as prescribed. Although insulin most commonly is administered I.V. to treat DKA, it may be given intramuscularly (I.M.) if I.V. access is not immediately available.
- ➡ **NurseALERT** Give only *regular* insulin by the I.M. or I.V. route. When giving it I.V., start with a bolus of 0.1 to 0.2 U/kg, followed by an infusion of 0.1 U/kg/hour, unless otherwise prescribed. Be sure to mix insulin in normal saline solution and then flush the I.V. tubing with about 50 ml of the insulin solution before administration. This will saturate the binding sites on the tubing and allow you to deliver insulin at the prescribed rate.
- ➡ **NurseALERT** Don't give insulin subcutaneously to treat DKA; the patient's dehydrated state will hinder its absorption, possibly causing a dangerous delay in delivering insulin to the bloodstream.
- Administer oxygen therapy, if indicated and prescribed.

WHAT TO DO NEXT

Once DKA therapy has started, continued care should include the following steps:

- Monitor your patient's blood glucose and serum electrolyte levels, arterial blood gas values, and vital signs hourly. As he stabilizes, you can check them less often.
- Continue fluid therapy with half-normal saline solution at a slower rate, as prescribed. Because most patients with DKA develop a total body potassium deficit, anticipate adding a potassium supplement to the solution. Remember that you may need to give the potassium supplement right away if your patient's serum potassium level drops below 2.5 mEq/L; otherwise, lethal cardiac arrhythmias could develop. (See *Detecting hypokalemia in a patient with DKA.*)
- When your patient's blood glucose level drops below 250 mg/dl, change the I.V. solution to dextrose 5% in half-normal saline solution, as ordered. Doing this will prevent hypoglycemia if his blood glucose level drops suddenly as it approaches normal limits.
- Make sure that the patient's blood glucose level doesn't drop by more than 100 mg/dl/hour. With a rapid drop, he could develop

DETECTING HYPOKALEMIA IN A PATIENT WITH D.K.A.

When caring for a patient with diabetic ketoacidosis (DKA), be aware that hypokalemia typically develops within the first 4 hours of DKA treatment. Why? Because total body potassium levels already are low from potassium lost through osmotic diuresis. Then, fluid replacement for DKA dilutes extracellular potassium and insulin therapy pushes potassium back into the cells.

Identifying hypokalemia early is essential to your patient's well-being and to ensure effective treatment for DKA. To detect hypokalemia, you'll need to:

- Obtain serum potassium levels as often as every hour.

- Use continuous cardiac monitoring to observe cardiac effects. Suspect hypokalemia if you see prolonged QT intervals, flattened or depressed T waves, and depressed ST segments on the cardiac monitor.
- Monitor your patient closely for signs and symptoms of hypokalemia: muscle weakness, an altered level of consciousness, abdominal distention or paralytic ileus, hypotension, and a weak pulse. Severe hypokalemia may even lead to respiratory arrest.
- If you detect hypokalemia, notify the physician right away and prepare to add a potassium supplement to the patient's I.V. solution.

D

cerebral edema when glucose pulls water along with it as it enters cells. Expect to decrease the insulin flow rate as your patient's blood glucose level approaches normal.
- Assess your patient every hour for evidence of fluid overload and for signs that DKA is resolving.
- Anticipate giving sodium bicarbonate if your patient's pH stays below 7.2 despite initial treatment.
- Withhold oral intake and prepare to insert a nasogastric tube if the patient begins to vomit or develops abdominal distention.

FOLLOW-UP CARE
- Monitor the patient's blood glucose level every 4 to 8 hours, or as ordered.
- Begin oral intake when the patient can tolerate liquids. Start with clear liquids, and progress to a soft diet and then a normal diet.
- Expect to stop giving I.V. fluids and insulin when the patient can maintain adequate oral intake and his blood glucose has stabilized at or near a normal level.
- Begin subcutaneous insulin therapy just before discontinuing I.V. insulin therapy, as ordered. Anticipate giving only regular insulin subcutaneously initially. Once the patient's blood glucose level stabilizes, the physician may add or substitute other insulin types.

SPECIAL CONSIDERATIONS
- To help determine what triggered DKA, evaluate the patient's knowledge about how to manage his prescribed diabetic treatment plan.
- As needed, instruct the patient on diabetes management. Include family members or significant others in your teaching.
- If the patient is noncompliant, try to find out why.

DIARRHEA, SEVERE

Nearly everyone knows firsthand how to recognize and define diarrhea. Simply put, it's an increase in the mass, frequency, and water content of stool. It leads to a typical daily fluid loss of about 200 ml. Commonly accompanied by abdominal and perianal pain, urgency, tenesmus, and incontinence, diarrhea clears up when the underlying cause resolves. (See *What causes diarrhea?*)

When diarrhea lasts too long or involves too much fluid loss, your patient is at risk for potentially serious problems. For instance, rapid movement of food through the intestines may impair her digestion and absorption, leading to malnutrition. Or, if diarrhea causes daily fluid loss of 10 to 15 L, she may suffer severe dehydration and imbalances of such crucial electrolytes as sodium, potassium, and bicarbonate.

Your response to severe diarrhea can make a dramatic difference in your patient's health and quality of life, particularly if she is already compromised by another illness.

WHAT TO LOOK FOR
Clinical findings in severe diarrhea may include:
- watery stools with excess mucus
- increased frequency and volume of stools
- complaints of urgency, anal discomfort, and cramping
- dry skin with poor turgor
- dry mouth and complaints of thirst
- dry mucous membranes
- increased respiratory rate
- oliguria with concentrated urine
- hypotension
- metabolic acidosis (blood pH below 7.35; partial pressure of carbon dioxide normal or low; bicarbonate level may be normal or low).

WHAT TO DO IMMEDIATELY
If your patient experiences severe diarrhea, notify the physician. Then take these measures:
- If you suspect enteral feedings as the cause of diarrhea, discuss with the physician and dietitian alternative enteral feeding products or the need to discontinue enteral feedings.
- Insert an I.V. line and give fluids, as prescribed.
- Record the patient's fluid intake and output; remember to count liquid stools as output.
- Check the patient's urine specific gravity.
- Withhold oral food and fluids for at least 4 hours because oral intake stimulates peristalsis.
- Administer prescribed antidiarrheal medications.
- Assess the amount, color, and consistency of the patient's bowel movements, and check for the presence of mucus. Look for evidence

WHAT CAUSES DIARRHEA?

Diarrhea can stem from a wide range of factors, including those listed below.

ENHANCED SECRETIONS

Secretory diarrhea occurs when chloride ions and water increase—commonly in response to a bacterial enterotoxin that the intestine's trying to expel (such as one produced by *Vibrio cholerae, Clostridium difficile,* or *Cryptosporidium*). Some drugs and hormones also may stimulate enhanced secretion. Secretory diarrhea persists even with fasting, and may produce 1 L or more of fecal output daily.

INCREASED SOLUTES

In *osmotic diarrhea,* the intestine holds increased amounts of poorly absorbable, osmotically active solutes, such as carbohydrates and magnesium sulfate. This increased osmolarity in the lumen pulls fluid out of intestinal cells in an attempt to dilute the solutes. Sodium follows, promoting even more water movement, and an ongoing cycle ensues. This is the mechanism of action for some laxatives and it's the primary reason behind diarrhea caused by enteral feedings.

Another cause of increased solutes is gastric resection (a condition called dumping syndrome), in which large amount of carbohydrates and other nutrients empty into the intestine at an abnormally fast rate. This influx changes the osmolarity, resulting in diarrhea. Osmotic diarrhea causes large stool volumes and may abate with fasting.

EXUDATION

When mucus, blood, and protein enter the intestinal lumen from a site of active mucosal inflammation, *exudative diarrhea* develops from the increased osmotic load and subsequent water shift. A type of osmotic diarrhea, exudative diarrhea typically occurs in inflammatory bowel diseases, such as Crohn's disease and ulcerative colitis.

INCREASED MOTILITY

When peristalsis speeds up, intestinal contents spend less time in contact with mucosal absorptive surfaces before reaching the rectum. Consequently, excess water remains in the fecal material. The volume and number of stools vary with the degree of absorption. However, stools typically are small and frequent. Increased motility occurs in such disorders as irritable bowel syndrome and excessive stress.

DISEASES

Any disease that causes malabsorption may do so, at least in part, by inducing diarrhea. Malabsorption may result from:

- lack of digestive enzymes, bile, or both
- decreased intestinal absorptive space
- changes in the intestinal lining (as from radiation)
- pancreatic and liver disorders, which decrease fat absorption, causing steatorrhea (in which stools are voluminous, foul-smelling, and fatty).

MEDICATIONS

Diarrhea may result from use of many medications, including certain antibiotics, chemotherapy agents, and liquid forms of such drugs as theophylline, acetaminophen, and isoniazid.

of blood in the stool—either bright red (from the lower intestine) or dark and tarry (from earlier bleeding in the upper GI tract). Keep in mind that because blood in the intestines can stimulate peristalsis, diarrhea may represent continued slow bleeding from the intestinal wall.

- Obtain and monitor the patient's laboratory values to help assess for dehydration, as indicated by increased serum osmolality, sodium, and blood urea nitrogen levels and increased hematocrit. Also make sure you watch for electrolyte imbalances, such as hypokalemia and decreased bicarbonate.
- Assess the patient's perianal area for redness, irritation, and excoriation.

WHAT TO DO NEXT

Once the patient's diarrhea begins to subside, take these steps:

* Try to determine what caused the diarrhea. Ask the patient about recent dietary intake, foreign travel, medication changes, and other potential contributing factors. Also ask whether family members or close friends have diarrhea. Find out when the patient last passed a normal stool.

➡ **NurseALERT** Know that fecal impaction or intestinal obstruction can lead to diarrhea if the blockage allows only liquids to pass.

* Check the patient's medication history. If she's taking a drug associated with diarrhea, such as an antibiotic, aminophylline, pyridostigmine (Mestinon), or quinidine (Quinora), notify the physician.

* When the patient resumes oral intake, offer small amounts of weak tea, bouillon, and flavored gelatin; these foods and beverages replace lost electrolytes without stimulating the intestines. Advance the diet as tolerated to a low-residue regimen that includes such foods as tender beef, veal, chicken, boiled or steamed rice, applesauce, and hard-boiled eggs. Avoid cold liquids, caffeine, and heavy sweets.

* Continue to give antidiarrheal drugs, as ordered. Administer these with caution because they may interfere with peristalsis and lead to drug interactions. Be aware that most antidiarrheals are given for a course of 24 to 48 hours. Evaluate their efficacy by assessing the number and consistency of the patient's stools.

* Provide perianal care after every bowel movement. (See *Providing perianal care.*)

* If diarrhea persists and the patient experiences repeated fecal incontinence, consider applying a fecal incontinence pouch to prevent severe perianal skin breakdown. The device also aids measurement of fluid loss and provides for safer containment of potentially infectious secretions. To apply the device correctly, ask for help from an enterostomal therapist.

➡ **NurseALERT** Be aware that although a rectal tube sometimes is ordered for persistent diarrhea, it may damage the rectal mucosa and sphincters. Use a rectal tube only on a short-term basis; inflate the balloon as little as possible and deflate it at least every 4 hours to prevent mucosal damage. If your patient is at high risk for bleeding or infection, don't use a rectal tube.

* Prepare the patient for possible rectal examination, lower GI barium studies, sigmoidoscopy, or colonoscopy, as appropriate.

FOLLOW-UP CARE

* Once diarrhea subsides, make sure the patient and her home caregivers know how to treat complications and prevent recurrence. As appropriate, teach them about fluid replacement, diet, medication use, and steps to take if diarrhea recurs. Reinforce the principles of good hygiene, including thorough and frequent hand washing, proper care of clothes and linens, and safe food preparation.

PROVIDING PERIANAL CARE

To provide perianal care to a patient with diarrhea, take these steps:
- Wipe the perianal area gently with soft toilet tissue.
- Clean the area carefully, using warm water and mild soap. Then rinse and pat dry.
- Apply a protective ointment, such as petroleum jelly.
- If irritation develops or persists despite this routine, wash with warm water, but no soap. Gently pat dry with absorbent cotton. Skip the ointment; it could foster irritation by blocking perspiration.

- Give sitz baths two or three times daily for 10 minutes at a time to promote healing and comfort.
- If needed, wipe the perianal area with a soft pad soaked in witch hazel (such as a Tucks pad) as an additional comfort measure.
- If the patient has leaking feces, try placing a piece of absorbent cotton over her anus and then holding it in place with snug underwear. The cotton allows air to reach the area and can be replaced easily and frequently, if needed.

D

SPECIAL CONSIDERATIONS
- Especially when accompanied by urgency and loss of bowel control, diarrhea can cause embarrassment. Be sensitive to the patient's need for privacy, and make sure her room is well ventilated and odor-free. Make it as easy as possible for her to get to the bedpan or toilet. If she needs your help to do so, respond as quickly as possible when she calls.
- Maintain a quiet, stress-free environment, and encourage the patient to rest to help minimize peristalsis.

DISSECTING ANEURYSM

An acute dissecting aneurysm can cause death almost instantly. This emergency develops when layers of the aortic wall separate, allowing blood to pass through a tear in the wall's innermost (intimal) layer to reach the middle (medial) layer. Because arterial pressure forces blood into the tear, a hematoma and false lumen form. Every time the heart contracts, more blood enters the false lumen and the dissection expands. (See *What happens in a dissecting aneurysm,* page 102.)

Life-threatening conditions may occur if the expanding hematoma compresses or occludes arteries that branch off from the aorta, such as those that supply the abdomen, spinal cord, brain, kidneys, and extremities. In another scenario, blood leaking into the pericardial sac may cause cardiac tamponade. In a third possibility, the dissection may rupture and hemorrhage into the mediastinal, pleural, and abdominal cavities.

Aortic dissection typically occurs at the point where stress from high-pressure blood flow is greatest: the thoracic aorta (ascending aorta, aortic arch, and descending aorta past the left subclavian artery). However, dissection can develop anywhere along the length of the aorta, including the abdominal portion.

PATHOPHYSIOLOGY

WHAT HAPPENS IN A DISSECTING ANEURYSM

In a dissecting aneurysm, blood flows through a tear in the artery's intimal layer, forcing it to separate from the medial layer, as shown in the illustration below.

Cross section of a tear in an artery

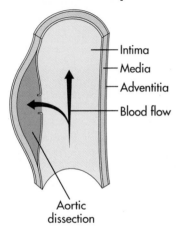

- Intima
- Media
- Adventitia
- Blood flow

Aortic dissection

Hypertension and other predisposing factors

Roughly 90% of dissecting aortic aneurysms occur in people who have hypertension. Other predisposing factors include:
- pregnancy
- complications of certain procedures (for instance, cardiac catheterization and intra-aortic balloon counterpulsation therapy)
- complications of such conditions as atherosclerosis, aortic coarctation or valve disease, Marfan's syndrome, cocaine use, and deceleration injuries.

WHAT TO LOOK FOR

Clinical evidence of dissecting aortic aneurysm may include:
- sudden, excruciating chest pain that radiates to the back, neck, shoulders, or abdomen; the patient may describe the pain as sharp, tearing, stabbing, or ripping
- hypertension (initially), which may mask signs and symptoms of shock
- tachycardia
- tachypnea
- altered level of consciousness, dizziness, and syncope
- weak or absent carotid and temporal pulses (if the dissection involves the aortic arch)
- sense of impending doom
- aortic regurgitation murmur from dissection of the ascending aorta and subsequent aortic valve insufficiency (see *Detecting aortic regurgitation murmurs*)
- dyspnea from severe aortic valve insufficiency, left ventricular failure, and pulmonary edema
- significant bilateral blood pressure and pulse differential in the arms (if the dissection involves one or both subclavian arteries)
- oliguria progressing to anuria as well as other signs of acute renal failure (if renal artery blood flow is affected)
- acute abdominal pain (if blood flow to the superior mesenteric artery is interrupted)
- pain, paralysis, paresthesias, and loss of one or more peripheral pulses in the lower extremities if the dissection extends down the descending aorta
- signs and symptoms of shock, such as pallor, diaphoresis, peripheral cyanosis, and restlessness (varying with the degree of blood loss, myocardial ischemia, and acute aortic regurgitation).

WHAT TO DO IMMEDIATELY

An unstable patient whose aneurysm ruptures is likely to die within 1 hour if he doesn't get emergency treatment. Prepare to transfer him to the critical care unit or surgery, as appropriate. Surgery may involve resection of the dissected aortic portion and replacement with a synthetic

TIPS AND TECHNIQUES

DETECTING AORTIC REGURGITATION MURMURS

Typically, dissection of the ascending aorta causes aortic regurgitation. In this condition, blood flowing back into the left ventricle through the aortic valve during diastole joins blood filling the left ventricle from the left atrium. Consequently, blood backs up into the pulmonary vasculature. With severe regurgitation, left ventricular failure and pulmonary edema may develop and death may ensue.

KEY ASSESSMENT QUESTIONS

To identify a murmur as that of aortic regurgitation, start by answering the following questions:

- *Location:* Where do you hear the murmur best—over the aortic, pulmonic, tricuspid, or mitral area?
- *Intensity:* How loud is the murmur? Use a grading such as the one below.

Grade	Description
I	Faint, barely audible
II	Quiet, but heard right away
III	Moderately loud, without thrill
IV	Loud, with palpable thrill
V	Very loud, with thrill; requires stethoscope to hear
VI	Like V, but audible with stethoscope off chest

- *Pitch:* Does the murmur have a high, medium, or low pitch? A high-pitched murmur is best heard with the diaphragm of the stethoscope; a low-pitched murmur, with the bell.
- *Shape:* Does the murmur increase in intensity, causing a crescendo waveform? Does it decrease, creating a decrescendo waveform? Does the intensity first increase and then decrease, creating a diamond-shaped waveform? Or does it stay at the same level, producing a plateau?
- *Quality:* Does the murmur sound harsh, rumbling, blowing, or musical?

- *Timing:* Does the murmur occur during systole, diastole, or both? To determine this, palpate the carotid artery while auscultating the heart. A murmur that accompanies the carotid pulse is systolic.
- *Radiation:* Does the murmur radiate to the axilla or neck, or down the left sternal border?
- *Position:* Can you hear the murmur best when the patient sits up, lies down, or leans forward?

MURMUR FEATURES

If your patient has an aortic regurgitation murmur, you'll hear it best at the second right (aortic area) or third left intercostal space along the left sternal border (Erb's point) as the patient leans forward and holds his breath at the end of expiration. The murmur occurs during diastole, immediately after S_2, and then decreases in intensity, as shown in this illustration.

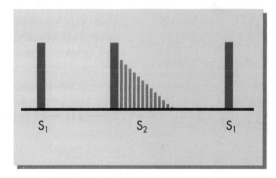

S_1 S_2 S_1

Because of its high pitch and blowing quality, a regurgitation murmur is best heard with the diaphragm of the stethoscope. Its intensity depends on the size of the blood leak. The aortic regurgitation murmur represented in this waveform begins during diastole and decreases in intensity. It's audible immediately after S_2.

graft or aortic valve replacement if the patient has severe aortic regurgitation. If possible, the surgeon may delay the operation so that localized edema can resolve and blood can clot in the false lumen.

If you suspect that your patient is developing a dissecting aneurysm, call for assistance. Ensure that the patient has an adequate airway, is breathing, and has adequate circulation. Then take the following actions:

- Check the patient's vital signs and neurologic status continuously or at least every hour.

- Prepare to assist with insertion of an arterial line (if one is not already in place). Continuously monitor blood pressure to assess vasodilator effectiveness.
- Begin continuous ECG monitoring to detect arrhythmias and ischemic changes, which signal reduced blood flow to the coronary arteries.
- Check peripheral pulses every hour, noting their absence or changes in quality.
- Administer I.V. nitroprusside (Nipride), as prescribed, to lower blood pressure rapidly. Expect to titrate the dose to achieve the desired blood pressure.
- ➡ **NurseALERT** Don't administer nitroprusside in doses above 10 µg/kg/min. It may lead to cyanide toxicity and renal failure and may drop the blood pressure too rapidly. To protect the solution from light, wrap the container in aluminum foil. Check for color changes and discard the solution if it's blue-green or dark red. During nitroprusside therapy, assess the patient for signs and symptoms of cyanide toxicity, including tinnitus, blurred vision, delirium, and muscle spasm.
- Expect to administer other drugs, including diuretics, beta blockers, and agents with both alpha- and beta-blocking properties (such as labetalol [Normodyne]). Propranolol, a beta blocker, lowers the force and velocity of myocardial contractions, reducing stress on the aortic wall and thus decreasing the force of ventricular ejection (which may be increased from nitroprusside therapy).
- Prepare your patient for surgery if he has dissection of the ascending aorta, a leaking dissection, occlusion of a major artery, or severe heart failure.
- Insert an indwelling urinary catheter, as ordered, to monitor hourly output. Note hematuria or decreased urine output, which indicates reduced renal perfusion.
- To decrease pain and anxiety, administer narcotic analgesics (such as morphine sulfate) and tranquilizers, as prescribed and tolerated.
- Administer blood and blood products, as prescribed. Keep in mind that if the patient has a dissecting aneurysm, his condition may quickly progress to circulatory shock and he'll need fluids administered quickly and early in treatment.
- Keep the patient on complete bed rest in semi-Fowler's position to minimize systolic blood pressure. Maintain a calm, quiet environment.

WHAT TO DO NEXT
Once the initial crisis has eased and the patient begins to stabilize, take the following actions:
- Monitor the patient's neurologic status, including level of consciousness and motor and sensory functions. (See *Five Ps of neurovascular assessment*, page 28.)

- Check for a new aortic murmur and for signs and symptoms of heart failure, such as a third heart sound (S_3), crackles, and tachycardia, which indicate aortic valve involvement. Be aware that widening pulse pressure may signal worsening aortic regurgitation.
- Assess for hemorrhaging and cardiac tamponade—possible consequences of bleeding from an ascending aortic dissection. Stay alert for signs and symptoms, such as narrowed pulse pressure, muffled heart sounds, and pulsus paradoxus. (See *Understanding pulsus paradoxus,* page 64.)
- Assess the patient's vital signs often, making sure that you take his blood pressure in both arms. Palpate pulses bilaterally in all extremities, and note any differences in quality.
- Assess bowel sounds. Administer stool softeners, as prescribed, to prevent constipation or straining.
- Monitor laboratory values, including hematocrit, blood urea nitrogen levels, and serum levels of creatinine, hemoglobin, and cardiac enzymes.

FOLLOW-UP CARE
- Continuously monitor the patient's blood pressure, and administer antihypertensive medication, as prescribed.
- Continue to assess his cardiovascular, neurologic, renal, and GI systems for evidence of complications.
- If your patient has been receiving prolonged nitroprusside therapy, monitor laboratory results for thiocyanate and cyanide levels, and assess for signs and symptoms of drug toxicity.
- After surgery, provide postoperative care and continue to assess the patient as described above. Monitor any drainage, such as from a chest or nasogastric tube.
- Assess for signs of hemorrhage. Monitor blood pressure carefully. Keep in mind that prolonged hypotension can result in aortic graft occlusion, whereas severe hypertension may place stress on the anastomoses.
- Inspect the incision site for hemorrhage and infection.
- To help prevent respiratory complications, turn and reposition the patient regularly and help him perform coughing and deep-breathing exercises. Teach him how to splint the incision when coughing. Begin early ambulation, as ordered, and provide pain control.

SPECIAL CONSIDERATIONS
- Watch for orthostatic hypotension, a possible effect of antihypertensive drugs. To avoid related injury, take safety precautions and instruct the patient to rise slowly to an upright position.
- Teach the patient about his condition and prescribed medications, including their names, purpose, dosages, dosing schedule, and adverse effects to report.
- Advise the patient which signs and symptoms of aortic dissection to report immediately.

DISSEMINATED INTRAVASCULAR COAGULATION

Also known as consumptive coagulopathy or intravascular coagulation-fibrinolysis syndrome, disseminated intravascular coagulation (DIC) is a perilous clotting disorder characterized by thrombosis, hemorrhage, and organ failure.

DIC is not a primary disorder but rather is triggered by some other disease or injury. Patients at risk for DIC include those who have suffered severe trauma, serious infection (especially with a gram-negative organism), neoplasm, acute respiratory distress syndrome, transfusion reaction, shock, or obstetric complications (abruptio placentae, amniotic embolus). For unknown reasons, these conditions activate the body's clotting mechanisms.

DIC begins as a clotting problem but manifests itself as a bleeding disorder. Usually, intrinsic anticoagulants, such as tissue plasminogen activator, keep the blood from clotting. However, in DIC, a precipitating factor, such as sepsis, causes accelerated clotting that results in the deposition of fibrin along the blood vessel walls and clots within the microcirculation. When these microclots impair circulation, tissue and organ ischemia follow. The overproduction of clotting factors ultimately depletes the supply faster than the liver is able to synthesize them. When clotting factors are depleted, bleeding and hemorrhage may ensue. Bleeding may worsen when fibrin degradation products (FDP) are released to break down fibrin clots.

Because DIC develops secondarily to such conditions as sepsis and shock, treatment must address the underlying cause in addition to the clotting disorder. Mortality from DIC ranges from 50% to 80%, so you'll need to quickly assess your patient and rapidly intervene.

WHAT TO LOOK FOR
Even though the underlying problem in DIC is excessive clotting, the major clinical sign is bleeding from multiple sites. The patient may exhibit:
- persistent oozing of blood from punctures, incisions, or old injuries
- overt bleeding from invasive lines, tubes (endotracheal or urethral catheters), drains, or wounds
- bruising and expanding hematomas
- bleeding from mucous membranes
- ecchymosis, purpura, petechiae
- scleral and conjunctival bleeding
- hematuria
- signs of GI bleeding, including tarry or bloody stools, hematemesis, hyperactive bowel sounds, and abdominal distention
- bleeding in joint spaces
- signs of pulmonary hemorrhage, including hemoptysis, dyspnea, tachypnea, and chest pain

- changes in neurologic status, indicating an intracerebral hemorrhage.

An occlusion in the microcirculation may manifest itself as organ dysfunction, such as:
- signs of acute tubular necrosis, such as oliguria or anuria and elevated creatinine and blood urea nitrogen levels
- signs of brain infarction, such as confusion, delirium, neurologic deficits, and coma
- signs of pulmonary infarction, such as dyspnea and chest pain
- signs of bowel infarction, such as abdominal pain, diarrhea, and GI hemorrhage
- signs of cutaneous thrombi, such as mottled and cold fingers, toes, and extremities.

D

Laboratory test results indicating DIC include:
- prolonged prothrombin time and activated partial thromboplastin time
- prolonged thrombin time
- low fibrinogen level
- low platelet count
- elevated FDP level.

(See *Laboratory findings in DIC*, page 108.)

WHAT TO DO IMMEDIATELY

If your patient develops DIC, you'll need to intervene immediately to control the bleeding and improve perfusion to the organs. Notify the physician. Then take these actions:
- Assess the patient's airway for patency. If he's having trouble breathing, prepare for endotracheal intubation.
- Apply pressure or pressure dressings to bleeding sites to prevent further blood loss.
- ➡ **NurseALERT** Avoid procedures likely to cause bleeding, such as venipuncture, complicated dressing changes, and shaving. Typically, the physician inserts a central venous catheter for fluid administration as well as a means of obtaining blood samples.
- Obtain a blood sample for typing and crossmatching, and make sure that blood is available.
- Correct the patient's hypotension and hemorrhagic shock by administering fluid, as prescribed. Anticipate insertion of a central venous catheter to monitor the patient's hemodynamic status and guide fluid resuscitation measures.
- Administer blood and blood products, as ordered, to correct coagulopathy.
- Administer medications and treatments, as prescribed, to treat the disease or problem that may have triggered DIC.

LABORATORY FINDINGS IN D.I.C.

To help evaluate a patient with suspected disseminated intravascular coagulation (DIC), you'll need to collect a blood sample and send it to the laboratory with an order for the panel of tests shown below.

UNDERSTANDING TEST RESULTS

Tests ordered to help assess DIC reveal the patient's clotting system activity. For example, the platelet count and fibrinogen level decrease in DIC because widespread clotting consumes these factors. Bleeding times increase from lack of available clotting factors.

Levels of fibrin degradation products rise from breakdown of excessive clots in the microcirculation. Antithrombin III, a plasma protein, prevents abnormal clotting by inhibiting coagulation factors. Some hospitals also test plasminogen levels; in DIC, these decrease, reflecting conversion of excess plasminogen to plasmin during fibrinolysis.

Test	Normal result	Result in DIC
Platelet count	150,000 to 400,000/mm^3	Decreased
Prothrombin time	11 to 16 seconds (varies among laboratories)	Increased
Activated partial thromboplastin time	25 to 38 seconds (varies among laboratories)	Increased
Thrombin time	14 to 16 seconds	Increased
Fibrinogen time	170 to 400 mg/dl	Decreased
Fibrin degradation products	≤ 10 µg (varies among laboratories)	Increased
D-dimer assay	≤ 200 mg/ml	Increased
Antithrombin III	80% to 120%	Decreased

WHAT TO DO NEXT

After taking initial steps, follow these guidelines:
- Administer antibiotics, if prescribed, to treat infection.
- Maintain a patent airway. Provide ventilatory support, if needed and ordered, and oxygen to correct metabolic or respiratory acidosis.
- Keep administering blood transfusions and normal saline solution, as prescribed, until blood and fluid loss are replaced.
- Monitor laboratory test results, especially hemoglobin, hematocrit, platelet, and coagulation factors. Monitor laboratory tests specific to the function of each organ. Also track lactate levels to assess for ischemic injury to organs.
- Prepare to administer heparin, if prescribed, to halt the clotting process. Use the patient's activated partial thromboplastin time to guide heparin therapy.
- Check the patient's peripheral pulses, and watch for signs of decreased perfusion, such as cool, pale limbs.

FOLLOW-UP CARE

- Monitor the patient's hemoglobin level and hematocrit closely; be aware that decreasing levels indicate continuing hemorrhage.

- Track his platelet count and coagulation factors. Decreasing platelet count or increasing clotting times suggest persistent coagulopathy.
- Continue to watch for bleeding from any site.
- If you're administering a heparin infusion, assess for complications, including worsening coagulopathy and increasing bleeding.
- Assess the patient's hemodynamic parameters and urine output to help monitor his hydration status.

SPECIAL CONSIDERATIONS
- Be aware that a platelet count below 20,000 is associated with spontaneous bleeding.
- ➡ **Nurse ALERT** Don't give antifibrinolytic agents, such as aminocaproic acid (Amicar), because they could cause a potentially fatal thromboembolism. Other therapies include exchange transfusions and plasmapheresis.
- Be alert for evidence of hemorrhagic shock that seems more severe than the patient's blood loss suggests. Remember that shock can lead to tissue hypoperfusion, lactic acidosis, and organ dysfunction.

DRUG TOXICITY

A toxic, or poisonous, substance can damage body structures or disturb normal body functions. Although drugs probably are the most common source of toxicity, the spectrum of toxic substances extends far beyond drugs.

Even if you don't know the source of a patient's drug toxicity, you'll need to react swiftly and accurately if she shows signs or symptoms of a toxicity-related problem. Your astute assessment may help identify the specific toxin correctly even when the patient can't or won't identify it for you. To help formulate an effective treatment plan, expect to integrate your clinical findings with data from the poison control center or other experts.

When caring for a patient with drug toxicity, remember that treatment focuses on the following goals:
- supporting the patient's vital functions
- identifying the toxin, if possible
- removing or neutralizing the toxin or reversing its effects
- speeding excretion of the toxin
- preventing or treating serious damage to body structures.

WHAT TO LOOK FOR
Clinical findings vary with the toxic drug involved. (See *Assessment findings and treatments in selected drug toxicities*, pages 110 and 111.)

WHAT TO DO IMMEDIATELY
If you suspect your patient is experiencing drug toxicity, notify the physician. Then take these actions:

ASSESSMENT FINDINGS AND TREATMENTS IN SELECTED DRUG TOXICITIES

Clinical findings in drug toxicity depend largely on the specific drug involved. This table describes the signs, symptoms, diagnostic findings, and treatments for some of the most common drug toxicities you'll encounter.

Toxin	Vital signs	Mental status	Signs and symptoms	Diagnostic findings	Treatment or antidote
Acetaminophen	• Normal	Altered level of consciousness (LOC), ranging from lethargy to coma	• Anorexia • Nausea and vomiting • Right upper quadrant tenderness • Jaundice	• Abnormal liver function tests • Elevated serum acetaminophen level	• Acetylcysteine
Alcohol—ethanol (grain)	• Hypotension • Tachycardia	Altered LOC, ranging from lethargy to coma	• Nausea and vomiting • Headache • Vertigo • Flushed skin • Diaphoresis • Abdominal tenderness	• ECG abnormalities • Ventricular arrhythmias • Elevated blood alcohol level	• Diazepam • Hemodialysis (in severe cases) • GI decontamination without activated charcoal and cathartics
Alcohol—isopropyl (rubbing)	• Hypotension • Hypoventilation	Altered LOC, ranging from lethargy to coma	• Intoxication • Hyporeflexia • Acetone breath odor	• Ketonemia • Ketonuria • Blood test positive for isopropyl alcohol and acetone	• Diazepam • Hemodialysis (in severe cases) • GI decontamination without activated charcoal and cathartics
Alcohol—methanol (wood)	• Hyperventilation • Hypotension	Altered LOC, ranging from lethargy to coma	• Blurred vision • Abdominal pain • Intoxication • Hyperemic disks	• Anion-gap metabolic acidosis • Increased osmolal gap • Blood test positive for ethanol and methanol	• Diazepam • Ethanol infusion • GI decontamination without activated charcoal and cathartics
Amino-glycosides	• Hypertension • Hypotension	Altered LOC, such as confusion	• Nausea and vomiting • Tinnitus • Dizziness • Ataxia	• Elevated blood urea nitrogen and creatinine levels • Oliguria • Proteinuria	• Hemodialysis
Amphetamines, hallucinogens	• Hypertension • Tachycardia • Hyperthermia	Hyperactivity, agitation, toxic psychosis	• Hyperalertness • Mydriasis • Hyperactive bowel sounds • Flushed skin • Diaphoresis	• Positive blood and urine toxicology screen	• Diazepam • Haloperidol • GI decontamination up to 4 hours after drug was taken
Barbiturates	• Hypotension • Hypoventilation • Hypothermia	Altered LOC, ranging from lethargy to coma	• Intoxication • Disconjugate eye movements • Hyporeflexia • Bullae	• Abnormal arterial blood gas values • Positive blood and urine toxicology screen	• Diazepam • GI decontamination up to 12 hours after ingestion with repeated doses of activated charcoal and cathartics

Toxin	Vital signs	Mental status	Signs and symptoms	Diagnostic findings	Treatment or antidote
Benzodiazepines	• Hypotension • Bradycardia • Depressed respiratory status	Altered LOC, ranging from confusion to somnolence to coma	• Diminished reflexes	• Increased urine and serum toxicology screen • Elevated liver function tests	• Flumazenil • Lavage if benzodiazepine was taken orally • GI decontamination
Cocaine	• Hypertension • Tachycardia • Hyperthermia	Altered LOC, including anxiety, agitation, and delirium	• Hallucinations • Mydriasis • Tremor • Diaphoresis • Seizures • Perforated nasal septum	• ECG abnormalities • Increased creatine kinase (CK) levels	• Diazepam • Haloperidol • Labetalol hydrochloride (for hypertensive crisis) • Propranolol
Cyclic antidepressants	• Tachycardia • Hypotension • Hyperthermia	Altered LOC, ranging from lethargy to coma	• Confusion • Dizziness • Mydriasis • Dry mucous membranes • Bladder distention • Flushed skin • Seizures	• Prolonged QRS complexes and cardiac arrhythmias on ECG	• GI decontamination if patient's alert • Activated charcoal and cathartic every 4 to 6 hours • Continuous nasogastric suction
Digoxin	• Hypotension • Bradycardia	Normal to altered LOC	• Nausea and vomiting • Anorexia • Confusion • Visual disturbances	• ECG abnormalities • Elevated serum digoxin level	• Digoxin immune Fab
Phencyclidine (PCP)	• Hypertension • Tachycardia • Hyperthermia	Altered LOC, ranging from agitation to lethargy to coma	• Hallucinations • Seizures • Miosis • Diaphoresis • Myoclonus • Blank stare • Nystagmus	• Myoglobinuria • Increased CK level • Positive PCP level • Positive blood and urine toxicology screen	• Diazepam • Haloperidol • GI decontamination up to 4 hours after PCP was taken; activated charcoal every 6 hours
Salicylates	• Hyperthermia • Hyperventilation	Altered LOC, ranging from confusion and agitation to lethargy to coma	• Tinnitus • Nausea and vomiting • Diaphoresis • Abdominal tenderness	• Anion-gap metabolic acidosis • Respiratory alkalosis • Abnormal liver function and coagulation tests • Positive blood salicylate level	• GI decontamination up to 12 hours after ingestion • Activated charcoal every 4 hours until stools are black
Sodium thiosulfate (antidote for cyanide)	• Hypotension	Decreased LOC	• Seizures • Cardiac arrhythmias • Pulmonary edema • Bright red venous blood • Decreased arterial venous oxygen level	• Cyanide level in arterial blood gas analysis • Abnormal hemoglobin (checking for methemoglobinuria)	• Supplemental oxygen • Cyanide antidote kit (containing amyl nitrite) • GI decontamination
Warfarin	• Normal to hypotension if bleeding has occurred	Normal or altered if patient has cerebral bleeding or severe hypotension	• Nausea and vomiting • Diarrhea • Abdominal cramps • Signs of abnormal bleeding (bruising, epistaxis, gum bleeding, GI bleeding)	• Prolonged clotting time • Elevated prothrombin and partial thromboplastin times	• Vitamin K

QUESTIONS TO ASK IN SUSPECTED DRUG TOXICITY

When assessing a patient with drug toxicity, use the information below to help identify the toxin and guide effective treatment.
- What is the chemical nature of the toxin?
- Did the patient ingest, inject, or inhale the drug, or take it by some other route?
- Is the patient's dose potentially lethal?
- Can the toxin rapidly be eliminated, neutralized, or counteracted to avoid further absorption? Will a binding agent work against it? What about activated charcoal, emesis, or lavage?

- Which organs does the toxin target? Where does the body store the toxin? Will metabolism of the toxin yield hazardous by-products?
- How is the toxin excreted? Can its elimination be hastened?
- Are laboratory tests available to determine the toxin's concentration, the patient's clinical status, or the course of organ injury?
- What concurrent problems has the patient been experiencing?

- Assess the patient's airway, breathing, and circulation. As needed, support her vital functions with basic and advanced life-support measures.
- Anticipate endotracheal intubation if the patient is unconscious and unable to maintain a patent airway or has evidence of respiratory failure.
- ➡ **NurseALERT** Remember to *treat the patient*, not the toxin. Only a few drugs have specific antidotes that dramatically relieve toxicity symptoms. More often, sound supportive care and aggressive attention to the patient's vital functions bring about a positive outcome.
- Establish I.V. access using a large-bore (18G to 20G) catheter.
- Obtain blood samples for toxicology testing, complete blood count, and arterial blood gas analysis and to measure blood urea nitrogen and serum electrolyte levels.
- Obtain a baseline ECG, as ordered, and institute continuous cardiac monitoring.
- Administer supplemental oxygen, as indicated and prescribed.
- Try to identify the toxic drug, if possible, to guide a specific plan of continuing treatment. (See *Questions to ask in suspected drug toxicity*.)
- If the patient has an altered level of consciousness, expect to give naloxone (Narcan) and dextrose I.V., as prescribed. Naloxone also can be effective if given by way of an endotracheal tube or sublingually if you can't gain I.V. access.
- ➡ **NurseALERT** Keep in mind that giving dextrose to a thiamine-deficient patient (such as an alcoholic) may induce Wernicke's encephalopathy. If your patient is an alcoholic or suspected of being one, give 100 mg of thiamine I.V. or intramuscularly as prescribed, before administering dextrose.

WHAT TO DO NEXT
Once the patient's vital functions have been stabilized, follow these guidelines:

- After the toxin has been identified, take steps to block further absorption of it or to hasten its excretion, if possible. (See *Reducing absorption, enhancing elimination*, page 114.)
- Administer a specific antidote for the toxic agent, if one is available.
- Provide further supportive measures, based on the patient's status.
- Place a hypotensive patient in Trendelenburg's position; as prescribed, administer I.V. fluids or vasopressor agents (such as dopamine or norepinephrine bitartrate [Levophed]).
- Give antihypertensive agents, if prescribed, to treat high blood pressure.
- Expect to administer antiarrhythmics to treat drug-induced cardiac arrhythmias.
- Keep in mind that drug-induced seizures may be hard to control or may not respond to anticonvulsant therapy. If a specific antidote is available to counteract a drug-induced seizure, administer it, as prescribed. (For example, isoniazid-induced seizures can be controlled with pyridoxine.)
- Be aware that for most causes of drug-induced seizures, no specific antidotes exist. Usually, you'll administer diazepam (Valium) I.V. to control seizures, followed by I.V. phenytoin (Dilantin), phenobarbital, or both, as prescribed.
- If seizures persist despite anticonvulsant therapy, anticipate more aggressive measures because prolonged seizures may lead to deterioration or even death. For instance, you may need to administer a paralyzing drug, such as pancuronium (Pavulon), to halt the muscle activity contributing to the seizure. If such treatment is necessary, prepare the patient for endotracheal intubation and mechanical ventilation.

FOLLOW-UP CARE
- Continue to monitor and support the patient's vital functions.
- Evaluate the effects of treatment and results of follow-up laboratory tests.
- Assess overall body organ and system function, staying alert for signs and symptoms of organ damage. Administer appropriate treatments, as prescribed.
- Try to determine the circumstances that brought about the drug toxicity. For instance, assess for suicidal ideation, and if indicated, take precautions to prevent a possible suicide.
- Discuss with the physician the need for a psychiatric evaluation of the patient.

SPECIAL CONSIDERATIONS
- If the toxic drug was prescribed for the patient, teach her how to avoid recurrence of toxicity.
- Evaluate the patient's ability to manage her medication program. Enlist the aid of family members, support people, and community resources, as necessary.

REDUCING ABSORPTION, ENHANCING ELIMINATION

Most treatments for drug toxicity focus on reducing absorption of the toxin or speeding its elimination. Here's an overview.

EMESIS FROM IPECAC SYRUP
Inducing emesis with ipecac syrup proves most effective when done within 30 minutes after toxin ingestion. Adults and children over age 12 require 30 ml of ipecac followed by 200 to 300 ml of water; children ages 1 to 12, 15 ml followed by 200 ml of water ; children ages 6 months to 1 year, 5 ml followed by 100 ml of water in a supervised setting. If you've given ipecac syrup, don't give activated charcoal within 2 to 4 hours (the emesis period). Be aware that in the emergency department, where gastric lavage can be performed and activated charcoal given immediately, ipecac is seldom used.

Ipecac syrup is contraindicated after ingestion of caustic or corrosive substances (such as acids and alkalis) and most petroleum distillates. It's also contraindicated during coma or impending coma, seizures or impending seizures, and other conditions that make vomiting dangerous (such as anatomic abnormalities, recent surgery, or a bleeding disorder).

ACTIVATED CHARCOAL
Activated charcoal absorbs most drugs and chemicals, making them unavailable for absorption into the bloodstream by way of the intestinal mucosa. Substances *not* absorbed by activated charcoal include acids, alkalis, boric acid, ethanol, ethylene glycol, iron tablets, mercury, and lithium.

Adults and adolescents typically receive 50 to 100 g; children, 1 to 2 g/kg of body weight, to a maximum of 50 g. Also, give at least 240 ml of a diluent (water or a cathartic) per 30 g of charcoal, as ordered. To enhance elimination of certain toxins, multiple doses may be administered.

CATHARTICS
Administered along with activated charcoal to hasten GI elimination of toxins, cathartics include the following:
- *Sorbitol.* Adults usually receive 1 to 2 g/kg of body weight per dose of 70% solution; children, 1 g/kg of body weight per dose of 35% solution.
- *Magnesium sulfate.* Adults receive 15 to 30 g/dose; children, 250 mg/kg of body weight per dose.
- *Magnesium citrate.* Usually, the patient receives 4 ml/kg of body weight per dose (up to 300 ml maximum).

Avoid giving a magnesium-based cathartic to a patient with renal failure or a sodium-based cathartic to a patient with heart failure. Use caution when giving repeat doses to any patient.

GASTRIC LAVAGE
In gastric lavage, the patient is placed in a left lateral decubitus position with the bed in Trendelenburg's position. Then tepid tap water or saline solution is instilled continuously through a large-bore orogastric or nasogastric tube until the effluent runs clear. Before or after lavage, the patient may receive activated charcoal through the lavage tube.

Gastric lavage may offer little benefit if performed more than 1 hour after toxin ingestion. Keep in mind that it may lead to esophageal perforation and aspiration of gastric contents. In a comatose patient, a cuffed endotracheal tube should be inserted before the lavage tube is inserted.

WHOLE-BOWEL IRRIGATION
This procedure may help neutralize certain substances, especially enteric-coated or sustained-release preparations and toxins not absorbed by charcoal (such as iron). For instance, a balanced electrolyte solution (Colyte, GoLYTELY) may be given by way of nasogastric tube until rectal effluent runs clear. Adults usually receive 1 to 2 L/hour; children, 400 ml/hour. Results are rapid because the GI tract clears in just a few hours. Be aware, however, that the large volume of solution required for irrigation may distend the stomach, causing vomiting and pulmonary aspiration.

DIURESIS
Occasionally, the physician may order diuretics to speed elimination of certain drugs—usually salicylates or phenobarbital. Know that forced diuresis raises the risk of fluid overload and renal failure.

HEMODIALYSIS
Hemodialysis isn't widely used to aid elimination of toxins, but it can be effective in some severe toxicities—possibly those involving salicylates, ethylene glycol, methanol, lithium, or theophylline. Hemodialysis also may prove useful in a patient with renal failure when the toxin's main elimination route is renal.

- Make sure mental health professionals are available to any patient who is experiencing suicidal thoughts or showing signs of clinical depression.
- Instruct parents to keep all potentially toxic substances out of children's reach, and discuss other childproofing strategies for the home.
- Inform all patients and family members of the toll-free phone number of their state's poison control hot line.

DYSPNEA

A sensation of shortness of breath or breathlessness, dyspnea is caused by a lack of sufficient oxygen, an increase in the work of breathing, or an alteration in ventilatory mechanics. Dyspnea associated with heavy exertion is normal in most people; dyspnea at rest or during light activity (such as dressing and bathing) suggests an underlying cardiac or respiratory problem.

Dyspnea frequently accompanies heart disease, lung cancer, and other respiratory conditions. Severe dyspnea of sudden onset may indicate one of a wide variety of disorders, ranging from anxiety or pain to respiratory failure, anaphylaxis, pneumothorax, pulmonary edema, cardiomyopathy, heart failure, and pulmonary embolism. Dyspnea of gradual onset typically indicates a slowly progressive respiratory disorder, such as emphysema. (See *Evaluating the cause of dyspnea,* pages 116 and 117.)

Prolonged dyspnea can lead to respiratory muscle fatigue and may even progress to respiratory failure. If your patient becomes dyspneic, you'll need to evaluate him quickly to help identify the underlying problem. Then expect to carry out interventions based on that problem, such as closely monitoring his vital signs, obtaining a chest X-ray, and administering oxygen.

WHAT TO LOOK FOR
Clinical findings associated with dyspnea vary with the underlying cause. The patient may have any of the following signs and symptoms:
- breathlessness during activity
- preference for high Fowler's position
- severe tachypnea (respiratory rate faster than 30 breaths/minute)
- use of accessory muscles for breathing
- pursed-lip breathing
- nasal flaring during inspiration
- uncoordinated or paradoxical breathing
- inspiratory or expiratory stridor (indicating airway obstruction)
- wheezing
- crackles (which suggest fluid in the lungs or opening of collapsed airways)

EVALUATING THE CAUSE OF DYSPNEA

Dyspnea can result from a wide range of cardiac, pulmonary, and other conditions. To help pinpoint the cause of your patient's dyspnea, take a detailed history and compare his dyspnea characteristics and associated findings with those listed in this chart.

Characteristics	Associated findings	Probable causes
• Gradual-onset dyspnea, beginning as exertional	• History of smoking • Minimal cough, usually nonproductive • Respiratory distress • Tachypnea • Prolonged, grunting expirations • Faint, high-pitched wheezes on end expiration • Diminished breath sounds • Carbon dioxide retention • Forward-leaning posture with arms extended • Accessory muscle use • Weight loss	• Emphysema
• Gradual-onset dyspnea • Paroxysmal nocturnal dyspnea (from increased sputum production)	• History of smoking, obesity, and frequent respiratory tract infections • Long history of cough and increased sputum production • Coarse crackles and wheezes, which change location and intensity with coughing • Cyanosis, finger clubbing, peripheral edema, neck vein distention, right ventricular failure, and cor pulmonale (late findings) • Carbon dioxide retention	• Chronic bronchitis
• Episodes of acute dyspnea	• Sensation of lump in throat • Hoarseness • Stridor and supraclavicular retraction on inspiration • Respiratory distress and failure	• Aspiration of food or foreign body • Allergic reaction (from angioedema) • Upper airway obstruction
• Exertional dyspnea that progresses to dyspnea at rest • Paroxysmal nocturnal dyspnea and orthopnea	• Coughing and wheezing • Feeling of suffocation or drowning • Moist inspiratory crackles • Tachypnea with gallop rhythms and heart murmurs • Jugular vein distention • Diaphoresis • Peripheral edema • Pleural effusions	• Heart failure • Myocardial infarction or ischemia • Valvular disease • Cardiomyopathy
• Dyspnea at rest	• Hyperventilation • Sharp, fleeting chest pain • Frequent sighing • Irregular breathing pattern with normal pattern during sleep	• Anxiety • Emotional stress

Characteristics	Associated findings	Probable causes
• Acute-onset dyspnea • Episodic occurrence, with individual attacks lasting minutes to hours • Common in children	• Coughing • Wheezing • Tachypnea with wheezing	• Asthma
• Dyspnea at rest • Sudden, unexplained breathlessness	• Sharp or stabbing pleuritic pain • Hemoptysis • Tachycardia and tachypnea • Accentuated pulmonic heart sounds • Hypotension • ST-segment changes on ECG • Pleural friction rub • Atelectasis after 24 hours from when pulmonary embolism occurred	• Pulmonary embolism
• Dyspnea at rest	• Cough that produces mucus, pus, or blood • Tachypnea • Decreased respiratory excursion and dullness to percussion on affected side • High-pitched, end-inspiratory crackles • Increased bronchial breath sounds • Increased tactile fremitus over consolidation area • Tachycardia • Fever • Chest pain • Confusion or disorientation (in elderly patient)	• Pneumonia
• Exertional, gradual-onset dyspnea	• Nonproductive cough • Dry crackles, usually at end of deep inspiration • Fatigue • Malaise • Pulmonary hypertension and finger clubbing (late findings)	• Interstitial fibrotic lung disease • Rheumatoid or collagen vascular disease • Sarcoidosis
• Gradual-onset dyspnea	• History of smoking • Productive cough • Wheezing • Stridor • Fever • Hemoptysis	• Pulmonary neoplasm (primary or metastatic)

D

- diaphoresis
- restlessness, irritability
- chest pain
- changes in level of consciousness
- anxiety, fear
- confusion
- cyanosis.

Don't confuse dyspnea with changes in a patient's respiratory pattern, such as rapid breathing (tachypnea); deep, rapid, or labored breathing in response to exercise or increased metabolism (hyperpnea); and a respiratory rate that exceeds the body's respiratory needs (hyperventilation).

WHAT TO DO IMMEDIATELY

If your patient experiences dyspnea, establish and maintain a patent airway, and call for help. Then follow these guidelines.

- Continuously monitor the patient's vital signs, especially his respiratory rate, depth, and character. Provide supplemental oxygen, as ordered.
- Help him to a position that facilitates breathing. Elevate the head of the bed to a high Fowler's position and help him sit upright in bed. If necessary, have him lean forward and rest his arms on an overbed table or on his knees for added support.
- To help identify the underlying cause of dyspnea, assess your patient for a possible airway obstruction and auscultate his lungs for crackles and wheezing. Also check for peripheral edema.
- Evaluate the patient's mental status; watch closely for subtle changes in his level of consciousness, which may indicate worsening hypoxemia.
- Assess his skin color, and check his oxygen saturation level by means of pulse oximetry.
- Obtain a blood sample for arterial blood gas (ABG) analysis to evaluate for hypoxemia, acidosis, and alkalosis. As ordered, also obtain samples for other laboratory tests, such as serum electrolytes, complete blood count, hemoglobin level, and hematocrit.
- Obtain an immediate chest X-ray, as ordered, to help identify the reason for dyspnea.
- Assess for complaints of chest pain.
- ➡ **NurseALERT** If your patient has chest pain along with dyspnea, suspect possible myocardial ischemia and anticipate the need for continuous cardiac monitoring, serum cardiac enzyme measurement, and nitroglycerin administration. Check his ECG frequently.
- Evaluate for relief of dyspnea after position changes.
- Encourage the patient to relax and breathe slowly and deeply. If he has a history of chronic obstructive pulmonary disease, encourage pursed-lip breathing to minimize air trapping.
- Administer diuretics, nebulizer treatments, or anxiolytics, if prescribed, for treatment of the underlying cause.

ASSISTING WITH ENDOTRACHEAL INTUBATION

The physician may order endotracheal intubation if your dyspneic patient deteriorates to respiratory decompensation. To assist with intubation, gather the necessary equipment and then follow these steps.

PREPARING THE PATIENT

- As ordered, preoxygenate the patient with 100% oxygen for at least 2 minutes, if possible. Administer prescribed drugs to decrease respiratory secretions (such as atropine) or to reduce anxiety (such as anxiolytics).
- Suction any copious secretions blocking the patient's pharynx and vocal cords.
- Place the patient in a supine position with his neck hyperextended to straighten the larynx and trachea.

DURING THE PROCEDURE

- Assist with insertion of the endotracheal tube, and help establish correct cuff pressure, as ordered.
- Check for correct tube placement by assessing air movement in and out of the tube, evaluating bilateral chest wall expansion, and listening for bilateral breath sounds.
- If the patient is unconscious, instill air into the endotracheal tube, using a manual resuscitation bag, and watch for his chest to rise. If bilateral breath sounds are absent, suspect that the tube is lodged in the mainstem bronchus. If you note abdominal distention and belching, suspect (and report) that the tube is in the esophagus.
- Obtain a chest X-ray to confirm tube placement. With correct placement, the end of the endotracheal tube appears 2 to 3 cm (¾" to 1") above the level of the carina.
- After tube placement is verified, note the marking on the tube where it exits the patient's mouth or nose, and secure the tube with tape to prevent dislodgment and minimize the risk of tracheal damage.
- Reposition the patient to promote comfort, taking care to avoid tube kinking and airway obstruction.

AFTERCARE

- Check tube placement often. Monitor endotracheal cuff pressure according to your facility's policy. To prevent tracheal necrosis, intracuff pressure shouldn't exceed tracheal capillary filling pressure (25 cm H_2O or 20 mm Hg).
- If you suspect a cuff leak, check to see whether the tube is still at the proper level by looking at the tube's exit mark. If the mark has moved, the tube will need to be repositioned. If possible, ask the respiratory therapist to check cuff pressure. If a leak is confirmed, gradually add about 0.5 to 1.0 cc of air until an adequate seal is achieved.
- Auscultate the patient's breath sounds, and observe for bilateral chest movement every 1 to 2 hours.
- Provide frequent mouth care, and suction as necessary to maintain airway patency and promote optimal gas exchange.
- Move the tube to the other side of the mouth every 8 hours to prevent breakdown of the oral mucosa.
- If necessary, apply soft hand restraints to reduce the risk of self-extubation (which can damage the vocal cords). Be sure to follow your facility's policy on restraints.

D

- Monitor for evidence that the patient is tiring, such as slow or shallow respirations and drowsiness. Be aware that slow respirations may progress to apnea. Keep equipment for endotracheal intubation and mechanical ventilation readily available in case the patient becomes unstable or slips into respiratory distress or arrest. (See *Assisting with endotracheal intubation.*)
- Stay calm and make sure you offer the patient reassurance to help relieve his anxiety.

WHAT TO DO NEXT

After taking initial steps, carry out these actions:

- Continue to monitor the patient's vital signs, and closely assess his respiratory rate, depth, and effort.

- Frequently evaluate his mental status; report confusion, drowsiness, lethargy, and change in level of consciousness.
- Assess his breath sounds every 1 to 2 hours until he's stable; report significant changes.
- Place the patient in semi-Fowler's to high Fowler's position to promote optimal lung expansion.
- Encourage frequent deep breathing, coughing, incentive spirometry, and pursed-lip breathing, as ordered and indicated.
- Continue to monitor the patient's pulse oximetry and ABG values; adjust the supplemental oxygen flow rate based on test results.
- Obtain blood samples for repeat laboratory tests, such as serum electrolytes, complete blood count, hemoglobin level, and hematocrit.
- Assess the patient's mucous membranes for dryness, and perform frequent oral hygiene. Be aware that a dyspneic patient who breathes through the mouth (in an effort to inhale more oxygen) is at risk for dry mucous membranes.
- Administer ordered treatments to correct the cause of dyspnea. For instance, expect to give analgesics if dyspnea results from pain, anxiolytics for anxiety.
- Continue to monitor the ECG, as indicated, and report changes.

FOLLOW-UP CARE
- Continue to assess the patient's vital signs and cardiopulmonary status. Auscultate his lungs at least every 4 hours, and report crackles or wheezing.
- Elevate the head of the bed 45 degrees to promote comfort and enhance lung expansion and aeration.
- Teach your patient how to perform incentive spirometry, use an inhaler, and breathe through pursed lips, as indicated.
- Monitor results of chest X-rays, blood tests, and ABG analysis; report abnormalities.
- Continue to assess the patient for pain and anxiety, and provide medication, as prescribed.

SPECIAL CONSIDERATIONS
- If your patient has pneumonia, keep supplies available for obtaining sputum specimens. Teach him how to produce a sputum specimen correctly—*not* by simply spitting into the culture cup. Be aware that a specimen can be obtained through voluntary coughing and expectoration, sputum induction by inhaling aerosol, nasotracheal or endotracheal suctioning, transtracheal aspiration, and bronchoscopy.
- Assess the patient's sputum for color, consistency, volume, and odor. Report foul-smelling sputum, production of more than 50 ml of sputum per day, and sputum that is not clear.
- Keep in mind that dyspnea may set off a vicious cycle, causing fear and anxiety—reactions that worsen the dyspnea and increase the patient's apprehension.

E, F, G

ENDOCARDITIS

An inflammation of the endocardium, the heart's inner layer, endocarditis usually results from infection with streptococcal or staphylococcal organisms. Less commonly, it's caused by a different type of bacterium or by a virus or fungus.

Because the endocardium is directly connected to the heart valves, the valves typically become infected too, possibly leading to serious complications. For example, vegetations made up of fibrin, leukocytes, platelets, and microbes may form on the valve leaflets, damaging them and their supporting structures. The result is valvular insufficiency (also called regurgitation or incompetence), which prevents the valve leaflets from closing properly and allows blood to leak backward through them. If this happens, the patient is at risk for heart failure. Vegetations also may embolize to the systemic circulation or pulmonary circulation, causing pulmonary embolism.

People at highest risk for endocarditis include:
- those with existing valve disease or mitral valve prolapse who undergo an invasive procedure, especially dental work
- those with damaged or malformed heart valves, prosthetic valves, rheumatic heart disease, congenital heart disease, Marfan's syndrome, hypertrophic cardiomyopathy, long-term I.V. or intra-arterial catheters, or prosthetic aortic grafts
- alcoholics
- I.V. drug users
- chronically ill and immunosuppressed patients.

Endocarditis can be acute or subacute. The acute form develops quickly in normal heart valves, causes severe damage (even in patients with no previous valve problem), and may be fatal unless treated. The subacute form typically affects heart valves with preexisting damage, progresses more slowly, and responds well to antibiotics. Patients with subacute endocarditis may develop acute endocarditis, and patients with acute endocarditis may resolve to subacute endocarditis.

One of your most important roles is to help determine which organism is causing your patient's disorder. Treatment consists of I.V. antibiotics based on the results of blood cultures. Delivery of antibiotics may be done on an inpatient or outpatient basis, depending on the severity of your patient's clinical condition. (See *Drawing blood for culture*, page 122).

E

TIPS AND TECHNIQUES

DRAWING BLOOD FOR CULTURE

Blood cultures are the mainstay of endocarditis diagnosis. To ensure accurate identification of the infecting organism, always draw samples carefully and correctly. Using standard precautions, follow the steps below:

- Explain the purpose of the test to your patient.
- Draw the first set of samples before antibiotic therapy begins. If this isn't feasible, draw the samples just before you give the next antibiotic dose, and use culture bottles that contain resin to bind the antibiotic.
- You'll draw two samples from each of three sites, so you'll need to collect six culture bottles—three aerobic and three anaerobic. (Don't use your patient's I.V. line to draw the samples.)
- Clean the patient's skin and the tops of the culture bottles with povidone-iodine, and let them air-dry.
- From each site, draw 10 to 15 ml of blood for each of the two bottles.

- Use a new sterile needle for each culture.
- Mix the culture bottles gently.
- On each bottle's label, write the patient's name, the date and time the cultures were drawn, and the name of any antibiotics the patient is receiving.
- Make sure the cultures go to the laboratory within 30 minutes after the samples are drawn.

FOLLOWING UP
- Check for a preliminary laboratory report of test results in about 24 hours.
- Begin giving appropriate antibiotics, as prescribed.
- Make sure to give all doses on time.
- Draw repeat blood cultures periodically to evaluate the effectiveness of therapy.

WHAT TO LOOK FOR
Clinical findings with an *infection* may include:
- chronic, intermittent, low-grade fever (subacute); marked temperature elevations to 103° F (39.4° C) and chills (acute)
- fatigue, malaise, headache
- anorexia
- elevated white blood cell (WBC) count
- elevated erythrocyte sedimentation rate.

Clinical findings with *heart valve involvement* may include:
- new aortic or mitral murmur
- heart failure (may have sudden onset in acute endocarditis), crackles in lung bases, peripheral edema, tachypnea, tachycardia.

Clinical findings with an *embolization* can vary, depending on the body system affected, but may include:
- petechiae (skin)
- splinter hemorrhages under the nails
- Osler's nodes (small, raised, tender, red or purple lesions on the pads of fingers and toes)
- Janeway lesions (small, flat, painless, red spots) on the palms and soles
- Roth's spots (round or oval retinal spots, consisting of coagulated fibrin, that may hemorrhage)
- arthralgia, myalgia (musculoskeletal)
- flank pain, hematuria (renal)
- headaches, visual disturbances (neurologic)

- chest pain, ischemic changes on ECG (cardiovascular)
- dyspnea, restlessness (respiratory).

WHAT TO DO IMMEDIATELY
If your patient develops signs and symptoms of acute endocarditis, follow these steps:
- Assess her vital signs. Auscultate heart and breath sounds. Be alert for heart murmurs, which may indicate valvular insufficiency, and adventitious breath sounds (crackles and wheezes), which may indicate heart failure.
- If the patient has a high fever or signs of heart failure, enforce bed rest to minimize oxygen demands. If you suspect heart failure, position her with the head of the bed elevated at least 30 degrees. Also implement measures to reduce fever, such as giving acetaminophen, as prescribed, to reduce the body's oxygen demands.
- Obtain blood cultures, as ordered.
- Assess the patient for chest pain. Be aware that reduced cardiac output or embolism of the coronary arteries or their branches may lead to myocardial ischemia.
- Obtain a 12-lead ECG, and evaluate for ischemic changes.
- Monitor the patient's arterial blood gas values or pulse oximetry. Give supplemental oxygen, if indicated and prescribed.
- Draw blood for cultures, as ordered, to identify the infecting organism. Expect to administer I.V. antibiotics based on blood culture results. Most patients undergo a 6-week course of therapy.
- If your patient has acute heart failure, administer a diuretic (such as furosemide [Lasix] or bumetanide [Bumex]) or another medication, as prescribed, to promote diuresis. Nitroglycerin or another nitrate also may be prescribed to reduce preload. Hydralazine (Apresoline) or enalapril (Vasotec) may be prescribed to reduce afterload. If your patient receives any of these medications, monitor her blood pressure closely for hypotension.
- Administer ordered drugs to increase myocardial contractility, such as digoxin (Lanoxicaps), dopamine (Intropin), dobutamine (Dobutrex), or amrinone (Inocor).

WHAT TO DO NEXT
After the initial crisis subsides, take these measures:
- Monitor laboratory test results. Remember that elevated blood urea nitrogen and serum creatinine levels indicate reduced renal perfusion, whereas elevations in the WBC count and erythrocyte sedimentation rate signal infection.
- Continue to monitor your patient's vital signs. Notify the physician of any fever (or if the patient's fever doesn't abate), and administer antipyretics, as prescribed.
- Assess for signs and symptoms of heart failure, which suggest worsening valve function. Auscultate the patient's heart and breath sounds for new murmurs and crackles, and watch for jugular vein distention.

E

FOLLOW-UP CARE

- Track the patient's blood culture results and WBC counts to assess antibiotic effectiveness.
- Monitor peak and trough serum antibiotic levels to prevent toxicity and assess therapeutic effectiveness. Obtain peak levels 30 minutes after I.V. administration and trough levels within 15 minutes before the next scheduled dose.
- If your patient is receiving a diuretic, check her serum potassium level regularly. If it drops below normal, anticipate giving a potassium supplement, if prescribed. Watch for signs and symptoms of hypokalemia, such as muscle weakness and arrhythmias.
- Monitor the patient's serum digoxin level and assess for signs and symptoms of digitalis toxicity, such as arrhythmias, nausea, vomiting, fatigue, and vision changes.

➡ **NurseALERT** If your patient is receiving digoxin, keep in mind that hypokalemia increases her risk of digitalis toxicity.

- Check the I.V. site for signs of infiltration, such as redness, warmth, tenderness, and pain. Change the I.V. tubing, solutions, and site according to your facility's policy.
- If your patient requires prolonged bed rest, perform passive or active range-of-motion exercises. Encourage her to perform frequent coughing and deep-breathing exercises, incentive spirometry, and position changes.
- Assess for adverse and toxic effects of prescribed antibiotics, and report them immediately.
- Continue to monitor cardiac and respiratory function. Be alert for the development of new heart murmurs and changes in existing murmurs.
- Provide nutritious meals; consult with a dietitian, if necessary.
- Provide diversionary activities if your patient faces a long hospitalization. Use volunteers to provide companionship, and encourage visits by family members and friends.
- Help the patient ambulate and stay as active as possible. Watch for signs and symptoms of activity intolerance, such as tachycardia and dyspnea. Plan rest periods to reduce her cardiac workload.
- If the patient shows signs of depression, arrange for counseling.
- Be aware that if the patient's valves have been seriously damaged, surgical repair or replacement may be needed after antibiotic therapy is complete and acute infection has resolved.

SPECIAL CONSIDERATIONS

- Be aware that a patient with endocarditis usually needs a 6-week course of antibiotic therapy and, therefore, is likely to be discharged on antibiotics. To promote an effective therapeutic outcome, begin discharge planning and medication teaching early in her hospital stay. Provide adequate discharge instructions, and make sure she has a home-care referral.

- Stress the need to take antibiotics before undergoing certain proce-dures, and make sure the patient understands the importance of telling all health-care providers about her history of endocarditis.
- Advise the patient to carry medical identification at all times.
- Give her a list of signs and symptoms that suggest infection and heart failure, and tell her to notify her physician at once if these occur. Make sure she knows how to take her temperature accurately.

EPIDURAL ANALGESIA PROBLEMS

Epidurally administered analgesia can be used to treat patients who have acute or chronic pain, especially cancer-related pain and severe, acute postoperative pain. The narcotic analgesic is delivered through a catheter inserted in the spinal epidural space below L2. The catheter can be used to give continuous or bolus medication doses. (See *What you should know about epidural analgesia*, page 126.)

Epidural analgesia has several advantages, including:
- smaller narcotic doses
- more consistent analgesia
- fewer systemic effects than with intramuscular or I.V. narcotic administration.

Despite these advantages, epidural analgesia can lead to serious prob-lems and complications. For instance, the catheter may become kinked, blocked, disconnected, or dislodged, preventing delivery of effective medication doses. Or the catheter may migrate into the subarachnoid space, raising the risk of meningeal infection or spinal anesthesia.

Infection at the catheter exit site, another possible complication, ne-cessitates catheter removal and anti-infective therapy. Also, the patient may become oversedated if the epidural narcotic diffuses from the injec-tion site (in the lumbar region) toward the opiate receptors in the medullary respiratory center of the brain, exposing him to the risk of life-threatening respiratory depression and hypotension.

Although an anesthesiologist inserts the epidural catheter, you're re-sponsible for assessing and monitoring the patient's response to analge-sia, checking for adverse effects, providing catheter care, and detecting and troubleshooting catheter problems. Swift action on your part may prove essential to your patient's well-being.

WHAT TO LOOK FOR
Clinical evidence of catheter *kinking, blockage, disconnection, dislodgment, or migration* includes:
- obvious kinking, disconnection, or dislodgment
- leakage of clear or blood-tinged fluid from the exit site or infusion tubing
- resistance to fluid instillation or aspiration

E

WHAT YOU SHOULD KNOW ABOUT EPIDURAL ANALGESIA

In epidural analgesia, an anesthesiologist inserts a flexible plastic catheter into the patient's spinal epidural space, which lies just above the dura. Cerebrospinal fluid (CSF) circulates in the subarachnoid space just below the dura. Medication deposited in the epidural space diffuses through the dura into the subarachnoid space, where it enters the CSF, which circulates around the spinal cord. There it binds to opiate receptors in the spinal cord and relieves pain by altering the patient's perception of it.

CATHETER PLACEMENT

As the illustration shows, the epidural catheter usually is inserted between the second and third or the third and fourth lumbar vertebrae and then advanced into the epidural space (between the dura mater and the walls of the vertebral canal). Once in place, the catheter may exit over the spine or it may be tunneled subcutaneously and exit over the abdomen or side.

EPIDURAL ANALGESICS

Special forms of morphine (Duramorph), fentanyl (Sublimaze), and hydromorphone (Dilaudid) may be delivered epidurally. Be aware that these forms aren't the same preparations typically found in the narcotic stock of a health-care facility.

These analgesics may be given in combination with a local anesthetic, such as bupivacaine (Marcaine). In case the patient needs emergency drugs, make sure he has a patent peripheral I.V. line during epidural analgesia.

CONTRAINDICATIONS

Epidural analgesia is contraindicated in patients with spinal arthritis or deformities, coagulopathy, hypotension, marked hypertension, or allergy to the prescribed medication.

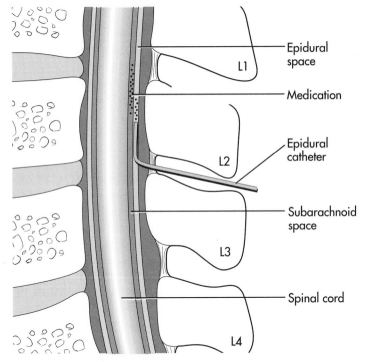

activation of the alarm on the infusion control device
- appearance of more than 0.5 ml of clear or discolored aspirate (with catheter migration)
- inadequate pain control.

With *infection* at the catheter exit site, clinical findings may include:
- elevated temperature
- pain and redness at the site
- purulent or increased drainage from the site
- pain when medication is infused or injected
- signs of meningeal infection, such as back pain, chills, fever, and central nervous system irritability.

With *oversedation,* your patient may exhibit:
• decreased level of consciousness
• respiratory rate below 10 breaths/minute.

WHAT TO DO IMMEDIATELY
If you suspect kinking, disconnection, blockage, dislodgment, or migration of your patient's epidural catheter, notify the physician. Then take these steps:
• Stop the epidural infusion.
• Inspect the infusion tubing to make sure all connections are secure. If you find a loose connection, try to reconnect it (using sterile technique), and notify the anesthesiologist immediately.
• If all tubing connections are secure, attempt to aspirate fluid from the catheter, if permitted by your facility; assess the aspirate for amount and color.
➡ **NurseALERT** If you aspirate more than 0.5 ml of clear or discolored fluid, suspect that the catheter has migrated into the subarachnoid space.
• If you can't aspirate any fluid, attach a syringe filled with preservative-free normal saline solution, and using strict sterile technique, gently try to instill 1 to 2 ml of the solution. If you meet resistance, suspect catheter blockage and notify the physician.
• If the catheter has become dislodged completely, place a sterile dressing over the exit site and notify the physician immediately.
• If the catheter is occluded or has migrated, discuss alternate pain-relief methods with the physician.

Dealing with infection
If you suspect an infection at the catheter exit site, carry out these interventions:
• Stop the infusion and prepare for catheter removal by the physician.
• Send the catheter tip and a specimen of exit site drainage for culture and sensitivity testing.

Managing oversedation
If you suspect your patient is oversedated from epidural analgesia, notify the physician. Then take these steps:
• Stop the epidural infusion.
• Monitor the patient's blood pressure and respiratory rate.
• Have naloxone (Narcan) ready to reverse sedative effects.
• If the patient experiences leg weakness or numbness, titrate the analgesic dose, as prescribed and necessary, to achieve adequate pain relief without producing excessive weakness. Assess the patient's motor and sensory functions every 2 to 4 hours.

WHAT TO DO NEXT
Once the patient has stabilized, take the following actions:
• Continue to monitor the patient for adverse analgesic effects for at

E

least 12 hours after the epidural infusion has been discontinued. (Remember that drugs in the epidural space are absorbed slowly).

- Assess the patient for pain, and provide alternate analgesia, as prescribed.

FOLLOW-UP CARE
- After catheter removal, assess for a possible dural tear, which can lead to cerebrospinal fluid (CSF) leakage. The dura may have been inadvertently punctured at the time of insertion or if the catheter has migrated. A patient with a CSF leak may complain of a headache that improves when he lies flat and worsens when he rises. Also stay alert for nausea, vomiting, muscle aches, visual changes, and hearing problems.
- If a CSF leak is suspected or confirmed, restrict the patient to bed rest for at least 24 hours to allow the dura to seal. If he continues to complain of headache, assist with a blood patch, if ordered. In this procedure, the physician withdraws about 10 ml of blood from a peripheral vein and instills it into the epidural space, where it clots over the dural defect.
- Continue to monitor the catheter site for signs and symptoms of infection.
- ➡ **NurseALERT** Watch for signs and symptoms of meningeal irritation, which could indicate meningitis. Patients with CSF leaks are at increased risk for meningitis.
- Perform meticulous skin care, using standard precautions.

SPECIAL CONSIDERATIONS
- Use aseptic technique when providing epidural catheter care.
- Change the dressing at the catheter exit site, as ordered.
- To help prevent catheter dislodgment and migration, apply tincture of benzoin to the patient's skin to improve adherence. Secure the catheter with sterile tape strips or hypoallergenic tape. Alternatively, loop a segment of the catheter under the dressing or tape it in place.
- ➡ **NurseALERT** Clearly label the epidural catheter's injection port to indicate that it is an epidural access site. This helps prevent serious errors that could occur if the epidural catheter is mistaken for a central venous or peripheral venous line.

EPIDURAL HEMATOMA

An epidural hematoma refers to bleeding into the epidural space—the potential space between the inner portion of the skull and the dura mater. Also called an *extradural hematoma* because of its location outside the dura, an epidural hematoma pushes the dura away from the inner table of the skull as it expands. This creates an oval mass that subjects underlying brain tissue to additional pressure. (See *Visualizing an epidural hematoma*.)

Because an epidural hematoma commonly results from trauma, suspect it in any patient with a skull fracture. A temporal bone fracture is es-

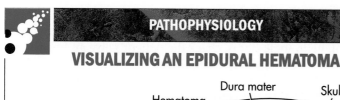

PATHOPHYSIOLOGY

VISUALIZING AN EPIDURAL HEMATOMA

An epidural hematoma, as shown in this illustration, develops in the space beneath the skull and above the dura mater.

With its swift onset and the rapid displacement of brain tissue and subsequent herniation, an epidural hematoma can quickly prove fatal.

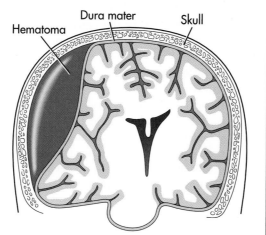

Hematoma   Dura mater   Skull

E

pecially likely to cause an epidural hematoma because it may lacerate the middle meningeal artery, which lies beneath the temporal bone.

If your patient has a large epidural hematoma, you'll need to act fast to avoid catastrophic consequences. With its swift onset and the rapid displacement of brain tissue and herniation that ensues, the condition quickly can prove fatal. If the patient shows signs or symptoms of increased intracranial pressure (ICP), she'll need emergency surgery (craniotomy) to remove the hematoma. Her outcome depends on her neurologic status before surgery and the time lag between symptom onset and intervention.

On the other hand, a small epidural hematoma may require only observation and serial computed tomography (CT) scans to check for lesion expansion. Usually, a small hematoma resorbs on its own.

WHAT TO LOOK FOR

A patient with an epidural hematoma may exhibit:
- momentary loss of consciousness, followed by rapid reawakening and a brief lucid period and then a swift, progressive decrease in consciousness, leading to coma
- changes in the respiratory pattern
- ipsilateral pupil dilation with a sluggish to fixed pupillary response to light
- headache
- seizures
- contralateral hemiparesis or hemiplegia
- decorticate or decerebrate posturing.

WHAT TO DO IMMEDIATELY

If you suspect that your patient has an intracranial hematoma and shows a deteriorating neurologic status, check the patient's airway, breathing, and circulation. Intervene appropriately and notify the physician at once. Then take these steps:

- Secure and maintain a patent airway. If the patient is unconscious, assist with endotracheal intubation and mechanical ventilation, as indicated.
- Maintain adequate oxygenation by administering supplemental oxygen, if prescribed. Monitor the patient's oxygen saturation using pulse oximetry or arterial blood gas analysis.
- Obtain an emergency CT scan, as ordered.
- Monitor the patient's vital signs and neurologic status carefully. Watch closely for signs of increasing ICP and impending irreversible herniation—elevated systolic blood pressure with widening pulse pressure and bradycardia (Cushing's triad), decorticate or decerebrate posturing, and unilateral pupil fixation and dilation.
- Prepare the patient for emergency surgery.

WHAT TO DO NEXT

When the patient returns from surgery, carry out the following interventions:

- Provide immediate postcraniotomy care. (See *Caring for your patient after a craniotomy*.)
- Continue to monitor the patient's vital signs and neurologic status.
- Maintain strict fluid intake and output records.
- Check the surgical dressing and drain (if present) for excessive drainage.
- ➡ **NurseALERT** A large amount of drainage after a craniotomy is not normal. If it occurs, notify the surgeon immediately.
- Administer osmotic diuretics, if prescribed, to help control ICP. Monitor serum osmolarity and electrolyte levels during diuretic therapy.
- Institute seizure precautions and closely observe the patient for seizures.
- Use cool compresses to decrease postoperative facial swelling.
- Assess for headache, and administer analgesics, as indicated and prescribed.
- ➡ **NurseALERT** Severe pain is not expected after a craniotomy. Notify the surgeon immediately if the patient complains of severe pain or a sudden increase in pain. This may indicate intracranial bleeding.
- Ensure adequate nutrition. If the patient can eat normally, maintain a calorie count initially. If she has trouble eating because of an altered level of consciousness or difficulty swallowing, the physician may order enteral or parenteral feedings. If so, be sure to weigh the patient at least every other day.
- Provide emotional support to the patient and family.

CARING FOR YOUR PATIENT AFTER A CRANIOTOMY

If your patient underwent a craniotomy to remove an epidural hematoma, focus your postoperative nursing care on:
- recognizing early signs and symptoms of increased intracranial pressure (ICP)
- maintaining hemodynamic monitoring
- preventing postoperative complications or detecting them early
- assisting with early rehabilitation planning.

To meet these goals, carry out the interventions described below.

PROVIDING BASIC CARE
- Monitor the patient's vital signs hourly, particularly her temperature and blood pressure.
- Watch closely for signs and symptoms of increased ICP during the first 72 hours after surgery. Cerebral edema can develop around the surgical site, leading to potentially life-threatening increases in ICP.
- Reposition the patient every 2 hours, maintaining good body alignment to help control ICP.
- Keep the head of her bed elevated between 15 and 30 degrees (depending on her blood pressure) to promote venous drainage. But keep in mind that a blood pressure drop could reduce cerebral blood flow, offsetting the benefits of drainage. Thus, be sure to tailor the degree of elevation to your patient's status.
- Ensure adequate oxygenation by administering supplemental oxygen, as indicated and prescribed. If necessary, perform nasotracheal suctioning to remove secretions that might impair gas exchange. Avoid routine suctioning because it can cause transient increases in ICP.
- Provide meticulous skin care every 2 to 4 hours, as appropriate.
- Assess the craniotomy dressing hourly. A large amount of drainage is *not* typical. Notify the surgeon if the dressing is saturated.

MONITORING NEUROLOGIC STATUS
- Assess your patient's neurologic status hourly. Report any change in level of consciousness immediately.
- A change in the patient's level of consciousness is the earliest sign of increasing ICP.
- If she has an ICP monitoring device in place, assess ICP readings. Correlate them with neurologic findings.

INSTITUTING SEIZURE PRECAUTIONS
- Observe the patient frequently for signs of seizure activity.
- As prescribed and indicated, administer anticonvulsants. To help prevent drug toxicity, monitor serum anticonvulsant levels closely.
- Maintain safety precautions, such as padding and raising the side rails, until the patient is fully awake and aware of her environment.
- Avoid restraints if possible. They may increase agitation in a patient with an altered level of consciousness and increase her ICP.
- As ordered, obtain an electroencephalogram.

ENSURING FLUID BALANCE AND BOWEL ELIMINATION
- Institute a bowel program early to prevent constipation. Provide adequate fluid and fiber intake, stool softeners, and laxatives. During the early postoperative period, make sure the patient avoids straining at stool because doing so increases ICP.

OTHER CARE MEASURES
- Care for the surgical incision as ordered. Inspect the site carefully for swelling, redness, and drainage.
- Advance the patient's activity level as soon as she shows stable vital signs.

E

FOLLOW-UP CARE
- Continue to assess the patient's neurologic status.
- Monitor carefully for signs and symptoms of infection related to surgery or the insertion of the ICP monitoring device (if one was used).
- Monitor closely for signs and symptoms of increased ICP, which could result from cerebral edema at the surgical site. The patient is at greatest risk for cerebral edema during the first 72 hours after surgery.
- ➡ **NurseALERT** To help control ICP, maintain a normal body temperature using hypothermia blankets and acetaminophen, as indicated and

prescribed. Take care not to cool the patient too much because shivering may raise her ICP.
- Begin rehabilitation therapy as soon as possible, if indicated.
- Make referrals to an acute or a subacute rehabilitation facility, if appropriate.

SPECIAL CONSIDERATIONS
- If your patient has an ICP monitoring device in place, be sure to use aseptic technique when changing the dressing; maintain a closed system to minimize the risk of infection.
- If the patient doesn't undergo a craniotomy, monitor her neurologic status carefully until the hematoma has stabilized. Stay alert for signs and symptoms of increased ICP, which indicate hematoma expansion.
- ➡ **NurseALERT** Know that the most sensitive indicator of increased ICP is a change in level of consciousness. Suspect increased ICP if your patient becomes irritable, restless, confused, or agitated, or if you detect an ipsilateral change in pupil size and light reaction. Be aware that vital sign changes are *late* indicators of increased ICP.
- ➡ **NurseALERT** Be aware that intracranial surgery is the most common cause of diabetes insipidus. Monitor the patient closely for signs and symptoms of this complication.

EPIGLOTTITIS

Epiglottitis is a rapidly progressing inflammation of the epiglottis, the cartilaginous flap that covers the larynx, and surrounding tissues. Because the swollen epiglottis may cause sudden and complete airway obstruction, always consider this condition an emergency. Until the threat of airway obstruction passes, the patient requires continuous observation, usually in the intensive care unit. (See *Epiglottitis airway occlusion.*)

You're most likely to encounter acute epiglottitis in children ages 2 to 7. However, it occasionally occurs in adults. Acute epiglottitis usually results from *Haemophilus influenzae* type B infection. Less often, another type of bacteria or a virus is responsible. The condition typically follows an upper respiratory tract infection.

WHAT TO LOOK FOR
Clinical findings in acute epiglottitis vary, depending on whether the patient is a child or an adult.

In a child
Clinical findings may include:
- sore throat
- fever
- difficulty breathing
- inspiratory stridor
- difficulty swallowing (which causes excessive drooling)

EPIGLOTTITIS AIRWAY OCCLUSION

In epiglottitis, the epiglottis becomes inflamed and edematous. With increasing edema, the lateral borders curl, which causes the tip of the epiglottis to protrude backward and downward. As the patient takes a breath, the swollen epiglottis is pulled, or sucked, over the larynx.

With severe edema, the epiglottis may completely occlude the laryngeal opening, causing acute airway occlusion. The illustrations below show a cross-section of a normal upper airway and how it compares to an airway with a swollen epiglottis.

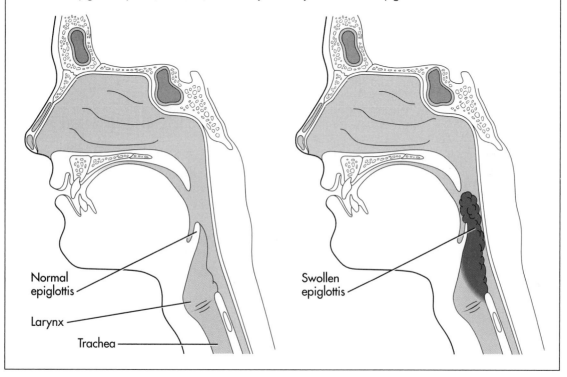

Normal epiglottis

Larynx

Trachea

Swollen epiglottis

- hoarseness
- tachypnea
- intercostal retractions
- cyanosis
- forward-leaning position with the neck hyperextended (an attempt to ease breathing)
- red, swollen epiglottis.

In an adult

Clinical findings are less dramatic but may include:
- difficulty swallowing
- severe burning or squeezing sensation during swallowing
- fever.

WHAT TO DO IMMEDIATELY

If you suspect that your patient has acute epiglottitis, notify the physician. Then follow these guidelines:

- Don't try to inspect the patient's throat visually. Visual inspection should be performed only by trained personnel, preferably in the operating room, with tracheotomy and intubation equipment on hand. An artificial airway may be inserted prophylactically.
- ➡ **NurseALERT** *Never* try to obtain a throat culture or gag the patient with a tongue blade. A swollen, inflamed epiglottis may obstruct the airway completely if it rises with the pressure of a tongue blade or culture swab.
- Bring emergency tracheotomy equipment to the bedside, and keep it on hand at all times in case of sudden, complete airway obstruction.
- Anticipate obtaining lateral neck X-rays or a sonogram to check for epiglottis enlargement.
- Assess the patient's oxygen saturation level using pulse oximetry.
- Administer oxygen, as prescribed, adding humidity to reduce epiglottal inflammation.
- Insert an I.V. line; as prescribed, administer I.V. antibiotics, such as chloramphenicol (Chloromycetin, effective against *H. influenzae*), until cultures identify the specific causative organism.
- Draw blood samples for laboratory tests, including complete blood count, white blood cell (WBC) count, and arterial blood gas (ABG) analysis, as ordered. However, you may need to delay venipuncture and other painful procedures that could make a child cry because crying could cause the swollen epiglottis to block the airway.
- Try to keep the child calm to prevent her from crying.

WHAT TO DO NEXT

Once acute epiglottitis has been confirmed, carry out these interventions:

- Prepare for possible tracheotomy or endotracheal intubation until epiglottal inflammation subsides (usually 24 to 48 hours) and the airway obstruction clears.
- Provide I.V. fluids, as prescribed, if the patient can't have oral intake because of difficulty swallowing.
- Assess the patient's vital signs and cardiopulmonary status frequently; report changes.
- Auscultate her breath sounds, and assess for an improved respiratory status, indicated by improved skin color, quiet breathing, relaxed body position, and absence of sternal retractions.
- Monitor WBC count, ABG values, and culture and sensitivity reports.
- Continue to give antibiotics, as prescribed. The physician may change to a different antibiotic or combination of antibiotics when culture and sensitivity reports become available.
- If the child has a tracheostomy or an endotracheal tube has been inserted, inform her parents that she won't make noise when she cries. Assure them that this is temporary.

- Avoid giving the patient a sedative because it could cause respiratory depression.

FOLLOW-UP CARE
- Regularly assess the patient for complications, such as otitis media, pneumonia, and bronchiolitis.
- Inform parents about the difference between croup and epiglottitis. They may wonder why epiglottitis requires hospitalization and a tracheotomy, whereas previous episodes of croup didn't. Explain that croup is an inflammation of the lower airways that doesn't involve the epiglottis.
- Teach parents how to give antibiotics at home. Stress the importance of completing the full course, even if the child appears well.
- Encourage the parents to participate in their child's care to promote a sense of control and provide emotional support. Urge them to help feed and bathe her and provide diversional activities, such as reading and playing games.

SPECIAL CONSIDERATIONS
- Assess the child's pain or discomfort level, watching for verbal expression, behavioral clues (such as facial expressions), and objective signs (including increased heart rate and blood pressure). Involve the parents in assessing their child's pain because they know her best.
- Be sure to keep pediatric-sized intubation and tracheotomy tubes readily available. A child's airway is shorter and smaller in diameter than an adult's, putting her at greater risk of airway obstruction from inflammation, edema, and mucous plugs.

ESOPHAGEAL VARICES, BLEEDING

Esophageal varices are enlarged, tortuous veins in the submucosa of the lower esophagus. If these varices bleed, particularly if the patient has underlying liver disease and coagulopathies, massive bleeding may develop and lead to hypovolemic shock and death, unless the patient receives immediate treatment.

Mortality from bleeding esophageal varices ranges from 50% to 80% for the first bleeding episode and rises with subsequent episodes. Be sure you know how to identify high-risk patients, how to recognize the signs and symptoms of this emergency, and how to respond appropriately.

How esophageal varices develop
Esophageal varices usually result from progressive liver disease (such as cirrhosis and cancer), which causes fibrotic changes and portal vein obstruction and elevates pressure in the portal system. Portal hypertension eventually causes collateral circulation to develop as a means of return-

LOOKING AT ESOPHAGEAL VARICES

When pressure in the portal vein increases, collateral channels develop in the lower esophagus as an alternative route for returning venous blood from the liver to the inferior vena cava.

As pressure continues to increase, more blood is diverted to these esophageal vessels, which begin to dilate from increased blood flow. This leads to the development of esophageal varices—enlarged, tortuous veins in the submucosa of the lower esophagus.

If these esophageal varices bleed, particularly if the patient has underlying liver disease and coagulopathies, massive bleeding may eventually develop and lead to hypovolemic shock and death—unless the patient receives immediate treatment.

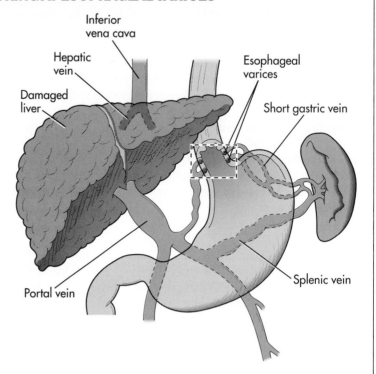

ing blood from the liver to the inferior vena cava. As pressure in the portal system rises, so does pressure within these collateral vessels. The distal esophageal veins, part of the collateral system, begin to bulge under pressure and may rupture. (See *Looking at esophageal varices*.)

Once varices develop, any increase in intra-abdominal pressure—such as from coughing, lifting, or straining—can cause these fragile vessels to bleed. Although the bleeding originates from veins, the high portal pressure causes forceful hemorrhage that resembles arterial bleeding.

WHAT TO LOOK FOR
Clinical evidence of bleeding esophageal varices may include:
• sudden, massive vomiting of bright red blood or profuse drainage of bright red blood from a nasogastric tube
• anxiety
• restlessness
• cool, clammy skin
• tachycardia

- hypotension
- hyperventilation
- decreased level of consciousness.

WHAT TO DO IMMEDIATELY

If you detect signs and symptoms of bleeding esophageal varices, establish and maintain an adequate airway, breathing, and circulation. Notify the physician, and then take these measures:

- If bleeding is profuse, call for emergency help, and if the patient's blood pressure can tolerate it, place him in semi-Fowler's position to prevent aspiration.
- Obtain the patient's vital signs, staying alert for changes that suggest developing hypovolemic shock. Keep in mind that systolic blood pressure below 100 mm Hg and a heart rate above 100 beats/minute indicate at least a 20% reduction in blood volume.
- Establish two I.V. lines with large-bore catheters, or verify that existing lines are patent. Then administer I.V. fluids, as prescribed, to maintain circulatory volume.
- Have the patient's blood typed and crossmatched. Then, as ordered, give transfusions of blood, fresh frozen plasma, platelets, and other blood products. If indicated, keep three units of packed red blood cells (RBCs) on hold at all times.
- Obtain blood samples, as ordered, to measure hematocrit; platelet count; prothrombin and activated partial thromboplastin times; liver function tests; serum electrolyte, hemoglobin, creatinine, and glucose levels; and blood urea nitrogen levels.
- Administer supplemental oxygen at 15 L/minute, as prescribed. Monitor oxygen saturation by means of pulse oximetry.
- Anticipate endotracheal intubation and mechanical ventilation if the patient is significantly obtunded or comatose or has evidence of respiratory failure.
- For patients with severe hemorrhage, prepare for arterial line insertion to allow continuous blood pressure monitoring and frequent blood sampling. Also expect the physician to insert a central venous line.
- To reduce bleeding, prepare to give an I.V. bolus infusion of vasopressin, 20 units in 100 ml of dextrose 5% in water, followed by a continuous infusion of 0.2 to 0.4 units/minute, as prescribed. Use an infusion pump to ensure the proper dose. As prescribed, increase the dose by 0.1 to 0.2 units/minute until bleeding stops or the dose reaches 1 unit/minute.
- As appropriate and ordered, gather equipment and supplies for nasogastric intubation or balloon tamponade intubation (suction device, irrigation supplies, or normal saline solution). Assist with either procedure, as indicated. (See *Options for managing bleeding esophageal varices*, page 138.)
- Administer isotonic fluids and blood products or plasma expanders, as ordered.

E

OPTIONS FOR MANAGING BLEEDING ESOPHAGEAL VARICES

A patient with bleeding esophageal varices may undergo one or more of the treatments described below to control acute, massive hemorrhage.

ENDOSCOPIC SCLEROTHERAPY OR LIGATION

The physician may attempt to repair a bleeding vessel endoscopically using sclerotherapy or ligation. In sclerotherapy, a sclerosing agent (such as sodium tetradecyl sulfate or ethanolamine oleate) is injected into the varices to harden and thicken them.

In endoscopic ligation, the physician places rubber bands on the bleeding vessel in a procedure resembling hemorrhoid ligation. Many patients undergo both sclerotherapy and ligation—a combination that has proved more effective than either treatment alone.

BALLOON TAMPONADE

Balloon tamponade controls bleeding by compressing the dilated vessels with two balloons, one esophageal and one gastric, as shown in the illustration. The Sengstaken-Blakemore tube is the most common choice for tamponade; it can be inserted either nasally or orally. This treatment is considered temporary, and its use is typically limited to 12 to 48 hours; otherwise, the patient risks potentially severe complications from the expanded balloons.

PHARMACOLOGIC THERAPY

To reduce blood loss, the physician may order drugs that decrease portal vein pressure. Such agents may include vasopressin or its analogue terlipressin, vasodilators used in combination with vasopressin, and somatostatin or its analogue octreotide.

Keep in mind that although vasopressin causes vasoconstriction, its effect isn't selective. To reduce the danger of widespread vasoconstriction, vasopressin therapy usually is limited to 24 or 48 hours. During therapy, watch for complications of ischemia in other vascular beds, including the heart. Also, the physician may order a concomitant vasodilator, such as nitroglycerin, to minimize constriction in other vessels.

The exact mechanism of somatostatin and octreotide in decreasing portal pressure is unknown. However, a 5-day course of these drugs has proved helpful in controlling hemorrhage.

SURGERY AND OTHER INVASIVE MEASURES

For a stable patient, the physician may consider more permanent measures, such as further sclerotherapy.

Liver transplantation may be an option, although donor organs are difficult to obtain.

More commonly, the patient undergoes surgery to shunt portal blood away from the liver. In transjugular intrahepatic portacaval shunt (TIPS), a relatively new procedure, the surgeon threads a catheter retrograde from the jugular vein to the portal vein. A stainless steel stent is then threaded through the liver parenchyma and connected to the portal vein. This procedure provides a means for blood to flow unobstructed from the portal vein to the hepatic vein and into the inferior vena cava. Performed radiologically rather than surgically, TIPS poses less risk to the patient.

Balloon Tamponade

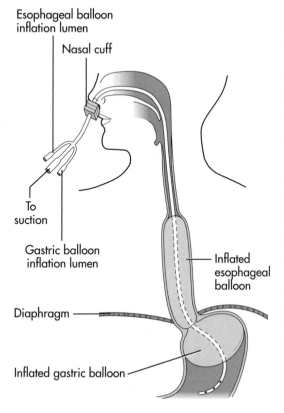

- Insert an indwelling urinary catheter, as ordered, to monitor hourly urine output.
- Stay with the patient at all times and provide reassurance and comfort measures, or make sure another staff member does.

WHAT TO DO NEXT
Once immediate measures have been taken, carry out these interventions:
- Monitor the patient's vital signs every 15 minutes, watching for tachycardia, hypotension, and other signs of worsening hypovolemia. If you suspect hypovolemic shock, alert the physician immediately and prepare to assist with pulmonary artery catheter insertion to monitor hemodynamic status.
- Assess the patient's level of consciousness for indications of cerebral ischemia.
- Assess urine output at least hourly. Watch for a decrease to less than 30 ml/hour. If urine output drops, notify the physician immediately.
- If a nasogastric tube has been inserted, begin lavage, as ordered. Expect to instill and aspirate 30 to 50 ml of tepid normal saline solution or tap water continuously. Note the color and consistency of the aspirant. Be sure to take lavage into account when monitoring fluid intake and output.
- If the patient is receiving vasopressin, observe for signs and symptoms of adverse effects related to vasoconstriction, such as angina, arrhythmias, abdominal colic, and limb pain.
- Maintain patent I.V. lines, and monitor the infusion of isotonic solutions, albumin, or blood products. Assess RBC count, hemoglobin values, and hematocrit to help detect hypovolemia and shock. Monitor arterial blood gas (ABG) values to evaluate the patient's oxygenation status.

If balloon tamponade is used
- Test the gastric and esophageal balloons for leakage before they are inserted by the physician. During insertion, keep the patient in a semi-Fowler's position and suction oral or nasal secretions, as needed.
- ➡ **NurseALERT** Complaints of sudden, sharp chest pain during balloon insertion or inflation suggest esophageal perforation.
- Maintain pressure on the oral or nasal tube by taping it securely to the patient's forehead or the chin guard of a football helmet or by applying orthopedic traction of up to 1 lb.
- Protect the patient's mouth or nares after tube insertion, such as by using foam "bumpers." Watch for excoriation, abrasions, and irritation around the nares or corners of the mouth. After cleaning these areas using normal saline solution, keep them dry.
- Monitor esophageal balloon pressure every hour. Report a reading over 40 mm Hg. The prescribed pressure is usually between 20 and

E

40 mm Hg. Irrigate the gastric tube, as ordered, and assess the gastric aspirate for consistency, color, and amount.

- Suction esophageal secretions as necessary, keeping in mind that your patient is at high risk for accidental aspiration because he can't swallow saliva while the balloon is inflated. If the balloon tube does not have a separate lumen for esophageal aspiration, you may use a separate nasoesophageal tube to suction the esophagus. Place a large, inflexible suction catheter at the bedside for suctioning thick secretions from the patient's oropharyngeal cavity.
- Realize that your patient may asphyxiate if the gastric balloon slides up into his esophagus. Keep a large scissors at the bedside; if the patient shows signs of asphyxiation (choking, respiratory distress), cut the entire tube (not just one "tail") with the scissors and then remove the tube as quickly as possible. Cutting the tube will cause both balloons to deflate. Be sure to cut the tube several inches from the patient's nose (or mouth if it's inserted orally), so that enough of the tube remains exposed for you to grasp it for removal.
- To prevent esophageal mucosal erosion— a possible complication of balloon tamponade—and to promote blood flow to the healthy mucosa, release the esophageal balloon frequently, such as by deflating it for 5 minutes every 4 to 8 hours.
- ➡ **NurseALERT** Never deflate only the gastric balloon or deflate the gastric balloon first; the resulting tension will pull the tube upward, causing severe esophageal damage and airway obstruction. To remove the tube, the physician first deflates the esophageal balloon, waits 8 to 24 hours, and then deflates the gastric balloon.

FOLLOW-UP CARE

- Be aware that depending on the amount of blood your patient has lost, he may remain hypovolemic even after esophageal bleeding is under control. Continue to monitor his vital signs and pertinent laboratory values, such as hemoglobin level and hematocrit.
- Assess the patient for signs and symptoms of continuing anemia, such as fatigue, pallor, dyspnea, tachycardia, and cool, clammy skin.
- Continue to assess his respiratory status and to monitor his oxygen saturation using pulse oximetry or ABG values. Recognize that hypoxemia (which causes dyspnea, abnormal breath sounds, and use of accessory muscles) may persist after an episode of massive bleeding.
- Maintain supplemental oxygen therapy, as necessary and prescribed; adjust the flow rate based on oxygen saturation and ABG values.

SPECIAL CONSIDERATIONS

- Provide emotional support to the patient and family, who are likely to be frightened by the massive bleeding.
- To prevent a recurrence of esophageal varices bleeding, instruct the patient to avoid activities that increase intra-abdominal pressure,

such as straining at stool, lifting heavy objects, and coughing vigorously. He should also avoid alcohol, caffeine, and food that can directly irritate the esophagus.
- Anticipate the use of beta blockers to decrease portal pressure and lactulose to decrease serum ammonia levels. Keep in mind that blood that enters the GI tract is a protein substance that breaks down into nitrogen, which the body converts into ammonia. Because the liver may not be able to convert the ammonia into urea for excretion by the kidneys, the patient may develop encephalopathy.

EXTRAVASATION OF A VESICANT

When a vesicant drug extravasates out of an I.V. line and into surrounding tissues, it can cause widespread damage, necrosis, and tissue sloughing. These problems may be severe enough to require tissue grafting or plastic surgery.

If you detect and correct extravasation quickly, you may be able to minimize the damage and preserve the patient's tissues. Corrective steps may involve trying to aspirate the drug, injecting an antidote (if one exists), and applying heat or ice.

Keep in mind that appropriate responses vary with geographical region, facility, and practitioner, so you'll need to check your facility's policy and follow it closely. In general, your response to an extravasated vesicant will be similar to the measures described below.

WHAT TO LOOK FOR
Clinical findings in extravasation may include:
- pain at the I.V. infusion site
- red, swollen area adjacent to the I.V. insertion site
- progressive blistering of the affected area
- localized tissue necrosis and sloughing.

WHAT TO DO IMMEDIATELY
If you detect extravasation, notify the physician. Then follow these steps:
- Stop the infusion.
- Assess the area around the venous access device for redness, swelling, firmness, and pain.

WHAT TO DO NEXT
Once you've stopped the infusion, take the following measures:
- Leave the I.V. access device in place.
- Try to aspirate a return from the I.V. access device and surrounding tissues.
- Obtain and administer the appropriate antidote, if one exists. If possible, give it through the I.V. access device. (See *Responding to extravasation*, page 142.)

TREATMENT OF CHOICE

RESPONDING TO EXTRAVASATION

The table below lists common vesicants and the treatments recommended to minimize damage if extravasation occurs.

DRUG	USUAL TREATMENT
amsacrine (Amsa P-D)	• Apply topical dimethyl sulfoxide (DMSO) as prescribed.
cisplatin (Platinol)	• Give 1/6 or 1/3 sodium thiosulfate into I.V. catheter or by subcutaneous injection into extravasated area. Use 2 ml for each 100 mg of vesicant extravasated.
dactinomycin (Cosmegen)	• Elevate the extremity or apply cold compresses. • Give hyaluronidase (Wydase) or a long-acting dexamethasone by subcutaneous injection into the extravasated tissue.
daunorubicin (Cerubidine), doxorubicin (Adriamycin)	• Apply ice packs or cold compresses every 15 minutes for 24 hours. • Give sodium succinate or hyaluronidase (Wydase) by subcutaneous injection into the extravasated tissue.
etoposide (VePesid)	• Give hyaluronidase 150 units/ml with 1 to 3 ml of normal saline solution into I.V. line. If patient doesn't have I.V. line, inject it or a long-acting dexamethasone subcutaneously into extravasated area. • Apply warm compresses.
idarubicin (Idamycin)	• Apply ice for 30 minutes immediately and then for 30 minutes four times daily for 4 days. • No antidote available.
mitomycin (Mutamycin)	• Apply topical DMSO every 6 hours for 14 days.
mechlorethamine hydrochloride (Mustargen)	• Give sodium thiosulfate into I.V. catheter or by subcutaneous injection into extravasated area. Use 2 ml for each milligram of vesicant extravasated.
norepinephrine bitartrate (Levophed)	• Give 5 to 10 mg of phentolamine (Regitine) and 10 to 15 ml of normal saline solution.
vinblastine (Velban), vincristine (Oncovin)	• Administer hyaluronidase 150 units/ml with 2 to 3 ml of normal saline solution into I.V. catheter or by subcutaneous injection into extravasated area. • Apply warm compresses.

• Remove the I.V. access device appropriately.
• If recommended for the vesicant involved, apply ice or heat.
• Document the medication that extravasated, the approximate amount, size of the tissue area involved (in centimeters), current condition of the area, and all actions you took to correct the problem.

FOLLOW-UP CARE
• Monitor the affected area closely every day, and document your findings.
• Watch for progressive tissue damage, which may continue for up to 4 weeks. Provide appropriate teaching to the patient and family.
• Administer additional treatment measures or dressings as required.

SPECIAL CONSIDERATIONS

- To prevent extravasation, don't use an existing I.V. line to administer a vesicant unless you can confirm the line's patency.
- When giving several medications, give the vesicant last.
- After administering a vesicant, give several milliliters of normal saline solution or dextrose 5% in water to flush the vesicant from the vein.
- Always respond immediately if a patient who is receiving a vesicant complains of pain at the I.V. site. Verify the line's patency often throughout the infusion through visual inspection and blood return.
- Know that many authorities recommend giving vesicants by the "side-arm" method to detect extravasation before much vesicant enters the tissues (any extravasation that does occur involves mostly fluid). To use this method, infuse an additive-free I.V. solution at a rapid rate through the I.V. access device. Then add the vesicant (it must be compatible with the solution) through the side injection port of the I.V. tubing and into the free-flowing fluid. Obtain a blood return after giving every 1 to 2 ml of vesicant, and monitor the site carefully for swelling.

F

FALLS

When it comes to patient falls, prevention is clearly the best strategy. That's because a patient who falls—from a chair or bed or during ambulation, for example—risks head, chest, and abdominal trauma in addition to musculoskeletal injuries. Depending on the patient's condition and the severity of the fall, some of his injuries may be life-threatening.

The patients at highest risk for falls include elderly patients and disoriented patients. Age-related musculoskeletal changes raise the risk of falls by impairing posture and gait. Also, elderly patients are more likely to experience nocturia and may fall when trying to reach the bathroom in the dark. Among disoriented patients, falls commonly result from attempts to get out of bed without help, sometimes by crawling over a side rail. In both cases, a darkened room and unfamiliar environment increase their risk of falling.

Although age and disorientation can be isolated easily as risk factors for falls, the truth is that many factors can raise your patient's risk of falling. A patient weakened by illness and immobility may fall even while you're at his side. (See *Is your patient at high risk for falls?*, page 144.)

Despite precautions, acute-care facilities report that more than 75% of incident reports involve patient falls. So you'll need to be ready to respond when the possible occurs. To help limit the extent of your patient's injuries and begin the appropriate treatment as soon as possible, you'll need to perform a rapid yet thorough assessment any time a patient falls, no matter how insignificant the accident seems.

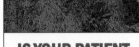

IS YOUR PATIENT AT HIGH RISK FOR FALLS?

Besides advanced age and disorientation, conditions that predispose a patient to falls include:

- neurologic disorders, such as cerebrovascular accident and transient ischemic attack
- paresthesias and peripheral neuropathy, as in longstanding diabetes mellitus
- cardiovascular problems, including arrhythmias, postural hypotension, and angina
- breathing problems, such as shortness of breath
- musculoskeletal problems, such as weakness, paralysis, tremors, and joint disease
- endocrine and metabolic problems, including hypoglycemia and electrolyte imbalances
- mental health disorders, such as acute psychosis
- certain medications, such as sedatives, analgesics, barbiturates, and antihypertensives.

WHAT TO LOOK FOR

Evaluate your patient's history and assessment findings for the following factors, which increase his risk for falls:

- confusion or agitation
- advanced age
- vision or hearing problems
- generalized weakness
- hypotension
- hypoxia (which can cause confusion)
- anemia
- impaired mobility
- impaired communication
- urinary incontinence or diuretic use
- cardiovascular, neurologic, or musculoskeletal disorders
- medical devices, such as indwelling urinary catheters, I.V. lines, and I.V. poles
- use of drugs that can cause confusion
- drug or alcohol withdrawal
- improper use of assistive devices, such as canes and walkers
- use of restraints.

➡ **NurseALERT** In the past, many health-care professionals believed that restraints could help prevent patients from falling. On the contrary, most experts now believe that restraints increase the risk of falls and may result in more serious injuries if a patient does fall.

WHAT TO DO IMMEDIATELY

If you see your patient fall or find him on the floor, take the following steps:

- Assess his airway, breathing, and circulation (ABCs); his fall may have resulted from cardiac arrest. If he isn't breathing and lacks a pulse, call for help and begin cardiopulmonary resuscitation (CPR) at once.
- If the patient's ABCs are normal, assess his level of consciousness and response to verbal stimulation.
- Perform a rapid head-to-toe assessment to check for injuries, such as lacerations, bruises, bleeding, and deformities. Using standard precautions, apply direct pressure to any active bleeding sites.
- If the patient is alert, ask him if he hurts and, if so, where the pain is located. If the painful area appears deformed, immobilize it, if possible (for example, with a splint).
- Stay with the patient and keep him warm and comfortable until help arrives.

Falls during ambulation

If your patient begins to fall while you're assisting him with ambulation, follow these steps:

- Try to break or cushion his fall, but *don't* try to hold him up. Gently slide him down to the floor as you support his body, especially his head and trunk. Call for assistance at once.
- Take the actions described above, starting with assessing his ABCs and performing CPR, if necessary.

WHAT TO DO NEXT

Once your patient is stabilized, carry out the following interventions:
- Help the patient back into the bed or chair, unless you suspect a fracture or head injury.
- Obtain his vital signs, especially heart rate and blood pressure.
- If you suspect a fracture, prepare the patient for an X-ray. For a head injury, prepare him for a computed tomography scan, as ordered, and perform a neurologic check (level of consciousness, pupil size and reaction, and extremity movement and strength).
- Continue to apply pressure to any active bleeding sites. Apply a pressure dressing, if indicated.
- To help identify what caused your patient to fall, try to determine the events that took place just before and during the fall. For instance, ask the patient if he felt dizzy or light-headed.
- ➡ **NurseALERT** If your patient is elderly, falling may be an early sign of acute illness, such as dehydration, or an exacerbation of chronic illness.
- If indicated, obtain a 12-lead ECG to evaluate the patient's cardiac status.
- Obtain samples for ordered laboratory tests, which may include serum electrolyte levels to detect electrolyte imbalances and hematocrit to assess for anemia.

FOLLOW-UP CARE

- Continue to monitor the patient's neurologic and cardiac status closely.
- Monitor his blood pressure for orthostatic changes.
- Clean and dress any wounds or other skin injuries.
- Based on diagnostic test results, prepare the patient for treatment, as indicated, such as cast application for a fracture or follow-up neurologic testing.
- Fill out an incident report. Be sure to include the name of the patient and any witnesses, all objective data about the fall (especially the patient's level of consciousness and mental status at the time of the fall), consequences to the patient, and interventions performed. Don't record any opinions, conclusions, assumptions, or suggestions about who or what might have been responsible.
- If the patient is disoriented, reorient him to his surroundings frequently. Try to determine the cause of any behavioral changes. Investigate his current medication history, noting any multiple medica-

tions prescribed by different physicians. Remember that a drug or drug combination may increase the risk of falls.

- Investigate for signs and symptoms of hypoxemia and fever.
- Assess the patient's risk for another fall, and institute fall precautions according to your facility's policy.
- Arrange for the patient to stay in a room within visual range of the nurses' station, if possible, to permit closer observation.
- If necessary, arrange for constant patient surveillance. For instance, contact his family and ask that someone sit with him.
- Make sure that side rails are up at all times unless the patient can ambulate without assistance. In this case, assess the need to keep the rails down or to use half rails. Keep the bed in the lowest position.
- Make sure the patient's call button is within easy reach. Encourage him to use it if he needs to get out of bed or a chair. Provide a night light to improve vision and orientation at night.
- Remove all obstacles from the patient's path, eliminate clutter from his room, and keep personal articles and care items within easy reach.
- Provide analgesics or nonpharmacologic pain relief, as indicated.
- Urge the patient to use ambulatory assistive devices, such as a walker or a cane, if needed. Teach him how to use these devices safely.
- If the patient has orthostatic hypotension, advise him to change position slowly and to sit at the edge of the bed for a few minutes before standing. Encourage him to ask for assistance with ambulation.
- If the patient is incontinent, help him to the bathroom or provide the bedpan every 1 to 2 hours.

SPECIAL CONSIDERATIONS
- Teach the patient about prescribed medications and their adverse reactions, especially orthostatic hypotension, dizziness, and drowsiness.
- Before discharge, instruct home caregivers about ways to make the home safe, such as by removing throw rugs and foot stools, avoiding wet floors, and improving lighting.

G.I. HEMORRHAGE

At least 300,000 Americans are hospitalized yearly for GI bleeding. Most such bleeding emanates from the upper GI tract, above the ligament of Treitz, where the duodenum joins the jejunum. In three patients out of four, it results from peptic ulcer disease. Other causes include bleeding esophageal varices, esophagitis, and Mallory-Weiss tears of the esophagogastric junction. Rarely, the cause may be cancer or an aortoduodenal fistula caused by repair of an aortic aneurysm.

GI hemorrhage can involve the lower tract as well. Typically, lower GI bleeding stems from the large intestine and is associated with such disorders as diverticulitis, polyps, ulcerative colitis, and cancer. It's usually slower and less massive than upper GI bleeding. Often, it stops on its own. For these reasons, upper GI bleeding poses a greater risk of hypovolemic shock than lower GI bleeding.

The degree of blood loss in GI hemorrhage and the hemodynamic effects that ensue depend largely on the underlying disorder. For example, inflammatory erosion of the esophageal or gastric mucosa produces slow, minor capillary bleeding. A bleeding peptic ulcer (especially a stress ulcer) can produce more significant blood loss. A Mallory-Weiss tear or esophageal varices can cause massive blood loss.

In an acute GI hemorrhage, the patient loses 25% or more of circulating volume (about 1,500 ml in adults). Overall, about 1 in 10 patients dies as a result of upper GI hemorrhage; among patients over age 55 who need emergency surgery, mortality is around 30%. If your patient has a GI hemorrhage, your rapid response could save his life.

WHAT TO LOOK FOR
Clinical findings in GI hemorrhage may include:
- hematemesis (vomiting of blood), which may look like frank red blood or like dark red, brown, mahogany, coffee-ground, or black vomitus
- hypotension (with acute, massive bleeding of more than 500 ml)
- confusion or decreased level of consciousness
- tachycardia
- diaphoresis
- nausea
- syncope
- pallor
- cold, clammy skin
- decreased urine output
- hyperactive bowel sounds
- melena (black, tarry, foul-smelling stools), which may accompany either upper or lower GI bleeding
- hematochezia (grossly bloody stools), usually seen with lower GI bleeding but sometimes occurs with rapid, massive upper GI bleeding
- rectorrhagia (passage of red blood from the rectum in the absence of feces), which typically signals anorectal disease.

Laboratory tests
Laboratory findings in GI hemorrhage may include:
- reduced red blood cell count
- decreased hemoglobin level and hematocrit (starting 6 to 8 hours after symptom onset)
- increased platelet and reticulocyte counts
- red blood cell indices indicating normocytic, normochromic cells
- elevated blood urea nitrogen level
- decreased serum iron levels and total iron binding capacity (with chronic GI bleeding)
- arterial blood gas values that indicate acidosis and hypoxemia
- positive fecal occult blood test.

WHAT TO DO IMMEDIATELY

If your patient has clinical evidence of GI hemorrhage, notify the physician. Then take these steps:

- Position a vomiting patient so he won't aspirate vomitus; also, elevate the head of the bed.
- Assess the patient's pulse rate and blood pressure.
- Evaluate the amount and color of any vomitus or stool.
- ➡ **NurseALERT** Keep in mind that blood darkens when exposed to gastric secretions; the longer blood stays in the stomach, the darker it is when passed. Vomitus that resembles coffee grounds reflects blood that has clotted in the stomach and been partially digested.
- If your patient has a nasogastric (NG) tube in place, begin gastric lavage, as ordered, by flushing the tube with cool saline solution or tap water. Instill the ordered solution into the NG tube 50 to 100 ml at a time, let it dwell for a short time, and then aspirate.
- If the patient doesn't have an NG tube in place, obtain the supplies needed for insertion. Make sure you collect the proper tube; the patient may need a special large-bore tube, which may be standard equipment on your facility's emergency carts. As appropriate, insert the tube or assist the physician with the procedure.
- Establish I.V. access and administer fluids, as prescribed.
- If prescribed, administer blood or packed red blood cells, using a large-bore I.V. catheter.
- Gather supplies for insertion of a central venous catheter to monitor hemodynamic status.
- Assess the patient's oxygen saturation; as prescribed, give supplemental oxygen.
- Insert or maintain an indwelling urinary catheter, as ordered, and monitor the patient's hourly urine output.
- Evaluate for evidence of tissue hypoxia, such as reduced urine output, arrhythmias, chest pain, confusion, and decreased level of consciousness.

WHAT TO DO NEXT

After taking these initial steps, carry out the following interventions:

- Prepare the patient for diagnostic endoscopy, if indicated, to determine the source of the bleeding. (See *Understanding endoscopy*.)
- Monitor his vital signs every 15 to 30 minutes.
- Continue with gastric lavage, as ordered, making sure to record intake and output and the quality and quantity of GI bleeding. Typically, gastric lavage is continued until the drainage is light pink or clear or is without clots.
- During fluid administration and if your patient is elderly or has cardiovascular disease, watch closely for signs and symptoms of fluid overload (decreased output, respiratory crackles, and dyspnea). If appropriate, record his central venous pressure every 1 to 2 hours.

UNDERSTANDING ENDOSCOPY

Endoscopy allows direct visualization of the inside of a body cavity after insertion of a lighted tube. For the upper and lower GI tract, endoscopy typically involves a flexible fiber-optic scope, which is more comfortable than the stiffer instruments previously used and reduces the risk of esophageal perforation. In 90% to 95% of cases, endoscopy reveals the source of GI bleeding.

PERFORMING THE TEST

Upper GI endoscopy may be done on an emergency basis to identify and treat the source of massive upper GI bleeding. Ideally, it's performed after an 8-hour fast to ensure optimal visualization and reduce the risk of aspiration. When done on an emergency basis, the patient's stomach contents are aspirated beforehand through a nasogastric tube.

Depending on the patient's status, he may receive an I.V. sedative, such as midazolam (Versed), to decrease anxiety before and during the procedure. To numb his throat, the physician swabs or sprays it with a local anesthetic or administers an anesthetic gargle.

After the gag reflex is suppressed, the patient assumes a lateral recumbent position. Then the physician passes the endoscope through the patient's mouth to the hypopharynx. The patient is instructed to swallow, and the scope is advanced further, as shown in the illustration. To enhance visualization, the physician insufflates air through the scope, distending the area to be examined.

During endoscopy, the physician may detect and photograph lesions (even small surface lesions that don't show up on X-rays), obtain biopsy specimens and brushings for cytologic examination, remove polyps and foreign objects, or treat bleeding vessels by electrocoagulation, laser, or heat probe.

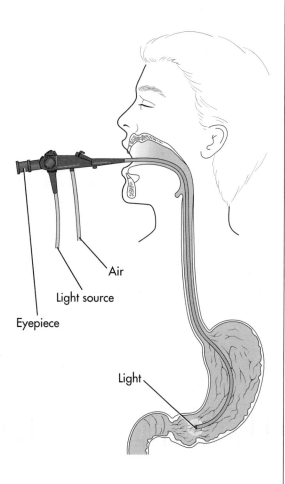

Air

Light source

Eyepiece

Light

G

Institute continuous cardiac monitoring, if indicated, to evaluate cardiac function.

- If your patient has lower GI bleeding, be prepared to administer saline enemas to remove blood from the intestines and prevent dangerous ammonia buildup.

FOLLOW-UP CARE

- Continue to monitor your patient's vital signs, cardiopulmonary status, and renal function closely. Inspect all drainage, vomitus, and stool for frank blood and test for occult blood.

- Continue administering ordered treatments to correct the underlying cause of GI bleeding.
- Anticipate surgery if your patient is still hemorrhaging after 24 hours or after receiving 6 to 8 units of blood or if she can't maintain adequate blood pressure despite transfusions. Be aware that such a patient is a poor surgical risk.

SPECIAL CONSIDERATIONS
- Teach the patient about prescribed antiulcer medications. If the physician prescribes iron supplements, teach the patient that taking them on an empty stomach increases absorption. Also tell her that she can take them with food if they upset her stomach. Mention that iron supplements may turn her stools dark green or black. Reassure her that this effect is harmless but may mask recurring lower GI bleeding.
- Teach the patient how to test her stool for occult blood. Tell her that she may detect blood for up to 3 weeks after a bleeding episode.

HEADACHE, SEVERE

Usually considered more annoying than dangerous, headaches can nevertheless raise concerns. That's because in rare cases, they result from a serious problem, such as a brain abscess or tumor, cerebrovascular hemorrhage, hypertension, meningitis, ruptured cerebral aneurysm, subdural hematoma, or trigeminal neuralgia.

Clearly, these more serious headaches require a rapid response. This means that you must be familiar with their signs and symptoms so you can help distinguish them from a headache caused by muscle tension, stress, depression, a sleep disturbance, vascular changes, or sinusitis. Your prompt, effective interventions may prevent a serious underlying problem from progressing. (See *Identifying common headaches*, page 152.)

WHAT TO LOOK FOR

When your patient complains of a headache, take a thorough history to help determine its cause. Be sure to review her medication history for medications that may cause headaches, such as nitrates. Pay close attention to how she describes the headache, including whether it's:
- sudden or gradual in onset
- unilateral or bilateral
- sharp, dull, excruciating, or throbbing
- constant or intermittent.

Also look for accompanying clinical findings that suggest a dangerous underlying cause for headache, such as:
- change in level of consciousness
- fever
- defects, crepitus, or tender spots on the head (detected through palpation)
- motor or sensory dysfunctions
- signs of increasing intracranial pressure, such as restlessness or irritability, decreased level of consciousness, elevated systolic blood pressure, and widened pulse pressure
- cranial nerve dysfunction, such as pupil abnormalities, extraocular palsies, and blurred vision
- abnormal reflexes
- signs of meningeal irritation, such as positive Kernig's or Brudzinski's signs, stiff neck, and photophobia

IDENTIFYING COMMON HEADACHES

Most headaches result from common, transient problems. Use the descriptions below to help identify them.

TENSION HEADACHE
A tension headache usually causes mild to moderate bilateral pain that may feel like a tight hat band. It isn't associated with nausea and doesn't worsen with activity.

MIGRAINE HEADACHE
A throbbing vascular headache, a migraine usually starts unilaterally and may be accompanied by other symptoms, such as nausea, sensitivity to light, and tingling of the face, lips, and hands. Typically, a migraine headache intensifies over several hours; it may last up to 72 hours.

CLUSTER HEADACHE
Cluster headaches tend to occur in groups and may strike up to eight times a day for several weeks. They cause severe, burning pain behind or around one eye, along with such autonomic symptoms as tearing, nasal congestion, runny nose, forehead and facial sweating, ptosis, and eyelid edema.

SINUSITIS HEADACHE
Typically, a sinusitis headache arises a week or so after the patient recovers from a cold. Commonly unilateral, it causes intense pressure and pain over the maxillary sinus. Antibiotics reduce both the pressure and the pain.

- elevated blood pressure
- nausea or vomiting
- seizures.

WHAT TO DO IMMEDIATELY

If you think your patient's headache may reflect a serious condition, notify the physician. Then take these steps:

- Take her vital signs. Pay close attention to subtle changes in level of consciousness and personality.
- ➡ **NurseALERT** Watch for irritability and restlessness, which are often the earliest signs of decreasing level of consciousness.
- Keep the patient on bed rest in a dark and quiet room. Elevate the head of the bed slightly.
- Administer analgesics, as prescribed, and observe for effectiveness. Codeine is the drug of choice for patients with moderate to severe pain of neurologic origin because it doesn't depress level of consciousness as much as other narcotic analgesics.
- Administer antiemetics to ease nausea or vomiting, as prescribed and indicated.
- Prepare the patient for diagnostic studies, such as computed tomographic scan of the brain, magnetic resonance imaging, and lumbar puncture.

WHAT TO DO NEXT

If the patient's headache results from a potentially serious problem, follow these guidelines:

- Continue to monitor vital signs and level of consciousness closely. Be alert for sudden changes or subtler trends.

- Administer analgesics, as prescribed, and monitor effectiveness.
- Notify the physician immediately if there's any change in the intensity, nature, or site of headache.
- ➡ **NurseALERT** Remember that a sudden increase in headache could indicate a new or an exacerbating intracranial hemorrhage.
- Prepare to treat the underlying cause, such as administering antibiotics for meningitis.
- If indicated, prepare the patient and family for surgery.

FOLLOW-UP CARE
- Once the source of the headache has been determined, teach the patient about the cause and the signs and symptoms that should be immediately reported to the physician.
- If the underlying cause of the headache can't be corrected or cured, teach the patient comfort measures to minimize the pain, including the use of prescribed analgesics.

SPECIAL CONSIDERATIONS
- ➡ **NurseALERT** Be aware that the classic first sign of a ruptured cerebral aneurysm is the sudden onset of an excruciating headache. Patients typically describe it as the worst headache they've ever had. Because a ruptured cerebral aneurysm is immediately life-threatening, always take such headache complaints seriously and notify the physician immediately.

HEART FAILURE

In heart failure, the heart can't pump enough blood to meet the body's metabolic and oxygen needs. Although the underlying problem may originate in the left or right side of the heart, heart failure eventually involves both sides. (See *Recognizing left- and right-sided heart failure,* page 154.)

Acute and chronic complications of heart failure include arrhythmias and sudden cardiac death, pulmonary edema, renal failure, activity intolerance, GI and metabolic problems, and thromboembolism. Your rapid response and expert nursing care for acute complications can improve your patient's outcome.

Pathophysiologic profile
Normally, when stroke volume decreases, the heart compensates by increasing its rate. In heart failure, the heart can't contract effectively enough to maintain adequate stroke volume. Consequently, stroke volume and cardiac output continue to diminish as the heart weakens from the increased workload or decreased oxygenation.

Decreasing cardiac output activates the renin-angiotensin-aldosterone and autonomic nervous systems, causing vasoconstriction and fluid retention by the kidneys, which attempt to return cardiac output to nor-

RECOGNIZING LEFT- AND RIGHT-SIDED HEART FAILURE

Early effects of heart failure depend on whether the left or the right ventricle is failing.

LEFT-SIDED FAILURE

When the left ventricle fails to empty completely, it impedes blood flow to the body tissues, causing blood to back up in the left atrium and pulmonary circulation. Fluid accumulates in the interstitial spaces of the lungs, leading to pulmonary edema with impaired gas exchange.

RIGHT-SIDED FAILURE

In right-sided heart failure, blood backs up into the systemic venous circulation, increasing right atrial, right ventricular end-diastolic, and systemic venous pressures. Peripheral tissues grow edematous, abdominal organs become congested, and the patient gains weight from fluid retention.

TREATMENT MAINSTAYS

With either type of heart failure, treatment typically involves use of angiotensin-converting enzyme inhibitors, vasodilators, diuretics, and digoxin, along with such measures as a low-sodium diet, exercise, and risk-factor reduction.

---

mal by increasing the blood volume returned to the heart. Unable to handle the increased blood return and peripheral vascular resistance, the ventricles dilate and hypertrophy. Eventually, cardiac output falls as myocardial fibers are stretched beyond their limits.

Causes of heart failure

Conditions that can lead to heart failure include:

- those that affect myocardial contractility, such as myocardial infarction
- those that alter myocardial relaxation, such as cardiomyopathy
- those that increase preload or afterload, including hypertension and valvular insufficiency
- those that markedly increase the heart's workload, such as anemia and thyrotoxicosis.

WHAT TO LOOK FOR

Early in heart failure, compensatory mechanisms work to maintain tissue perfusion and cardiac output. At this point, the patient may experience symptoms only when he increases his activity.

As compensatory mechanisms fail, the patient experiences symptoms with less and less activity or even at rest. Changes in vital signs may include:

- narrow pulse pressure
- weak pulse (decreased pulse amplitude)
- tachycardia
- hypotension.

Findings in left-sided failure

A patient with left-sided heart failure may have:

- dyspnea and orthopnea

- activity intolerence, dyspnea on exertion, fatigue
- tachypnea
- crackles
- wheezes, especially expiratory
- dullness over the lung bases (if they're fluid-filled)
- dry cough or cough that produces frothy, pink sputum
- paroxysmal nocturnal dyspnea
- anxiety
- confusion
- diaphoresis
- cool, clammy skin
- cyanosis of the nail beds and lips
- enlarged or displaced apical impulse
- pulsus alternans
- gallop heart sounds (S_3 and S_4).

Findings in right-sided failure
A patient with right-sided heart failure may have:
- neck vein pulsations
- jugular vein distention
- dependent edema
- ascites
- nausea
- abdominal pain and distention
- shifting abdominal dullness
- hepatomegaly
- splenomegaly
- positive hepatojugular reflux (increased neck vein distention after 30 seconds of pressing over the liver)
- elevated central venous pressure.

WHAT TO DO IMMEDIATELY
If you suspect your patient has heart failure, notify the physician. Then take these steps:
- Obtain baseline arterial blood gas (ABG) measurements, as indicated.
- Give supplemental oxygen, as prescribed. Assess the patient's oxygen saturation by way of pulse oximetry or ABG values.
- Begin continuous cardiac monitoring to detect arrhythmias and myocardial ischemic changes.
- Establish a peripheral I.V. line. If fluids are prescribed, use an infusion-control device to prevent fluid overload.
- Administer angiotensin-converting enzyme (ACE) inhibitors, if prescribed, to relax blood vessels and ease the heart's work of pumping. (See *Administering ACE inhibitors*, page 156.)

H

ADMINISTERING A.C.E. INHIBITORS

By relaxing blood vessels and making it easier for the heart to pump blood, angiotensin-converting enzyme (ACE) inhibitors can improve the functional ability of a patient with left systolic ventricular dysfunction.

If the physician prescribes an ACE inhibitor for your patient, expect to begin therapy at a lower dose and titrate upward toward the maximal dose while closely monitoring your patient's blood pressure. For recommended dosages of specific agents, see the chart below.

Know that ACE inhibitors are contraindicated in patients with hyperkalemia, symptomatic hypotension, or a history of intolerance or adverse reactions to these drugs. Also be aware of their adverse effects—hypotension, hyperkalemia, coughing, and renal insufficiency. To help prevent or minimize these adverse effects, read what follows.

MANAGING HYPOTENSION
Before starting your patient on an ACE inhibitor, anticipate correcting any volume depletion to help minimize hypotension. When drug therapy begins, start with a low dose and monitor the patient closely for weakness and dizziness. Advise him to rise slowly and to call the physician immediately if he feels light-headed.

PREVENTING HYPERKALEMIA
Because ACE inhibitors inhibit potassium excretion, they may cause hyperkalemia. During therapy, monitor your patient's serum potassium level carefully, and watch for signs of hyperkalemia, such as diar-

rhea, nausea, and muscle weakness or cramping. Avoid giving potassium-sparing diuretics or potassium supplements unless the patient has hypokalemia.

COPING WITH COUGH
Although ACE inhibitors may cause a dry, persistent, nonproductive cough, heart failure itself can have the same effect. Therefore, you'll need to assess your patient for signs and symptoms of pulmonary congestion, such as increasing dyspnea and crackles.

Your patient may be tempted to stop taking his medication if his cough becomes bothersome. Instruct him to talk with his physician before stopping the drug or reducing the dose on his own.

AVERTING RENAL INSUFFICIENCY
To evaluate your patient's renal function, monitor his serum creatinine level during ACE inhibitor therapy, and report any elevation. If his renal function is impaired, you may need to administer a reduced dose. Also be sure to assess his fluid volume status to make sure he's not hypovolemic.

DEALING WITH OTHER ADVERSE EFFECTS
Angioedema (swelling of the face, throat, hands, and feet) is a rare but potentially serious adverse effect of ACE inhibitors. If your patient experiences pharyngeal edema, immediately stop the drug, call the physician, and prepare to give emergency care. Tell your patient to report any difficulty swallowing immediately.

If your patient develops a rash, report it to the physician. If the rash doesn't resolve on its own, the dose may need to be adjusted.

If the patient reports altered taste sensation, reassure him that this should resolve with continued therapy. If it doesn't, the physician may switch him to a different ACE inhibitor.

ADVISING YOUR PATIENT
Teach your patient about signs and symptoms to report to the physician, and explain the need for periodic blood tests during ACE inhibitor therapy. Also stress the importance of not stopping the medication abruptly and taking any over-the-counter medications unless the physician approves.

ACE inhibitor	Initial oral dosage	Target dosage	Recommended maximum dosage
captopril	6.25 to 12.5 mg t.i.d.	50 mg t.i.d.	100 mg t.i.d.
enalapril	2.5 mg b.i.d.	10 mg b.i.d.	20 mg b.i.d.
lisinopril	5 mg daily	20 mg daily	20 to 40 mg daily
quinapril	5 mg b.i.d.	20 mg b.i.d.	20 to 40 mg b.i.d.

Source: U.S. Department of Health and Human Services, AHCPR Publication No. 94-0612.

➡ **NurseALERT** Keep in mind that ACE inhibitors can cause hypotension and hyperkalemia. During therapy, monitor your patient's blood pressure and serum potassium level closely while titrating the ACE inhibitor to the desired dose.

• Expect to give diuretics, as prescribed, if your patient has fluid volume overload with pulmonary congestion.

- Anticipate administering digoxin to strengthen myocardial contractility if your patient has severe heart failure or continues to experience symptoms with ACE inhibitors and diuretics.
- If your patient develops acute pulmonary edema, prepare to give I.V. diuretics, nitrates, morphine sulfate, and oxygen, as prescribed. Provide mechanical ventilation, if necessary and ordered.

WHAT TO DO NEXT

After the initial crisis subsides, follow these guidelines:

- Administer vasodilators, as prescribed. If your patient can't tolerate ACE inhibitors, he may receive hydralazine (Apresoline). If he has advanced heart failure, you may need to give nitrates concomitantly with ACE inhibitors or hydralazine.
- Give beta-adrenergic blockers, if prescribed.
- ➡ **NurseALERT** Although previously contraindicated in heart failure, beta blockers may be used to improve left ventricular function, hemodynamic and functional status, and exercise tolerance.
- Monitor your patient's vital signs, fluid intake and output, and daily weight.
- Perform frequent cardiopulmonary assessment for S_3 and S_4 heart sounds, heart rate and rhythm, jugular vein distention, crackles, dependent edema, dyspnea, skin color and temperature, capillary refill, respiratory rate and depth, and activity tolerance.
- Assess for arrhythmias; administer antiarrhythmic medications, as needed and prescribed.
- ➡ **NurseALERT** Be aware that because many antiarrhythmics depress left ventricular function and may themselves induce arrhythmias, their routine use isn't recommended in patients with heart failure.
- Administer ordered treatments to correct the underlying cause of arrhythmias, such as hypoxemia, hyperkalemia, and hypomagnesemia.
- If your patient has atrial fibrillation or another risk factor for embolism, expect to give anticoagulants, as prescribed.
- Implement interventions to correct any condition that may aggravate heart failure. For example, make sure the patient takes prescribed antihypertensive medication and follows the prescribed low-sodium diet.

FOLLOW-UP CARE

- If your patient is receiving digoxin, watch for signs and symptoms of digitalis toxicity, such as arrhythmias, nausea, vomiting, diarrhea, blurred vision, and yellow-green halos around visual images.
- Monitor laboratory test results, including prothrombin time, white blood cell count with differential, blood urea nitrogen level, and serum creatinine, electrolyte, and digoxin levels. Report abnormal values.
- Teach your patient about the pathophysiology of heart failure, how diet and medications can help him feel better, and ways to reduce risk factors (such as smoking cessation). Instruct him to weigh him-

H

self daily and to maintain adequate nutrition. Urge him to limit his alcohol intake because it can depress myocardial contractility. Tell him which signs and symptoms to report to the physician.
- Discuss a home care referral with your patient and the physician.

SPECIAL CONSIDERATIONS
- Explain to your patient and his family that heart failure increases the risk of lethal arrhythmias and sudden cardiac death. Encourage family members to learn cardiopulmonary resuscitation, and make sure they know how to activate the emergency medical service in their community.
- Explain the benefits of exercise, and encourage the patient to exercise as recommended by the physician. Advise him that exercise will improve his functional status, increase his activity tolerance, and prevent deconditioning. Assess his level of activity intolerance and help him plan appropriate rest periods.
- Keep in mind that noncompliance is a major problem in patients with heart failure. Provide the patient and family with plenty of information to convince them of the benefits of compliance. Also consider a multidisciplinary care team and referrals to educational programs and support groups.
- If your patient has advanced heart failure, advise him to consider completing an advance directive and to discuss his wishes for future care with his family and health-care providers.

HEMATURIA AND HEMOGLOBINURIA

Both hematuria (blood in the urine) and hemoglobinuria (free hemoglobin in the urine) produce urine that takes on some shade of red. Hematuria commonly results from a urinary tract infection, glomerulonephritis, kidney trauma, renal calculi, bladder cancer, or a urinary obstruction from benign prostatic hyperplasia. Hemoglobinuria tends to result from a transfusion reaction, hemolytic anemia, severe burns, or infection. (See *How bleeding changes urine color.*)

Differential diagnosis
The timing of blood's appearance in the patient's urine stream may provide clues to the source of her bleeding. For example, blood that appears at the start of the urine stream (seen most easily in male patients) usually signals bleeding from the anterior urethra. Blood that appears throughout voiding signals a bleeding source above the bladder neck. And blood that appears only at the end of the urine stream suggests a source in the posterior urethra or bladder neck.

Blood clots have significance too. Large clots in the urine typically indicate bleeding in the bladder, whereas elongated, strandlike clots suggest upper urinary tract bleeding.

HOW BLEEDING CHANGES URINE COLOR

Your patient's description of her urine color—or your observation of it—may provide clues to the severity of her bleeding. Use the chart below to help assess the significance of her urine color.

Urine color	Bleeding rate
Cranberry or cherry colored	Minimal
Cherry-red, port-wine, or cola colored	Minimal to moderate
Tomato-soup or muddy red appearance	Moderate to severe
Thick clots, bright red appearance	Severe to critical

No matter what the cause of your patient's bloody urine, you'll need to intervene immediately; this sign could reflect a serious underlying disease. Remember—the amount of blood doesn't necessarily indicate the severity of the underlying problem. Even a minute amount of blood in the urine warrants prompt attention.

H

WHAT TO LOOK FOR

With *hematuria*, clinical findings may include:
- gross macroscopic hematuria (a large amount of blood clearly visible in the urine)
- cloudy red urine, possibly containing blood clots
- microscopic hematuria (blood not visible in urine; red blood cells detected on microscopic examination).

With *hemoglobinuria*, clinical findings may include:
- clear red urine (although hemoglobin may be difficult to detect even with a microscope).

WHAT TO DO IMMEDIATELY

If your patient has blood-tinged urine, take the following actions:
- Assess her urine for general appearance, color, and clots. Ask her when the blood first appeared and whether she's been experiencing pain, fever, and urinary urgency, hesitancy, or frequency.
- Review the patient's medication history for substances that can change urine color, such as phenazopyridine (Pyridium) and large doses of vitamin C; also check for anticoagulants, which may cause spontaneous urinary tract bleeding.
- Find out if the patient has had hematuria before or if she's had a renal, urologic, or coagulation disorder. Also ask if she has recently experienced trauma. (Ask a male patient if he has a history of prostate disorders.)
- Palpate and percuss the patient's abdomen, flank, and costovertebral angle.
- Notify the physician and report your assessment findings.

➡ **NurseALERT** Suspect a renal neoplasm if the patient has gross hematuria accompanied by dull, aching flank pain and a smooth, firm, palpable flank mass.

- Obtain a urine specimen for analysis, as ordered. Anticipate withdrawing the specimen from a urinary catheter to ensure a sterile specimen (for example, if the patient is menstruating).

WHAT TO DO NEXT
When your patient is stable, carry out these interventions:
- Monitor her vital signs every 2 to 4 hours; report significant changes.
- Evaluate her urine for the amount and pattern of hematuria. During therapy, obtain spot urine specimens and check for occult bleeding.
- Monitor her fluid intake and output.
- To prevent clots from obstructing urine outflow, increase her oral fluid intake. If she can't tolerate oral intake, give I.V. fluids, as prescribed. Anticipate continuous bladder irrigation if the clots persist to obstruct urine outflow.
- Prepare her for diagnostic tests to determine the cause of hematuria. They may include additional blood and urine studies, kidney-ureter-bladder radiography, excretory urography, cystoscopy, and, possibly, renal biopsy.
- If she complains of pain, administer analgesics, as prescribed.

FOLLOW-UP CARE
- Carry out ordered treatments to correct the underlying cause of hematuria.
- Continue to assess the patient's urine output and evaluate her laboratory test results.

SPECIAL CONSIDERATIONS
- Keep in mind that beets, berries, and foods containing red dye may tint the urine red, causing *pseudohematuria*. Be sure to ask the patient about recent intake of these foods.
- Therapy or treatments that involve urinary tract instrumentation or manipulation may cause hematuria.

HEMOPTYSIS

If your patient produces blood when she coughs, she may have a serious respiratory or GI problem. If the problem turns out to be respiratory, it's called hemoptysis, and it may stem from a wide range of injuries (such as violent coughing and tracheal irritation after extubation) or disorders. (See *Performing the litmus test*.)

Typically, these disorders occupy one of three categories:
- airway disease, such as bronchitis, bronchiectasis, and bronchogenic carcinoma

- parenchymal disease, such as infection, tuberculosis, lung abscess, and pneumonia
- vascular lesions, such as pulmonary embolism, pulmonary infarction, pulmonary edema, and arteriovenous malformation.

Whatever its category, hemoptysis may indicate a pressing problem, one that may rapidly progress to airway obstruction, asphyxiation, and respiratory and cardiac arrest. If your patient is coughing up blood from her airways, you'll need to assess her quickly and thoroughly, and then take appropriate actions.

WHAT TO LOOK FOR
If your patient has hemoptysis, associated findings may include:
- apprehension and fear
- panicked appearance, feeling of impending doom
- altered level of consciousness (which may indicate hypoxemia or hypercapnia)
- acute dyspnea
- oxygen saturation below 90%
- coughing, possibly violent
- gagging (which may result from clots with severe bleeding)
- tachycardia
- tachypnea
- hypotension
- diaphoresis
- pallor
- cyanosis (with severe bleeding)
- shock.

WHAT TO DO IMMEDIATELY
If you detect hemoptysis, notify the physician. Then take these measures.

For mild hemoptysis
- If the patient has blood-streaked sputum (mild hemoptysis), provide humidified supplemental oxygen, as prescribed. Monitor her closely for signs and symptoms of respiratory distress.
- ➡ **NurseALERT** Always use standard precautions whenever you anticipate contact with a patient's sputum.
- Obtain your patient's vital signs, and assess her level of consciousness for changes that suggest hypoxemia or hemorrhage.
- Assess oxygen saturation by way of pulse oximetry or arterial blood gas values. Give supplemental oxygen, as ordered and needed.
- Insert a large-bore I.V. catheter if one isn't in place already, and administer I.V. fluids, as prescribed, to maintain fluid volume.
- For severe bleeding, anticipate blood transfusions.

PERFORMING THE LITMUS TEST

If blood is coming from your patient's mouth, you'll need to quickly determine whether it's from her respiratory system (hemoptysis) or her GI system (hematemesis). Here's how to tell the difference.

HEMOPTYSIS
Blood expectorated from the lungs is bright red or pink. It may be frothy and mixed with sputum. And it doesn't change the color of litmus paper (the paper remains blue).

HEMATEMESIS
Blood vomited from the stomach is dark red and may look like coffee grounds. It's usually mixed with food, and it turns litmus paper pink.

H

- Obtain blood samples for laboratory tests, as ordered, including complete blood count, hematocrit, and serum electrolyte and hemoglobin levels . Evaluate the results and report significant findings.

For severe hemoptysis
- If the patient has severe hemoptysis with frank bleeding or clots, place her in a semirecumbent position.
- Assess the secretions to verify that the bleeding source is respiratory (hemoptysis) rather than gastric (hematemesis).
- Prepare your patient for bronchoscopy, as indicated. (See *Assisting with bronchoscopy*.)
- Prepare to administer emergency medications, such as atropine, epinephrine, and lidocaine, as prescribed.
- Keep resuscitation equipment (manual resuscitation device, suction, and backboard) nearby in case the patient's respiratory status deteriorates. Suction as necessary.
- Prepare the patient for possible emergency surgery to cauterize bleeding sites.

WHAT TO DO NEXT
Once you've taken initial steps, follow these guidelines:
- Monitor the patient's vital signs and cardiopulmonary status closely—every 15 minutes to 1 hour—if indicated. Watch for tachycardia because subtle changes in heart rate may signal bleeding. Also report hypotension, tachypnea, and respiratory distress.
- Assess the patient's mental status for subtle changes that suggest hypoxemia (from decreased cardiac output secondary to bleeding).
- Maintain high-humidity airflow with supplemental oxygen, as prescribed. Continuously monitor the patient's oxygen saturation level.
- Administer ordered treatments to correct the underlying cause of hemoptysis.
- Ask the patient if she has ever had similar bleeding before; if so, ask about its frequency, duration, consistency, quantity, and color. To help her estimate the quantity of coughed-up blood, tell her to describe it in familiar terms, such as number of teaspoons or shot glasses per day.

FOLLOW-UP CARE
- Continue to monitor the patient's cardiopulmonary status frequently, watching for changes in vital signs and mental status. Assess breath sounds every 2 hours or more frequently if indicated.
- Continue to administer humidified oxygen, as ordered, and provide adequate hydration to liquefy secretions and lessen the need for vigorous coughing.
- Keep the head of the bed elevated 45 degrees to promote optimal lung expansion.
- Provide frequent oral hygiene to prevent drying of mucous membranes.

ASSISTING WITH BRONCHOSCOPY

A patient with hemoptysis may need to undergo bronchoscopy to identify the source and cause of the bleeding. This procedure may be performed with a flexible or rigid bronchoscope. The flexible fiber-optic bronchoscope is used most often because it allows the physician to view more of the patient's airway, particularly the right upper lobe. What's more, the physician can perform this procedure at the bedside, and in addition to being inserted through the nose, the bronchoscope can be inserted into a tracheotomy or endotracheal tube. A rigid bronchoscope, a hollow metal tube with a light at its end, is used most often to remove a foreign body or thick secretions or to examine the airways with massive hemoptysis. Familiarize yourself with this procedure and the nursing care your patient will require before, during, and after it.

ABOUT THE PROCEDURE
During bronchoscopy, a flexible fiber-optic scope is inserted through the patient's nose and larynx and into the tracheobronchial airway, allowing direct visualization (see illustration). A rigid bronchoscope is inserted through the patient's mouth. The examiner can locate the source of bleeding, remove foreign bodies and secretions, obtain sputum specimens, or remove a specimen of lung tissue for cytologic examination.

PREPARING THE PATIENT
- Explain the procedure to the patient.
- Remove the patient's dentures, eyeglasses, or contact lenses to keep them safe during the procedure.
- Administer medications, such as sedatives and local anesthetics, as prescribed.
- Bring resuscitation and suction equipment to the bedside.

DURING BRONCHOSCOPY
- Assist with the procedure, as necessary.
- Monitor the patient's vital signs and respiratory status closely throughout bronchoscopy.

AFTERCARE
- Monitor the patient's vital signs every 15 minutes for the first hour, every 30 minutes for the next hour, every hour for the next 4 hours, and then every 4 hours—or according to your facility's policy.
- Assess the patient for laryngospasm and respiratory distress caused by the local anesthetic given during bronchoscopy and for edema from the procedure.
- Withhold oral intake until the anesthetic has worn off and the patient is stable. Make sure the patient's gag reflex has returned before offering any oral fluids—even ice chips.
- Monitor the color and character of the patient's secretions. Although blood-tinged secretions are normal for several hours after bronchoscopy, notify the physician if sputum becomes grossly bloody.
- Although some hoarseness is normal after bronchoscopy, report persistent hoarseness. Provide warm saline rinses and lozenges to relieve sore throat.
- Immediately report signs and symptoms of complications, including a persistent cough, bloody or purulent sputum, wheezing, dyspnea, difficulty breathing, stridor, and chest pain.

H

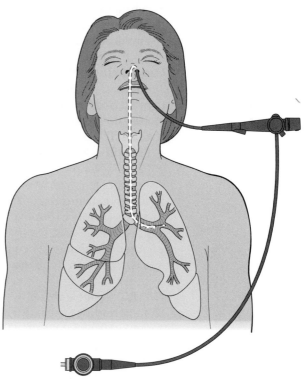

SPECIAL CONSIDERATIONS
- Teach the patient about signs and symptoms of the underlying disorder. Urge her to notify the physician at once if hemoptysis recurs to help prevent progression to severe bleeding.

HEMORRHAGE

By definition, hemorrhage means that a patient loses a large amount of blood over a short period from his arteries, veins, or capillaries or from a combination of vessels. In an *internal* hemorrhage, blood leaves the vessels but remains inside the body. In an *external* hemorrhage, blood leaves the body through a wound or an orifice.

Although internal and external hemorrhages commonly stem from wounds created by traumatic injury, they also can result from invasive procedures, such as:
- arterial catheter placement
- arterial puncture (such as for arterial blood gas measurement)
- central venous catheter placement
- emergency transvenous or transthoracic cardiac pacing
- percutaneous intra-aortic balloon pump insertion
- pericardiocentesis
- subclavian, femoral, or internal jugular vein catheterization
- surgery
- umbilical artery or vein catheter placement.

Classifying hemorrhage
Typically, a hemorrhage is classified according to the severity of the patient's blood loss:
- Class I—up to 15% of total blood volume lost
- Class II—15% to 30% of total blood volume lost
- Class III—30% to 40% of total blood volume lost
- Class IV—more than 40% of total blood volume lost.

A massive hemorrhage (called an exsanguinating hemorrhage) can progress rapidly to hypovolemic shock and death. It can be either internal or external and requires immediate surgical intervention. Clearly, your rapid response to hemorrhage can mean the difference between life and death for your patient.

WHAT TO LOOK FOR
Clinical findings vary with hemorrhage severity, as described below.

Class I
With a class I hemorrhage, findings typically include:
- blood loss of up to 750 ml

- pulse less than 100 beats/minute
- normal or slightly increased pulse pressure
- respiratory rate of 14 to 20 breaths/minute
- anxiety.

Class II
With a class II hemorrhage, clinical findings may include:
- blood loss of 750 to 1,500 ml
- pulse above 100 beats/minute
- normal blood pressure
- decreased pulse pressure
- respiratory rate of 20 to 30 breaths/minute
- anxiety.

Class III
With a class III hemorrhage, expect:
- blood loss of 1,500 to 2,000 ml
- pulse above 120 beats/minute
- decreased blood pressure
- reduced pulse pressure
- respiratory rate of 30 to 40 breaths/minute
- anxiety and confusion.

Class IV
With a class IV hemorrhage, clinical findings may include:
- blood loss greater than 2,000 ml
- pulse above 140 beats/minute
- decreased blood pressure
- reduced pulse pressure
- respiratory rate above 35 breaths/minute
- confusion and lethargy.

WHAT TO DO IMMEDIATELY
If your patient is hemorrhaging, notify the physician. Then focus on stabilizing the patient and stopping the bleeding. Follow these guidelines:
- Assess the patient's airway, breathing, and circulation. Begin cardiopulmonary resuscitation, if indicated.
- Using standard precautions, apply direct pressure to control external bleeding.
- If bleeding persists despite direct pressure, apply indirect pressure over a vascular area proximal to the wound. If the bleeding source is a distal extremity, apply a blood pressure cuff proximal to the bleeding site and inflate it.
- Anticipate applying elastic compression dressings to control bleeding from a venous or an arterial injury or applying a proximal tourniquet to a pulsating hemorrhage of an upper or a lower extremity.

H

FLUID REPLACEMENT OPTIONS

The physician may order one of the following types of fluid replacement therapy for a hemorrhaging patient.

I.V. FLUID THERAPY

A patient who's hypotensive from hemorrhage usually receives I.V. fluids. The fluid of choice is a balanced solution, such as lactated Ringer's injection. For an adult, expect to give an initial bolus of 1 to 2 L as rapidly as possible. Use a large-bore catheter, short I.V. tubing, and a rapid-infuser device.

BLOOD COMPONENT THERAPY

A patient who doesn't respond to I.V. fluids typically receives type-specific, crossmatched blood. If that's not available and he needs immediate resuscitation, the second choice is O negative blood. If that's scarce, a male patient may receive O positive blood (males seldom have plasma anti-D antibodies). A premenopausal woman of unknown blood type typically won't receive O positive blood because it could cause problems if she's pregnant.

Give warmed blood and warmed normal saline solution through a large-bore catheter using a filtering device designed to trap clots, such as a microaggregate filter.

➡ **NurseALERT** Use a tourniquet to stop bleeding *only* as a last resort—and then for no longer than 2 hours.

- In rare cases, you may need to assist with the application or management of a pneumatic antishock garment to control massive soft-tissue bleeding and raise the patient's blood pressure.
- Try to determine the cause of the hemorrhage. If you suspect a fracture, immobilize the injured area.
- Place the patient in a supine position, with the head of the bed elevated 20 to 30 degrees.

➡ **NurseALERT** Keep in mind that although the Trendelenburg position (legs elevated higher than the torso) may raise venous pressure, it has several drawbacks: It increases afterload, boosts myocardial oxygen demands, and may lead to or worsen respiratory compromise.

- Expect to transport the patient to the operating room promptly for exploration and repair or ligature of bleeding vessels.
- Evaluate the patient for evidence of hypotension and shock by assessing his heart rate, respiratory rate, and blood pressure every 15 minutes. To evaluate cardiac output, assess his level of consciousness, skin temperature, and peripheral pulses. Report indications of shock immediately, and institute ordered measures to raise blood pressure and treat shock.
- Provide I.V. fluid volume replacement therapy, as prescribed. To deliver fluids rapidly, use a large-bore I.V. catheter. Anticipate the possible need for a second I.V. access site or central venous catheter. (See *Fluid replacement options.*)
- Assess the patient's oxygen saturation by way of pulse oximetry and arterial blood gas (ABG) values; administer supplemental oxygen, as prescribed and indicated. Be aware that he may need endotracheal intubation and mechanical ventilation if his respiratory status deteriorates.
- Obtain laboratory tests, such as blood typing and crossmatching, complete blood count, hematocrit, blood urea nitrogen (BUN) level, and serum creatinine, hemoglobin, and electrolyte levels, to establish a baseline and guide therapy.

WHAT TO DO NEXT

After the patient is stabilized initially, take the following steps:

- As ordered, assist with insertion of a pulmonary artery or central venous catheter to evaluate the patient's hemodynamic status and an arterial line to monitor blood pressure continuously and directly.
- Insert an indwelling urinary catheter, as ordered, and assess the patient's urine output at least every hour. Monitor fluid intake and output closely, and report significant changes.

- Insert a nasogastric tube, as ordered, to prevent gastric distention. Check drainage from the tube for frank or occult bleeding, and be sure to include drainage when measuring output.
- Begin continuous cardiac monitoring; evaluate the patient's ECG for ischemic changes and life-threatening arrhythmias.
- Continue to monitor the patient's respiratory status, including respiratory rate, breath sounds, and oxygen saturation.
- If indicated and ordered, prepare the patient for surgery to control the hemorrhage.

FOLLOW-UP CARE
- Continue to assess all physiologic indicators, including cardiopulmonary status, blood pressure, respiratory rate, and hemodynamic values.
- ➡ **NurseALERT** Stay alert for signs and symptoms of stress ulcers and subsequent GI hemorrhage. Stress ulcers may result from ischemia of the gastric mucosa caused by the physiologic stress response to massive hemorrhage.
- Continue to administer I.V. fluids and blood replacement therapy, as prescribed.
- Regularly assess the patient's level of consciousness, skin temperature, and peripheral pulses to evaluate his circulatory status.
- Continue to monitor his fluid intake and output to evaluate renal function.
- Keep a close watch on laboratory test results, including hematocrit, ABG values, BUN level, and serum creatinine, hemoglobin, and electrolyte levels; report significant changes.

SPECIAL CONSIDERATIONS
- Be aware that delayed hemorrhage may occur from the same causes as the initial hemorrhage, but for some reason, bleeding temporarily stopped, such as from a tamponade effect that is no longer present. Delayed hemorrhage may also signal the development of an infection, which can erode a suture line or a vein graft. Remember, too, that occult bleeding may present as a delayed hematoma or a pseudoaneurysm. Therefore, even after resuscitation has been initiated and normal blood pressure is restored, be sure to evaluate your patient every 1 to 2 hours initially and every 4 hours thereafter.

HEPATIC FAILURE, ACUTE

The liver can sustain a great deal of damage before hepatic failure sets in. In fact, only a few symptoms may appear until about 70% of liver tissue is damaged, and the liver can perform all its normal functions until about 90% of its tissues are damaged. Consequently, liver disease may

H

progress slowly, over years, before the patient develops signs and symptoms of hepatic failure. In this case, the patient has chronic hepatic failure, which typically results from cirrhosis, cancer, or metabolic disorders. Acute hepatic failure develops suddenly when severe injury or disease causes widespread necrosis of hepatic cells, leading to hepatic failure and hepatic encephalopathy in a patient without previous liver disease. Acute hepatic failure is frequently caused by viral hepatitis but may also be caused by exposure to hepatotoxins (carbon tetrachloride, certain mushrooms) as well as by drug reactions and profound shock.

As hepatic failure advances, the patient risks developing a number of associated conditions, including hepatic encephalopathy, bleeding esophageal varices, ascites, hypovolemia, electrolyte imbalances, respiratory distress, hepatorenal syndrome, and sepsis. Hepatic failure and the conditions it causes deserve your expert rapid response. (See *Consequences of hepatic failure*.)

WHAT TO LOOK FOR

Clinical findings in hepatic failure may include:
- jaundice (the hallmark of acute hepatic failure)
- nonspecific flulike symptoms, such as malaise, anorexia, nausea, vomiting, weight loss, and dull pain in the right upper abdominal quadrant
- liver enlargement and tenderness (however, with significant necrosis, the liver becomes small, hard, and nonpalpable)
- bleeding diathesis, indicated by prolonged bleeding after venipuncture, bleeding from gums, and excessive bruising
- palpable ascites, visible in the lower abdomen when the patient sits upright
- dependent edema in the lower extremities and sacral area
- dyspnea and hyperventilation
- disorientation, confusion, or irrational behavior
- signs and symptoms of sepsis, including fever, decreased blood pressure, and rapid pulse rate
- hematemesis or bleeding from a nasogastric tube
- evidence of poor nutrition, including dry, flaky skin; dull, fragile hair; and thin extremities
- decreased urine output (less than 200 ml in 24 hours).

Laboratory tests

Laboratory test results may show:
- increased serum bilirubin, ammonia, and sodium levels
- decreased serum albumin and potassium levels
- increased levels of liver enzymes (aspartate aminotransferase, alanine aminotransferase, and lactate dehydrogenase)
- prolonged prothrombin and partial thromboplastin times.

CONSEQUENCES OF HEPATIC FAILURE

Hepatic failure can lead to a number of associated conditions that require expert care, including those discussed below.

HEPATIC ENCEPHALOPATHY

As ammonia and other noxious elements normally cleared by the liver build up in the blood and cross the blood-brain barrier, they can damage brain tissue. Hepatic encephalopathy typically progresses through four clearly demarcated stages.

- *Stage 1:* The patient exhibits subtle personality changes and reduced mental status. Other effects of hepatic failure may mask these signs.
- *Stage 2:* The patient is confused and disoriented and may become aggressive and combative. You may observe asterixis—involuntary flapping motions of the hands when extended.
- *Stage 3:* Confusion, lethargy, and somnolence worsen.
- *Stage 4:* The patient lapses into a coma or becomes unresponsive. Mortality in this stage is nearly 100%.

ESOPHAGEAL VARICES

When pressure increases in the portal circulation, fragile esophageal vessels swell from backflow pressure. If they burst, the patient probably will lose massive amounts of blood; in fact, bleeding esophageal varices usually prove fatal.

ASCITES AND EDEMA

As the liver stops producing adequate amounts of albumin, plasma oncotic pressure decreases. Fluid then moves into the interstitial space, where it accumulates and leads to ascites and profound dependent edema. These conditions in turn can cause relative hypovolemia, diminished venous return, reduced cardiac output, and, possibly, circulatory collapse. If ascites causes diaphragmatic elevation, respiratory distress may arise.

HEPATORENAL SYNDROME

An ominous development in late-stage hepatic failure, hepatorenal syndrome involves unexplained kidney dysfunction with oliguria and low urinary sodium concentration. Usually sudden in onset, the syndrome seldom responds to treatment.

SEPSIS

Normally, Kupffer cells help rid the body of microorganisms and infectious debris. As these cells cease functioning, bacteria may enter the systemic circulation, causing sepsis.

H

WHAT TO DO IMMEDIATELY

If your patient develops signs or symptoms of acute hepatic failure, notify the physician. Then follow these guidelines:

- Monitor your patient's vital signs at least every hour and more often if indicated.
- Assess his mental status frequently. If possible, have him write his name in his chart every day to help track the progress of hepatic encephalopathy. Expect to administer lactulose (Cephulac) if the patient is obtunded.
- Position the patient to maximize the effectiveness of his respiratory effort—usually in semi-Fowler's or high Fowler's position.
- Establish I.V. access and give I.V. fluids, as prescribed.
- ➡ **NurseALERT** Take care not to give excessive fluids because a patient with hepatic failure is predisposed to fluid retention.
- Insert an indwelling urinary catheter, as ordered, to monitor hourly urine output.
- Thoroughly inspect the patient's skin, especially edematous areas around the sacrum and lower extremities.

- If indicated, obtain supplies for paracentesis to drain ascitic fluid and relieve pressure on the diaphragm. Assist with the procedure, as appropriate. (See *Assisting with paracentesis*, page 204.)

WHAT TO DO NEXT

After taking these initial steps, carry out the following interventions:
- Continue to monitor your patient's vital signs, level of consciousness, respiratory status, urine output, and laboratory values.
- Maintain I.V. therapy by administering prescribed albumin, antibiotics, and diuretics.
- If your patient has ascites, expect to give diuretics, salt-poor albumin infusions, or both. Assess his response by evaluating urine output, skin turgor, and other hydration markers. Be aware that poor hydration may indicate overly vigorous fluid restriction.
- After paracentesis, monitor the puncture site for excessive bleeding and oozing of ascitic fluid.
- If your patient has hepatic encephalopathy, administer prescribed therapy to reduce his serum ammonia level, such as lactulose and neomycin (Mycifradin) given orally or as a retention enema. Make sure rectal tubes and medications are readily available. Also anticipate the possible need for dialysis to reduce his serum ammonia level.
- If the patient becomes irrational and combative, take steps to prevent injury, such as padding and raising the side rails, keeping sharp objects out of his reach, and placing mittens on his hands to prevent scratching. Use restraints only if necessary, making sure to follow your facility's policies and procedures.
- Prepare the patient for percutaneous liver biopsy, if indicated, and provide the appropriate care during and after the procedure. (See *Understanding percutaneous liver biopsy*.)

FOLLOW-UP CARE

- Maintain meticulous skin and mouth care.
- Provide a high-carbohydrate, low-protein, low-sodium diet, as ordered. If the patient can't tolerate oral intake, administer appropriate enteral or parenteral feedings.
- If indicated, prepare the patient for surgery to shunt portal circulation away from the liver. Be aware that a patient with hepatic failure is a poor surgical risk.

SPECIAL CONSIDERATIONS

- Know that hepatic coma signals the terminal phase of hepatic failure.
- Although some patients may be candidates for liver transplantation, this option isn't recommended for those who have widespread liver cancer or chronic hepatitis (the disease may recur in the transplanted organ). Other considerations include the patient's chance of surviving the procedure, organ availability, and long-term prognosis.

UNDERSTANDING PERCUTANEOUS LIVER BIOPSY

If your patient has hepatic failure, he may undergo a liver biopsy to help reveal the source of his problem—such as cirrhosis, hepatitis, primary or metastatic liver cancer, or another disease. For diffuse disease, he'll probably have a closed biopsy, in which a physician uses a needle to extract liver tissue for microscopic examination. Here's what you should do before, during, and after the procedure.

BEFORE THE PROCEDURE
- Advise the patient to avoid aspirin, nonsteroidal anti-inflammatory drugs, and anticoagulants for at least 2 weeks before the procedure.
- Have the patient fast for 6 hours before the test.
- Check the patient's most recent coagulation studies, and obtain his baseline vital signs.
- Administer a sedative and an analgesic, such as diazepam or midazolam, as ordered.

DURING THE PROCEDURE
- Help the patient onto his left side (or into a supine position) and have him raise his right arm over his head.

- After establishing a sterile field around the area to be punctured, the physician numbs the area with local anesthetic and asks the patient to exhale and then to hold his breath as the biopsy needle is inserted. The physician then extracts a small liver specimen and removes the needle.
- Place a pressure dressing over the insertion site.

AFTER THE PROCEDURE
- Have the patient lie on his right side for 2 hours.
- Monitor his vital signs every 15 to 30 minutes for the first 2 hours and every hour for the next 4 hours, or according to your facility's policy.
- Observe the pressure dressing for bleeding, and assess for pain in the patient's right upper abdominal quadrant.
- Assess the patient's respiratory status for indications of pneumothorax, a possible complication of biopsy.
- Have the patient lie as flat as possible for 12 to 24 hours.

HYPERCALCEMIA

Hypercalcemia refers to an abnormally high level of calcium in the blood (greater than 10.6 mg/dl). Because calcium profoundly influences contraction and relaxation of cardiac muscle, a calcium excess can lead to cardiac arrhythmias—including blockage of all supraventricular impulses to the ventricles, possibly leading to a loss of cardiac output. (See *About calcium*, page 172.)

Hypercalcemia usually arises secondary to another condition, such as hyperparathyroidism and cancer (most commonly, cancer of the breast or lung, multiple myeloma, and squamous cell carcinoma of the head, neck, or esophagus). It can also result from the use of thiazide diuretics and from other conditions, including renal failure, hyperthyroidism, granulomatous disease (such as sarcoidosis, tuberculosis, and histoplasmosis), hypophosphatemia, metabolic acidosis, milk-alkali syndrome, and excessive calcium or vitamin D intake.

To avert the potentially life-threatening consequences of hypercalcemia, make sure you know how to recognize its signs and symptoms and how to take the appropriate actions. Your rapid, knowledgeable response may help your patient avoid cardiac arrest and death.

ABOUT CALCIUM

A cation (a positively charged ion), calcium has many physiologic functions. For example, through its influence on membrane permeability and the firing level of excitable cells, it's responsible for the resting membrane potential of nerve and skeletal muscle cells.

Calcium concentration also affects membrane permeability in the GI tract and in the heart's pacemaker cells, where it alters the cells' firing rate. Calcium also:
- facilitates normal muscle contraction
- aids blood clotting
- promotes hormone secretion and acid-base balance
- hardens and strengthens bones and teeth (in conjunction with phosphate).

Nearly all the body's calcium (99%) exists in the bones. The remaining 1% is found in the blood; of this amount, about 45% is in active ionized (free) form, 40% binds to albumin, and about 15% forms complexes with carbonate, citrate, phosphate, and other ions.

CALCIUM MOVEMENT
Calcium constantly moves from the extracellular fluid (ECF) into the intestine by secretion. Through reabsorption, it moves from the intestine back into the ECF.

The kidneys also continually filter calcium, reabsorbing it into the ECF. Calcium constantly moves into bone through mineralization and out of bone through resorption.

CALCIUM REGULATION
Calcium is regulated through the interactions of three hormones:
- parathyroid hormone (PTH), produced by the parathyroid glands
- calcitriol (1,25 dihydroxycholecalciferol), a vitamin D metabolite produced by the kidneys
- calcitonin, produced by the thyroid gland.

PTH causes calcium to move into and out of the bone, GI tract, and kidneys in response to extracellular ionized calcium.

Calcitriol, the most active form of vitamin D_3, promotes calcium absorption from the intestine, bone resorption, and renal tubular reabsorption of calcium, all of which increase serum calcium concentration in the ECF and help prevent hypocalcemia.

Calcitonin plays the opposite role in maintaining calcium balance. It increases urinary excretion of calcium and inhibits bone resorption, both of which can lower the serum calcium level. It can contribute to the opposite imbalance, hypocalcemia, by lowering the serum calcium level and increasing urinary calcium excretion.

CALCIUM-PHOSPHATE LINK
A patient's serum phosphate level influences his serum calcium level: As the phosphate level increases, the calcium level declines, and vice versa.

WHAT TO LOOK FOR
Signs and symptoms of hypercalcemia vary with the severity of the imbalance, the speed of its onset, and the underlying cause. Clinical findings may include:
- personality changes
- confusion and psychotic behavior
- altered level of consciousness, ranging from lethargy to coma
- depressed deep tendon reflexes
- profound fatigue
- muscle weakness and irritability
- anorexia
- nausea and vomiting
- peptic ulcer disease
- constipation
- hypoactive bowel sounds

- arrhythmias
- paralytic ileus
- sinus bradycardia
- ECG changes, including shortened QT interval and shortened ST segment
- hypertension
- polyuria
- dehydration
- polydipsia
- renal calculi
- kidney damage, impaired renal function
- bone pain.

WHAT TO DO IMMEDIATELY

If you suspect that your patient may have hypercalcemia or if laboratory results confirm it, notify the physician. (See *Confirming hypercalcemia*, page 174.) Then take the following measures:

- Obtain blood samples, as ordered, for repeat measurement of ionized serum calcium and total serum calcium, albumin, other serum electrolytes (such as potassium and magnesium), blood urea nitrogen (BUN), and creatinine. Be aware that the patient's renal function must be assessed before hydration therapy begins.
- ➡ **NurseALERT** When drawing a blood sample for ionized calcium measurement, use an anaerobic tube with minimal heparin, place the tube on ice at once, and send it to the laboratory immediately.
- Establish I.V. access. For severe hypercalcemia, expect to administer normal saline solution or isotonic saline solution I.V., as prescribed, to restore intravascular volume. Some physicians may prescribe alternating infusions of half-normal saline solution and normal saline solution.
- ➡ **NurseALERT** To help prevent heart failure and fluid overload from cardiac or renal insufficiency, assess the patient's cardiovascular and renal function before starting I.V. fluid therapy.
- As indicated, place the patient on continuous cardiac monitoring, and observe his ECG for such changes as shortened QT intervals and arrhythmias (including sinus bradycardia).
- Check the patient's blood pressure, pulse and respiratory rates, and mental status every 5 to 15 minutes; stay alert for signs of circulatory overload, such as crackles and dyspnea.
- Monitor the patient's hourly fluid intake and output. As indicated, also measure urine specific gravity.
- ➡ **NurseALERT** Be aware that decreased urine output may signal circulatory overload. Closely monitor the patient with decreased output for crackles and dyspnea. Prepare to assist with insertion of a central venous line for continuous evaluation of fluid status. Administer a diuretic, as prescribed, to prevent fluid overload and hasten calcium excretion.

H

CONFIRMING HYPERCALCEMIA

To confirm hypercalcemia, the physician may want to measure your patient's ionized calcium and serum albumin levels, as well as his total calcium level. That's because calcium exists in the body in various forms. For example, inactive calcium is stored in bones, lending them strength and remaining ready for use when the body's other calcium stores are depleted.

Calcium in the intravascular space either binds to protein (primarily albumin) or floats freely in ionized form. Ionized calcium is essential for maintaining cell membrane permeability and for normal neuromuscular activity, including cardiac function. As a result, measuring a patient's ionized calcium level is the best way to evaluate his calcium status.

HOW CALCIUM RELATES TO ALBUMIN
The amount of ionized calcium in serum depends partly on the amount of albumin: As serum albumin increases, ionized calcium begins to bind with albumin, and ionized calcium levels fall. Conversely, as serum albumin falls, calcium detaches from albumin, and ionized calcium levels rise. Thus, the serum albumin level is closely associated with the amount of free calcium in circulation.

EXPECTED TEST RESULTS
Most facilities consider 8.5 to 10.5 mg/dl to be the normal range for serum calcium. Values below and above this range reflect hypocalcemia and hypercalcemia, respectively.

Several methods are used to correct measured calcium concentration for albumin changes. You should check with your facility's laboratory to find out which method is used. However, keep in mind that you can determine your patient's corrected calcium level by adding 0.8 to the calcium level for each 1g/dl the albumin has dropped below the normal range.

WHAT TO DO NEXT
Once your patient is stable, take these actions:
- Monitor serial measurements of BUN and serum electrolytes, albumin, and creatinine every 4 hours, as ordered. Immediately report significant changes to the physician. Abnormal BUN or creatinine values may indicate renal impairment and a possible need for dialysis or other treatments to remove toxins from the blood.
- As prescribed, administer a diuretic, such as furosemide (Lasix), once the patient's intravascular volume has been restored. Diuretics help prevent fluid overload and increase calcium excretion.
- Assess your patient's vital signs every hour during I.V. fluid therapy.
- Continue to monitor his hourly fluid intake and output.
- Keep watching the ECG for arrhythmias and shortened QT intervals.
- Closely monitor the patient's neurologic status, checking for personality changes, confusion, disorientation, and loss of consciousness.
- Check the I.V. site for signs of infiltration, such as redness, swelling, warmth, and pain. If any occur, discontinue the I.V. line, apply warm soaks, and start a new line.
- Withhold oral intake in case the patient needs dialysis. If indicated, prepare him for the procedure.

Alternate therapy
If your patient's condition doesn't improve with administration of furosemide and saline solution or if these treatments are contraindicated, be prepared to take these steps:

- Administer calcitonin, if prescribed, to further inhibit bone resorption and increase urinary calcium excretion. Monitor the patient closely for the first 24 to 48 hours of calcitonin therapy; his serum calcium level should start to fall about 2 hours after the initial dose.
- If prescribed, administer pamidronate (Aredia), etidronate disodium (Didronel), alendronate (Fosamax), or plicamycin (Mithracin; destroys osteoclasts and thus reduces bone resorption).
- ➡ Nurse**ALERT** Be aware that plicamycin is nephrotoxic and hepatotoxic and must be used cautiously in patients with impaired renal function. Monitor renal function and liver enzymes closely.
- If prescribed, administer glucocorticoids to help inhibit bone resorption and decrease calcium absorption in the GI tract. Because glucocorticoids have a slow onset, the physician may combine them with other treatments if your patient has severe hypercalcemia.

FOLLOW-UP CARE
- Regularly monitor the patient's BUN and serum electrolyte, albumin, and creatinine values.
- Continue to record his fluid intake and output.
- For the duration of I.V. fluid therapy, monitor urine specific gravity and continually assess all indicators of renal function for changes that suggest renal insufficiency or the need for dialysis.
- Assist the patient with ambulation. (Prolonged immobility may contribute to hypercalcemia.)
- Obtain a complete patient history to help identify the underlying cause of hypercalcemia and guide long-term treatment.

SPECIAL CONSIDERATIONS
- As indicated, keep emergency equipment, such as a defibrillator and an emergency cart, readily available in case of respiratory or cardiac insufficiency.
- ➡ Nurse**ALERT** If your patient has been receiving digitalis glycosides, be aware that calcium potentiates digitalis effects, putting him at risk for digitalis toxicity, which can lead to cardiac arrest. Immediately report signs and symptoms of digitalis toxicity (arrhythmias, nausea, visual changes, and fatigue).
- Be aware that treatment for hypercalcemia may raise the patient's risk of hypocalcemia. Watch for signs and symptoms of hypocalcemia, such as muscle twitching, cramps, carpopedal spasm, tingling sensations, seizures, irritability, memory impairment, bradycardia, diarrhea, and hypotension. The physician may prescribe electrolyte replacement or alternative therapy to treat a serious calcium deficit.

H

HYPERCAPNIA

Hypercapnia refers to a state of excess carbon dioxide (CO_2) in the blood, expressed in arterial blood gas (ABG) values as a partial pressure of carbon dioxide ($Paco_2$) greater than 45 mm Hg. This condition reflects respiratory insufficiency (inadequate gas exchange during normal activity) or respiratory failure (cardiopulmonary inability to maintain adequate gas exchange at the alveolar level).

Normally, CO_2 production and elimination are balanced to maintain the blood's CO_2 content. Any condition that interferes with CO_2 elimination may cause hypercapnia. Reduced CO_2 elimination may occur when gas exchange in the lungs is disrupted, as from:

- lung disease (emphysema, asthma)
- lung infections
- metabolic acidosis
- damage to the brain stem's respiratory center, such as from trauma or brain stem stroke or as a result of increased intracranial pressure
- low cardiac output.

Because CO_2 is a potent vasodilator and central nervous system depressant, the effects of hypercapnia extend beyond the respiratory system. In fact, hypercapnia also impairs renal, neurologic, and cardiovascular function and alters acid-base balance. If its underlying cause isn't corrected, the patient may slip into a deadly sequence of events. Breathing becomes increasingly difficult, causing respiratory muscle fatigue. This condition in turn triggers decompensation, which worsens ventilation and oxygenation. Eventually, respiratory failure and death ensue. Clearly, this condition requires a rapid, expert response.

WHAT TO LOOK FOR

Most signs and symptoms of hypercapnia reflect the potent vasodilatory and sedative effects of CO_2. Thus, clinical findings may include:

- rapid, deep respirations (an early sign that reflects the body's attempts to "blow off" CO_2)
- depressed respiratory rate and depth (late signs that accompany respiratory center depression)
- changes in mental status and level of consciousness, such as drowsiness, lethargy, confusion, and coma
- flushed skin
- diaphoresis
- bounding pulses
- increased blood pressure
- tachycardia and other arrhythmias
- asterixis
- irritability.

WHAT TO DO IMMEDIATELY

If your patient's signs and symptoms or ABG values suggest hypercapnia, notify the physician. Then take these measures:

- Assess her cardiopulmonary status and vital signs closely; report abnormalities.
- Evaluate her level of consciousness for changes. Remember that subtle level of consciousness changes may be the first sign of CO_2 retention.
- Obtain immediate ABG values to determine the degree of hypercapnia and establish a baseline for later comparison.
- Initiate continuous cardiac monitoring, and observe the patient's ECG for ischemic changes and arrhythmias.
- Elevate the head of the patient's bed 45 degrees to promote lung expansion.
- Assess her oxygen saturation by way of pulse oximetry or ABGs; administer supplemental oxygen, as indicated and prescribed.
- ➡ **NurseALERT** Normally, elevated $Paco_2$ provides the stimulus to breathe. But if your patient has chronic hypercapnia, keep in mind that hypoxia stimulates her breathing because she's developed a tolerance for increased CO_2. Thus, be sure to administer controlled, low-flow oxygen carefully; giving her a high oxygen concentration may lead to diminished respirations and increased hypercapnia, producing CO_2 narcosis.
- Administer bronchodilators, as prescribed, to dilate smooth muscles of the large airways and thus decrease airway resistance.
- If the patient doesn't respond to initial treatments and begins to decompensate, expect to prepare her for endotracheal intubation and mechanical ventilation. Keep suction and emergency equipment at hand. Anticipate starting end-tidal CO_2 ($ETCO_2$) monitoring. (See *Confirming hypercapnia*, page 178.)
- Obtain laboratory tests, as ordered, including complete blood count, hematocrit, and serum electrolyte and hemoglobin levels; report abnormal results.

WHAT TO DO NEXT

Once your patient is stabilized, follow these guidelines:

- Continue to assess her cardiopulmonary and mental status at least every hour; report significant changes.
- Continue to assess the patient's oxygen saturation by way of pulse oximetry. Continue to give supplemental oxygen, as prescribed, at the appropriate flow rate. Monitor serial ABG values for improvement or worsening of hypercapnia; obtain $ETCO_2$ measurements, as ordered.
- Monitor her ECG for cardiac rhythm, rate, arrhythmias, and ischemic changes.
- Obtain a chest X-ray, as ordered, to help determine the underlying cause of hypercapnia.
- Keep the head of the bed elevated 45 degrees.

H

CONFIRMING HYPERCAPNIA

Arterial blood gas (ABG) analysis and end-tidal carbon dioxide monitoring (ETCO$_2$) are used to confirm hypercapnia. Familiarize yourself with these important studies.

ARTERIAL BLOOD GAS ANALYSIS

ABG values provide information about the patient's ventilation status by measuring the pH, partial pressures of oxygen and carbon dioxide (Pao$_2$ and Paco$_2$), oxygen saturation, and bicarbonate (HCO$_3^-$) levels of an arterial blood sample. The sample may be withdrawn from an arterial line or from percutaneous puncture of the radial, brachial, or femoral artery.

Implications of results

In hypercapnia with acute respiratory failure, Pao$_2$ drops suddenly to 60 mm Hg or lower (as the patient breathes room air), Paco$_2$ rises to 50 mm Hg or higher, and blood pH measures about 7.35.

END-TIDAL CARBON DIOXIDE MONITORING

Also called capnometry, ETCO$_2$ monitoring is a noninvasive, continuous method for evaluating CO$_2$ concentration in the airway. Using a photo detector, the monitoring device measures the amount of infrared light absorbed by airway gases during inhalation and exhalation. Elevated CO$_2$ concentrations, as in hypercapnia, cause increased light absorption. The monitor converts the amount of light absorbed into a numerical value shown both in units (mm Hg) and as a graphic waveform (capnogram).

If the patient is intubated, the ETCO$_2$ sensor (which resembles nasal prongs used to administer oxygen) is placed between the endotracheal tube and breathing circuit tubing. Otherwise, it's placed in the patient's airway.

Implications of results

Normally, ETCO$_2$ measures between 36 and 44 mm Hg. It may rise in fever and sepsis and drop in hypothermia, muscle relaxation, and increased depth of anesthesia.

Because of dead-space ventilation, the ETCO$_2$ value typically measures about 5 mm Hg less than the Paco$_2$ value. Increased ETCO$_2$ measurements above 44 mm Hg suggest an increase in Paco$_2$.

- Continue to monitor laboratory results and to report abnormal values.
- Avoid giving the patient sedatives or narcotics because they exacerbate respiratory depression. Also avoid giving cough suppressants because they may cause mucus to remain in airway passages.
- Encourage frequent turning, coughing, and deep breathing; teach your patient how to use the incentive spirometer and perform pursed-lip breathing.
- If the patient is on a mechanical ventilator, provide endotracheal tube care and evaluate ventilator function regularly.

FOLLOW-UP CARE

- Assess the patient's cardiopulmonary status every 2 to 4 hours, as indicated.
- Continue to give bronchodilators, antibiotics, or other medications, as prescribed and indicated.
- Maintain bed rest and limit your patient's activity until her respiratory status and hemodynamic status stabilize. Keep the head of her bed elevated 45 degrees.
- Compare follow-up laboratory test results with baseline values to evaluate for improvement or deterioration.
- Continue to encourage the patient to cough, deep breathe, and perform incentive spirometry and pursed-lip breathing.

- Have your patient ambulate as soon as she's stable and can tolerate being out of bed. During activity, monitor her oxygen saturation and, as needed, adjust her activity level. Note whether activity causes dyspnea, tachypnea, tachycardia, headache, or dizziness.
- As the patient's condition improves, prepare her for weaning from the ventilator and for endotracheal extubation if present, according to your facility's policy.

SPECIAL CONSIDERATIONS
- If your patient has chronic hypercapnia, teach her ways to maintain adequate respiratory function, including complying with drug therapy, performing breathing exercises, preventing disease exacerbation, and minimizing exposure to irritants and infection. Urge her to keep all follow-up medical appointments.
- Keep in mind that a patient with chronic hypercapnia may develop acute respiratory failure when a secondary problem, such as infection, overtaxes her already compromised pulmonary function.
- Know that the patient's serum potassium level may fall as hypercapnia and subsequent respiratory acidosis improve, but watch for an excessive drop, which indicates hypokalemia.

H

HYPERGLYCEMIA

Defined as an excess of glucose in the blood, hyperglycemia results from insufficient insulin or the inability of the body to use insulin effectively. Associated with diabetes mellitus, a hyperglycemic episode may cause life-threatening metabolic abnormalities and other complications that necessitate a rapid response by the health-care team.

Because glucose can't enter most cells without insulin's help, it accumulates in the blood and quickly can rise to a dangerous level in a diabetic patient. In response to the increasing blood glucose level, the kidneys try to compensate by filtering glucose from the blood and excreting it in the urine. However, because glucose is a large molecule, it draws excess water and electrolytes with it. This leads to increased urine volume, which in turn causes fluid and electrolyte imbalances. If severe, these imbalances can produce hypovolemic shock and life-threatening cardiac arrhythmias.

To make matters worse, cells deprived of glucose—their normal energy source—must seek alternative sources, such as protein or fat. However, fat and protein metabolism are ineffective, and fat breakdown may lead to other problems, such as ketoacidosis.

WHAT TO LOOK FOR
Clinical findings in hyperglycemia mirror those of uncontrolled diabetes mellitus and include:
- polyuria

- polydipsia
- polyphagia
- glycosuria
- sudden, unexplained weight loss
- weakness
- fatigue
- blurred vision
- dry mucous membranes
- poor skin turgor
- tachycardia
- hypotension.

WHAT TO DO IMMEDIATELY

If your patient develops hyperglycemia, notify the physician. Then take these steps:

- Double-check the patient's blood glucose level.
- Measure her vital signs, including temperature.
- Obtain specimens of blood, urine, sputum, and drainage for culture, as needed.
- ➡ **NurseALERT** Be aware that because infection commonly causes hyperglycemia in diabetics, antibiotic therapy may begin right away.
- Investigate the patient's diabetes management program, including the time and dose of her last hypoglycemic medication.
- Begin fluid replacement, as prescribed, to combat dehydration. For severe hyperglycemia, establish an I.V. line for fluid administration. Expect to give isotonic saline solution at a rate sufficient to offset fluid lost through urination.
- Monitor the patient's fluid intake and output to help determine her fluid replacement needs.
- Administer regular insulin subcutaneously, intramuscularly, or I.V., as prescribed. Anticipate giving a short-acting insulin preparation because it lowers the blood glucose level quickly.

WHAT TO DO NEXT

After initiating ordered treatments for hyperglycemia, take these steps:

- Monitor your patient's blood glucose level at least every 4 hours.
- Check her urine for ketones at least every 4 hours.
- ➡ **NurseALERT** Notify the physician immediately if you detect urine ketones. Their presence may signal diabetic ketoacidosis, a life-threatening complication of diabetes mellitus.
- Encourage the patient to drink calorie-free fluids to help offset fluids lost through excessive urination.
- Continue to give insulin, as prescribed, and watch closely for signs and symptoms of the opposite imbalance, hypoglycemia. If they appear, expect to stop giving insulin immediately and to administer rapid-acting glucose, as prescribed.

- Implement interventions to address the underlying cause of hyperglycemia, such as administering prescribed antibiotics to treat
infection.

FOLLOW-UP CARE
- Check your patient's blood glucose level before each meal and at
bedtime or as prescribed.
- Evaluate the patient's and family's understanding of the prescribed
diabetic treatment regimen. Correct any misconceptions and provide
instructions, as indicated.
- Urge the patient to see her physician on a regular basis.

SPECIAL CONSIDERATIONS
- Try to determine what caused your patient's hyperglycemic episode
and help her take steps to avoid a recurrence.
- If possible, question family members or significant others when assessing the patient's knowledge of diabetes and disease management
skills. Remember that hyperglycemia can cloud her judgment and
impair her ability to manage diabetes.

H

HYPERGLYCEMIC HYPEROSMOLAR NONKETOTIC SYNDROME

An acute metabolic condition most often seen in non–insulin-dependent
(type II) diabetics, hyperglycemic hyperosmolar nonketotic (HHNK) syndrome refers to a condition in which the blood glucose level exceeds 600
mg/dl, accompanied by little or no ketotic neurologic dysfunction. Although the cause of HHNK syndrome is unknown, it's associated with insulin deficiency and some precipitating factor that raises the blood glucose level. Most precipitating factors fall into four general categories:
- certain drugs, such as glucocorticoids, beta-adrenergic blocking
agents, and diuretics
- certain therapeutic procedures, including dialysis, hyperosmolar ali-
mentation, and surgery
- chronic illness, such as kidney disease, heart disease, and loss of the
thirst mechanism
- acute illness, such as infection, burns, myocardial infarction, and
cerebrovascular accident.

Although HHNK syndrome resembles diabetic ketoacidosis, it tends to
make the patient more seriously ill. Also, HHNK syndrome causes minimal to no ketosis despite extremely high blood glucose levels, possibly
because the type II diabetic secretes some insulin—perhaps enough to
block fat breakdown (the origin of ketosis). However, not enough insulin is produced to stop counterregulatory hormones, such as glucagon
and growth hormone, from producing massive amounts of glucose in
response to a stressor.

DETERMINING SERUM OSMOLARITY

An index of the patient's hydration status, serum osmolarity normally ranges from 280 to 295 mOsm/kg. Values above 295 mOsm/kg indicate dehydration; values below 280 mOsm/kg reflect overhydration.

If your patient has hyperglycemic hyperosmolar nonketotic (HHNK) syndrome, you may want to use her serum osmolarity level to track resolution of her dehydration and evaluate the effectiveness of fluid replacement therapy.

If you know your patient's serum electrolyte and blood glucose levels, you can easily figure out her serum osmolarity. Just use this formula:

$$\text{Serum osmolarity} = 2(Na^+ + K^+) + \frac{\text{glucose mg/dl}}{18} + \frac{\text{blood urea nitrogen mg/dl}}{2.8}$$

The following example uses figures typical of HHNK syndrome:

$$2(130\,\text{mEq/L} + 5\,\text{mEq/L}) + \frac{1{,}044\,\text{mg/dl}}{18} + \frac{28\,\text{mg/dl}}{2.8} = 338\,\text{mOsm/kg}$$

In HHNK syndrome, serum osmolarity exceeds 330 mOsm/kg. However, with fluid administration, your patient's osmolarity gradually should return to normal.

No matter how it develops, HHNK syndrome is a dire condition marked by severe dehydration and acute neurologic dysfunction. HHNK syndrome has a high mortality rate; if you suspect your patient has HHNK syndrome, you'll need to take quick action to keep her alive.

WHAT TO LOOK FOR

Clinical findings in HHNK syndrome, which reflect severe dehydration and hyperglycemia, may include:
- extreme polyuria
- glycosuria
- dry mucous membranes
- poor skin turgor
- longitudinal wrinkles in the tongue
- decreased salivation
- hypotension
- tachycardia
- grand mal or focal seizures
- aphasia
- homonymous hemianopia
- depressed sensorium, ranging from confusion to coma
- serum blood glucose level above 600 mg/dl
- serum osmolarity above 330 mOsm/kg (see *Determining serum osmolarity*).
- ➡ **NurseALERT** Despite the extreme rise in the blood glucose level, don't expect to see Kussmaul's respirations because the patient isn't in ketosis. She may not have polydipsia either because, despite extreme polyuria, neurologic deficits may alter her ability to respond to thirst.

WHAT TO DO IMMEDIATELY

If you suspect your patient has HHNK syndrome, notify the physician. Then take these actions:

- Double-check your patient's blood glucose level, using a venous sample.
- Begin continuous cardiac monitoring.
- If your patient is confused or comatose, establish a safe environment.
- Establish I.V. access; as prescribed, begin I.V. fluid replacement with normal saline solution (1 L/hour) until the patient's urine output reaches 60 ml/hour and her blood pressure is normal. If she's hypernatremic, you may need to give half-normal saline solution instead.
- Begin insulin therapy. Expect to administer only regular insulin at a rate of 0.1 unit/kg/hour, unless otherwise prescribed. Mix the insulin in normal saline solution and then flush the I.V. tubing with about 50 ml of the resulting solution before giving the dose. This method saturates binding sites on the I.V. tubing, ensuring that the patient receives the full amount of insulin.
- ➡ **NurseALERT** Don't give insulin by the subcutaneous or intramuscular route for HHNK syndrome because the patient's severe dehydration will hinder insulin absorption and may delay its arrival in the bloodstream.
- Be prepared to intubate the patient and provide mechanical ventilation, as indicated.
- Initiate seizure precautions, such as padding and raising the side rails and bringing an artificial airway to the bedside.
- If the patient is comatose, insert a nasogastric tube to prevent aspiration.
- Begin hemodynamic monitoring; as indicated, track the patient's central venous pressure, pulmonary artery wedge pressure, and pulmonary artery pressure.

WHAT TO DO NEXT

Once you've started therapy for HHNK syndrome, follow these steps:

- Monitor your patient's blood glucose and serum electrolyte levels hourly.
- Check her vital signs every 15 minutes until she's stable.
- Continue giving I.V. fluids, as prescribed. If you started with normal saline solution, expect to switch to half-normal saline solution to avoid excessive sodium intake. Also expect to adjust the flow rate according to your patient's response.
- When the patient's blood glucose level falls below 250 mg/dl, change the I.V. solution to dextrose 5% in half-normal saline solution. Doing so will prevent hypoglycemia as her glucose level approaches normal.
- Give a potassium supplement in the I.V. fluid, as prescribed, to replace potassium lost through osmotic diuresis.
- Maintain the insulin flow at a rate sufficient to reduce your patient's blood glucose level by no more than 100 mg/dl/hour. Remember that a rapid blood glucose drop may cause cerebral edema (because

glucose pulls water with it as it enters cells). Expect to discontinue insulin when your patient's glucose level falls within the range of 250 to 300 mg/dl.
- Obtain hemodynamic monitoring measurements hourly.
- Assess your patient every hour for evidence of fluid overload and resolution of HHNK syndrome.
- Begin ordered therapy to treat the condition that precipitated HHNK syndrome, if known.

FOLLOW-UP CARE
- Monitor the patient's blood glucose level every 4 to 8 hours or as ordered.
- Begin oral intake once the patient's neurologic dysfunction resolves and her nasogastric tube has been removed. Start with clear liquids and progress to a soft diet and then to a house diet, as tolerated.
- Anticipate discontinuing I.V. fluids when the patient can maintain adequate oral intake and her glucose has stabilized within or near normal levels.
- Expect the physician to add an oral hypoglycemic to the patient's regimen if the patient can't manage her diabetes with diet alone.

SPECIAL CONSIDERATIONS
- Try to determine what caused HHNK syndrome. Help the patient learn how to manage the prescribed diabetic treatment plan so she can avoid a recurrence.
- Keep in mind that about half the patients who develop HHNK syndrome don't know they have diabetes.
- Include family members or significant others when assessing the patient's knowledge level and diabetes management skills.

HYPERKALEMIA

Hyperkalemia refers to an abnormally high concentration of potassium in the blood. A normal serum potassium level is between 3.5 and 5.0 mEq/L. Hyperkalemia exists when the serum potassium level is greater than 5.0 mEq/L. Keep in mind that normal potassium levels may vary slightly with different laboratories.

Hyperkalemia may result from:
- acute or chronic renal failure, which raises the serum potassium level by reducing urinary potassium excretion
- aldosterone deficiency
- excessive intake of salt substitutes or potassium supplements
- high-dose penicillin potassium salts
- malignant cell lysis
- metabolic acidosis
- potassium-sparing diuretics, such as spironolactone (Aldactone), triamterene (Dyrenium), and amiloride (Midamor)

TREATMENT OF CHOICE

ABOUT POTASSIUM

A cation (positively charged ion), potassium is the most abundant electrolyte in the intracellular fluid (ICF). Besides helping to maintain acid-base balance, potassium plays a major part in regulating cell excitability because, unlike most other ions, it can permeate cell membranes. Potassium movement greatly affects ICF composition and concentration.

POTASSIUM MOVEMENT AND CELL POLARIZATION
Normally, some potassium ions leave the cell and some enter at all times, diffusing into or out of the cell with the concentration gradient. As more positively charged potassium ions leave, the cell grows more negative. Attracted by the cell's negative charge, potassium ions eventually move back inside the cell, and the cell's charge becomes more positive.

If potassium concentration in the extracellular fluid (ECF) rises, as in hyperkalemia, fewer potassium ions leave the cell; the cell then becomes less negative and more excitable. If the ECF potassium concentration decreases, as in hypokalemia, more potassium ions leave the cell; the cell becomes more negative and less excitable.

Changes in the potassium concentration affect all excitable cells—especially the specialized cardiac cells that trigger the heart's electrical activity and conduct impulses through the heart.

POTASSIUM REGULATION
In a healthy person, normal renal function and dietary intake closely regulate the serum potassium level. The kidneys excrete about 80% of the body's potassium stores every day; the other 20% leaves the body through bowel movements and sweat glands. Because our bodies lack reserves of potassium, we must consume potassium through our daily diet.

H

- rapid I.V. infusion of potassium solutions
- rapid transfusion of aged blood
- severe tissue damage, such as from crush injury or burns.

Hyperkalemia can lead to pronounced cardiac changes, which eventually may induce cardiac arrest, respiratory arrest, and death. (See *About potassium*.) If your patient is at risk for this electrolyte imbalance, you'll need to stay alert for the signs and symptoms and be prepared to act quickly.

WHAT TO LOOK FOR
Clinical findings in hyperkalemia may include:
- anxiety
- irritability
- personality changes, especially a flat affect
- numbness, tingling, and paresthesias
- muscle weakness
- ascending paralysis, (starting in the legs and progressing to involve the trunk, arms, and, finally, facial and respiratory muscles)
- bradycardia
- postural hypotension
- characteristic ECG changes, such as peaked, narrow T waves and shortened QT intervals; as the potassium level continues to climb, PR intervals become prolonged, P waves disappear, and QRS complexes widen (see *ECG changes in hyperkalemia*, page 186)
- ventricular arrhythmias, which may trigger cardiac arrest
- nausea and vomiting

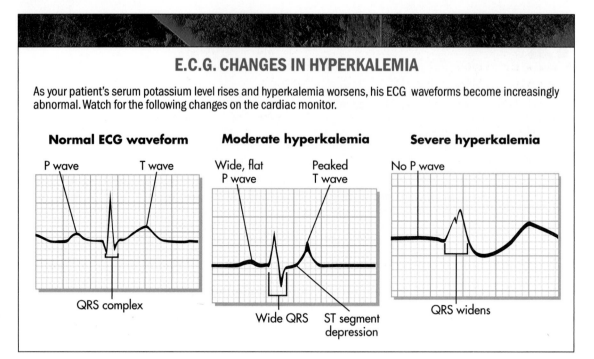

E.C.G. CHANGES IN HYPERKALEMIA

As your patient's serum potassium level rises and hyperkalemia worsens, his ECG waveforms become increasingly abnormal. Watch for the following changes on the cardiac monitor.

Normal ECG waveform

P wave   T wave

QRS complex

Moderate hyperkalemia

Wide, flat   Peaked
P wave   T wave

Wide QRS   ST segment
depression

Severe hyperkalemia

No P wave

QRS widens

- abdominal cramps
- diarrhea
- oliguria.

WHAT TO DO IMMEDIATELY

If your patient shows signs or symptoms of hyperkalemia or if his serum potassium level exceeds 5.2 mEq/L, notify the physician. Then take these actions:

- Place the patient on continuous cardiac monitoring and watch for ECG evidence of hyperkalemia. Suspect *severe* hyperkalemia if P waves are absent, T waves are peaked, and QRS complexes are broad.
- Establish I.V. access. Administer I.V. sodium bicarbonate solution, as prescribed, to promote shifting of potassium from extracellular to intracellular fluid.
- As prescribed, administer I.V. insulin (which lowers the serum glucose level, promoting potassium influx into cells) and I.V. glucose (which counteracts the serum glucose drop and prevents hypoglycemia and insulin shock).
- Anticipate the administration of oral or nasogastric sodium polystyrene sulfonate (Kayexalate) to reduce serum potassium, as prescribed.
- If your patient has severe hyperkalemia and needs immediate myocardial stabilization, anticipate administering I.V. calcium gluconate (typically, 10 to 12 ml of 10% solution).
- ➡ Nurse**ALERT** Before giving calcium gluconate, check the patient's medication history for digoxin use. Calcium gluconate enhances

digoxin's effects and increases the risk of toxicity. If you must administer calcium to a patient on digoxin, watch closely for evidence of toxicity, including nausea, fatigue, vision changes, and arrhythmias.

➡ **NurseALERT** A too-rapid infusion of calcium gluconate can cause bradycardia. Monitor the patient's ECG continuously.

- Don't administer calcium gluconate together with a bicarbonate solution; combining the two causes an instant interaction that produces a precipitate of white sediment.
- Obtain blood samples for repeat measurements of serum potassium and other electrolytes as well as blood urea nitrogen (BUN) and creatinine levels (to evaluate renal function). To ensure accurate results, don't withdraw blood above the site of a potassium infusion, and don't leave the tourniquet on the patient's arm for a prolonged period before drawing the blood. Also, instruct the patient not to clench and unclench his fist before you withdraw blood.
- Check the patient's blood pressure and pulse and respiratory rates every 5 to 15 minutes.
- Evaluate his neuromuscular function every 5 to 15 minutes, including assessing for paralysis and paresthesias of the leg and trunk muscles.
- Keep a manual resuscitation bag, endotracheal intubation set, defibrillator, and emergency medications on hand in case of cardiac arrest. Prepare to assist with cardiopulmonary resuscitation if the patient's heart or respiratory muscles fail.
- Administer supplemental oxygen, if prescribed.
- Monitor oxygen saturation levels using pulse oximetry or arterial blood gas analysis.
- Withhold all oral intake and prepare for endotracheal intubation and mechanical ventilation, if indicated, for respiratory distress.

WHAT TO DO NEXT

Once you've taken initial steps, carry out these measures:

- Continue to monitor the patient's BUN and serum electrolyte and creatinine levels.
- Frequently monitor his blood pressure and pulse and respiratory rates.
- Regularly observe his ECG for bradycardia and other arrhythmias.
- Continue to monitor the patient's neuromuscular function for improvement of paralysis or paresthesias.
- Check the I.V. site for signs and symptoms of infiltration, such as redness, swelling, warmth to the touch, and pain. If infiltration occurs, discontinue the I.V. line, apply warm soaks, and start a new line.
- For the duration of insulin and glucose therapy, obtain fingerstick blood glucose levels frequently and assess the patient for signs and symptoms of hypoglycemia, such as muscle weakness, excessive hunger, diaphoresis, changes in mental status, and loss of consciousness.
- Monitor the patient's fluid intake and output hourly.

- Anticipate the possible need for dialysis—either as a last resort or as an early treatment for a patient with kidney disease. If dialysis is ordered, help prepare the patient.

FOLLOW-UP CARE
- Continue to monitor the patient's BUN and serum electrolyte and creatinine levels.
- Keep a close watch on his cardiac status, including heart rate, ECG characteristics, and blood pressure.
- Carefully record the patient's hourly fluid intake and output.
- Continue with regular checks of the patient's neuromuscular status, assessing extremities for paralysis or paresthesias.
- Restrict your patient to bed rest until his serum electrolyte levels return to normal. Be aware that until then, he may experience weakness, paresthesias, and some degree of paralysis.
- Obtain a complete patient history to help identify the underlying cause of hyperkalemia and to guide treatment.

SPECIAL CONSIDERATIONS
- Make sure you send the patient's blood samples to the laboratory immediately. For accurate electrolyte measurement, serum must be separated from cells within 1 hour after withdrawal. Suspect poor blood withdrawal technique if laboratory results show a high serum potassium level in a patient without characteristic ECG changes. If in doubt about the accuracy of test results, obtain another blood sample, using a centrally inserted catheter, if possible .
- Keep in mind that treatment for hyperkalemia may lead to hypokalemia. Watch for such signs and symptoms as dizziness, hypotension, characteristic ECG changes (flattened T wave, elevated U wave, depressed ST segment), nausea, vomiting, diarrhea, reduced peristalsis, muscle weakness and fatigue, leg cramps, polyuria, irritability, confusion, speech changes, decreased reflexes, and respiratory paralysis.
- Be aware that although calcium gluconate temporarily protects the heart, it doesn't lower the serum potassium level.

HYPERNATREMIA

An abnormally elevated serum sodium level (greater than 145 mEq/L), hypernatremia represents a deficit of extracellular fluid (ECF) volume relative to ECF sodium content, and can occur with normal, decreased, or increased ECF volume. (See *About sodium.*)

It's most common in infants, debilitated elderly people, and seriously ill patients of all ages. Infants are at risk because they can't ask for fluids when thirsty; elderly people, because osmotic stimulation of thirst and the kidneys' ability to conserve water diminish with age.

Hypernatremia occurs when sodium gains exceed water gains or when water losses exceed sodium losses, as in the following conditions:

- burns (second- or third-degree)
- decreased fluid intake or lack of access to fluids
- diabetes insipidus
- excessive adrenocortical hormones
- excessive salt ingestion
- excessive parenteral administration of sodium-containing fluids (such as hypertonic 3% or 5% saline solution), sodium bicarbonate given to treat cardiac arrest or lactic acidosis, or normal saline solution used to treat primary fluid loss
- fever
- GI sodium losses (as through diarrhea, vomiting, or naso-gastric suctioning)
- high-protein feedings without adequate water intake
- hyperalimentation or other hypertonic fluid administration
- hyperventilation
- osmotic diuresis
- potent diuretic therapy without sufficient water replacement
- profuse perspiration
- renal conditions, such as renal failure, acute tubular necrosis, postobstructive uropathy, and hypokalemic or hypercalcemic nephropathy.

ABOUT SODIUM

The most abundant cation (positively charged ion) in extracellular fluid (ECF), sodium plays a major role in fluid and electrolyte balance, maintaining the distribution of water and ECF volume. Sodium also:
- aids transmission of nerve impulses
- facilitates muscle contraction
- maintains ECF serum osmolarity
- affects electrolyte concentration, absorption, and excretion (through its interaction with chloride, potassium, and other electrolytes)
- helps maintain acid-base balance.

A number of factors, such as systolic blood pressure, extracellular osmolarity, and adrenal and pituitary hormones, work together to influence kidney excretion or reabsorption of sodium to maintain normal sodium and water balance.

In severe hypernatremia, increased plasma osmolality causes water to shift out of the cells. This shift induces brain cell dehydration, which may lead to cerebral edema and, ultimately, death. Your quick response may prevent your patient's condition from progressing to seizures, coma, and permanent neurologic damage.

WHAT TO LOOK FOR
Signs and symptoms of hypernatremia commonly include:
- irritability
- altered level of consciousness, ranging from lethargy to coma (depending on the speed of hypernatremia's onset)
- disorientation, delusions, or hallucinations (with severe hypernatremia)
- weakness
- muscle irritability and twitching
- hyperreflexia
- seizures
- postural hypotension (with fluid volume depletion)
- pulmonary edema and increased venous pressure (with fluid volume excess)
- flushed skin
- dry, swollen tongue
- dry, sticky mucous membranes

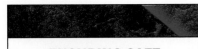

ENSURING SAFE SODIUM CORRECTION

When administering I.V. fluids to correct your patient's hypernatremia, remember that slower is better. An overly rapid fall in the serum sodium level may cause cerebral edema, seizures, permanent neurologic damage, and death.

That's because with prolonged hypernatremia, the brain adapts to a hyperosmolar state by increasing its osmolality. Once cerebral adaptation has occurred, a rapid decrease in the serum sodium level creates an osmotic gradient that allows water to move back into the brain cells. This in turn causes intracellular cerebral edema, which may progress to death.

MONITORING SODIUM REDUCTION

To ensure safe reduction of the serum sodium level, record the time I.V. fluid therapy was initiated and monitor your patient's repeat serum sodium measurements closely. The sodium level should drop to normal over no less than 48 hours. Also monitor and document the I.V. infusion rate and the patient's serum osmolality values.

- thirst
- fever
- decreased urine output.

WHAT TO DO IMMEDIATELY

Notify the physician if your patient shows signs or symptoms of hypernatremia or if she has a serum sodium level above 145 mEq/L, serum osmolality above 295 mEq/L, and urine specific gravity above 1.030. (Double-check your facility's specific reference values.) Then take the following actions:

- Obtain blood samples for repeat measurements of serum sodium, chloride, and osmolarity.
- Obtain a urine specimen to determine urine osmolality and sodium concentration.
- Establish I.V. access. As prescribed, administer a hypotonic electrolyte solution (0.2% or half-normal saline solution) or a salt-free solution. To help prevent hyponatremia, alternate these solutions, if ordered.
- Administer dextrose 5% in water I.V., as prescribed. Because this solution causes diuresis, be sure to monitor the patient's urine output and urine specific gravity closely.
- Record your patient's fluid intake and output accurately to prevent overly rapid fluid infusion. Remember that reduced output may lead to cerebral edema and circulatory overload.
- Monitor the patient for telltale signs of cerebral edema, including lethargy, headache, nausea, vomiting, bradycardia, and hypertension.
- Record the time I.V. therapy was initiated to help ensure a gradual reduction of the patient's sodium concentration.

➡ **Nurse**ALERT To avoid catastrophic cerebral changes, hypernatremia must be corrected gradually, not rapidly. (See *Ensuring safe sodium correction.*)

- Place the patient on continuous cardiac monitoring, as indicated. Monitor the ECG for changes in heart rate.
- Initiate seizure precautions, such as padding and raising the side rails, and keep emergency airway equipment on hand. Protect the seizure-prone patient from self-injury and loss of I.V. access. If a seizure occurs, maintain a patent airway, notify the physician, and administer anticonvulsants, as prescribed. After the seizure, assess the patient and immediately obtain a blood sample to evaluate her fluid and electrolyte status.
- Assess the patient's blood pressure and pulse and respiratory rates every 5 to 15 minutes. Monitor for bradycardia and hypertension.
- Evaluate the patient's level of consciousness every 5 to 15 minutes, noting agitation, confusion, or disorientation. Be aware that loss of consciousness may signal permanent neurologic damage.

WHAT TO DO NEXT

Once your patient is stable, take the following actions:

- Monitor the patient's vital signs and mental status every hour. As her serum sodium level decreases, expect an improving level of consciousness and increasing muscle strength.
- Continue to monitor the I.V. fluid infusion rate to ensure gradual correction of hypernatremia.
- Monitor the patient's serum sodium, chloride, and osmolality levels.
- Continue to monitor urine specific gravity, osmolality, and other ordered urine tests.
- Continue to monitor her hourly fluid intake and output.
- Maintain seizure precautions, as indicated. If the patient is receiving anticonvulsants, check for therapeutic serum levels.
- Observe the I.V. site for signs of infiltration, such as redness, swelling, warmth, tenderness, and pain. If any occur, discontinue the I.V. line, apply warm compresses, and restart therapy at new I.V. site.

FOLLOW-UP CARE

- Continue to monitor the patient's serum and urine laboratory test results for the duration of I.V. fluid therapy.
- Continue to document her fluid intake and output carefully.
- Regularly assess her mental status, including level of consciousness and orientation to time, place, and person.
- Maintain seizure precautions, as needed. As the patient's electrolyte imbalance improves, her risk for seizures decreases.
- Restrict your patient to bed rest until her serum electrolyte values normalize. Otherwise, she may be weak and confused and may experience orthostatic hypotension.
- Obtain a complete patient history to help identify the underlying cause of hypernatremia and guide long-term treatment.

SPECIAL CONSIDERATIONS

- Keep in mind that elderly patients may not experience the thirst sensation that often accompanies hypernatremia, so frequently remind them to drink water and remain vigilant in recording intake and output.
- To prevent excessive sodium intake, teach the patient and family members to avoid processed foods, over-the-counter medications with high sodium content, and using table salt for cooking.

HYPERTENSIVE CRISIS

Hypertensive crisis refers to a sharp increase in diastolic blood pressure (to above 120 mm Hg) that comes on suddenly, over a few hours or days, with the patient showing signs and symptoms of organ damage. A medical emergency, hypertensive crisis requires prompt recognition and intervention with I.V. drugs to avoid further damage to the brain, heart, blood vessels, kidneys, and retinas and reduce the risk of death.

The sharp increase in blood pressure may damage the arteriolar linings, resulting in necrosis of the tunica intima and tunica media. These arteriolar changes may in turn damage target organs, particularly the kidneys and retinas, possibly causing renal failure and blindness.

Some patients in hypertensive crisis experience hypertensive encephalopathy, in which extremely high blood pressure impairs the autoregulatory mechanisms of cerebral arterioles. Consequently, cerebral blood flow greatly increases, leading to cerebral edema, rupture of tiny cerebral vessels, and microinfarcts. Without immediate intervention, the patient may suffer irreversible brain damage.

Causes of hypertensive crisis

Conditions that may precipitate hypertensive crisis include:
- chronic, uncontrolled hypertension
- subarachnoid or cerebrovascular hemorrhage, cerebral infarction
- pheochromocytoma
- acute or chronic renal failure
- eclampsia or preeclampsia
- monoamine oxidase (MAO) inhibitors taken with tyramine-containing foods
- abrupt withdrawal of antihypertensive medication
- use of cocaine or crack.

WHAT TO LOOK FOR

Along with the abrupt rise in diastolic pressure to a level above 120 mm Hg, clinical findings in hypertensive crisis may include:
- severe headache
- blurred vision or diplopia
- dizziness
- tinnitus
- vertigo
- epistaxis
- muscle twitching
- tachycardia or other arrhythmias
- narrowed pulse pressure
- distended neck veins
- nausea and vomiting
- irritability, confusion, or stupor.

Findings in hypertensive encephalopathy

A patient with hypertensive encephalopathy may have:
- decreased level of consciousness, ranging from lethargy to coma
- disorientation, confusion
- severe headache

- seizures
- fluctuating focal neurologic deficits, including cortical blindness, hemiparesis, and unilateral sensory deficits.

Retinal findings
If hypertensive crisis involves the retinas, signs may include:
- acute retinopathy and hemorrhage (on fundal examination)
- retinal exudates
- papilledema.

Renal findings
If the severe blood pressure elevation affects kidney function, clinical findings may include:
- hematuria
- reduced urine output
- increasing blood urea nitrogen (BUN) and serum creatinine levels.

Cardiopulmonary findings
With cardiopulmonary involvement, signs and symptoms may include:
- chest pain
- tachycardia
- pedal edema
- ECG changes that suggest ischemia or infarction
- orthostatic dizziness
- indications of heart failure (including S_3 and S_4 heart sounds, crackles, dyspnea, and jugular vein distention)
- changes in cardiac enzyme levels that suggest myocardial infarction.

Neurologic findings
If the central nervous system is involved, clinical findings may include:
- altered level of consciousness (irritability, drowsiness, confusion, or coma)

WHAT TO DO IMMEDIATELY
If you suspect that your patient is in hypertensive crisis, notify the physician. Then take these actions:
- Establish and maintain a patent airway. Remember—hypertensive crisis commonly causes decreased level of consciousness, which can lead to airway occlusion.
- Begin continuous blood pressure monitoring. Be prepared to use an automatic blood pressure cuff. As ordered, assist with insertion of an intra-arterial line for direct pressure monitoring.
- Determine the patient's mean arterial pressure (MAP) by using the following formula:

$$MAP = \frac{\text{diastolic pressure} + (\text{systolic pressure} - \text{diastolic pressure})}{3}$$

H

- Watch carefully for signs and symptoms of hypertensive encephalopathy.
- ➡ **NurseALERT** Be aware that neurologic signs and symptoms may mimic those of cerebrovascular accident.
- Assess the patient's oxygen saturation level using pulse oximetry or arterial blood gas (ABG) analysis. Administer supplemental oxygen, as indicated.
- Begin continuous cardiac monitoring.
- Start an I.V. line, and administer antihypertensive medications, as prescribed.
- ➡ **NurseALERT** Keep in mind that although your initial goal is to reduce the patient's MAP by 25% to 30%, lowering blood pressure too fast can cause cerebral ischemia by reducing cerebral blood flow.
- Administer nitroprusside sodium (Nitropress), as prescribed. (See *Giving nitroprusside sodium safely.*)
- Prepare to give other I.V. vasodilators, such as nitroglycerin (Nitro-Bid), diazoxide (Hyperstat), nicardipine (Cardene), or hydralazine (Apresoline), as prescribed.
- Administer adrenergic inhibitors (such as phentolamine [Regitine], labetalol [Trandate], and methyldopa [Aldomet]) and ACE inhibitors (such as enalapril [Vasotec]), if prescribed.
- If your patient is retaining sodium and water, expect the physician to prescribe diuretics.
- Titrate drug doses to achieve the target blood pressure set by the physician while continuously monitoring your patient's blood pressure. Reduce or stop the medication if his blood pressure falls below the target range.

WHAT TO DO NEXT
After the initial crisis eases and your patient becomes stable, take these measures:
- Monitor his blood pressure at least every hour, as ordered.
- Obtain vital signs frequently, and assess heart and breath sounds. Check his ECG for arrhythmias and ischemic changes.
- Monitor fluid intake and output hourly to assess renal function and response to diuretics (if given). Also check for hematuria.
- Assess the patient frequently for a decreasing level of consciousness or deteriorating mental status. Ask him about the severity of his headaches, and administer analgesics, as needed and prescribed.
- Ask the patient if he is having vision problems.
- Report seizures immediately.
- ➡ **NurseALERT** If your patient shows signs of hypertensive encephalopathy, institute seizure precautions, such as raising and padding the side rails.
- Monitor the patient for signs and symptoms of heart failure, such as S_3 and S_4 heart sounds, jugular vein distention, tachycardia, crackles, and dyspnea.

TREATMENT OF CHOICE

GIVING NITROPRUSSIDE SODIUM SAFELY

With its fast onset and short duration of action, nitroprusside sodium is the most effective and potent treatment for hypertensive emergency. By relaxing arteries and veins, it decreases arterial and venous pressures and lowers systemic vascular resistance.

You'll need to monitor your patient carefully during nitroprusside sodium therapy. Ideally, the drug should be given only in a critical care setting. If you need to administer it, follow these guidelines:

- Dilute 50 mg of nitroprusside sodium in 2 to 3 ml of dextrose 5% in water (D_5W), and then dilute this in 250 to 1,000 ml of D_5W, as ordered. For hypertensive emergency, the physician typically orders an I.V. infusion of 0.3 to 10.0 µg/kg/minute. Always use an infusion pump for more accurate delivery.
- Wrap the container of nitroprusside sodium solution in aluminum foil to protect it from light.
- Change the solution every 12 to 24 hours, according to your facility's policy. Discard the solution if it turns blue, green, or dark red.
- Monitor the patient's blood pressure directly by way of an intra-arterial catheter.
- Assess for adverse drug effects, including nausea, vomiting, muscle spasms, dizziness, headache, hypotension, sweating, and restlessness.
- Watch for evidence of thiocyanate and cyanide toxicity. Toxicity may arise because the liver converts cyanide (the metabolic product of nitroprusside) to thiocyanate, which the kidneys then eliminate. Serum bicarbonate and anion gap offer the earliest evidence of cyanide toxicity.

PRECAUTIONS
- Always give nitroprusside sodium as a separate I.V. infusion. Never mix it with other drugs in solution.
- Remember that a patient with hepatic or renal insufficiency is at risk for drug toxicity if he receives nitroprusside sodium for more than 2 days. Signs and symptoms of thiocyanate toxicity, most common at blood drug levels of 5 to 10 mg/dl, include fatigue, nausea, anorexia, rash, headache, disorientation, and psychotic behavior. Blood levels above 20 mg/dl are dangerous.
- Nitroprusside is generally contraindicated for patients with increased intracranial pressure or impaired cerebral circulation.

H

- Maintain a quiet environment and administer sedatives, as prescribed, to reduce your patient's anxiety.

FOLLOW-UP CARE
- Administer oral antihypertensives, as ordered, once your patient's blood pressure stabilizes.
- Continue to monitor his blood pressure.
- Monitor laboratory test results for thiocyanate and cyanide levels if the patient is receiving nitroprusside sodium. Also monitor his cardiac enzymes, hematocrit, BUN, and serum creatinine and electrolyte levels. Report any abnormalities.

SPECIAL CONSIDERATIONS
- Keep in mind that antihypertensives can lead to hypotension, including severe orthostatic hypotension. Continue to monitor your patient's blood pressure carefully, and urge him to rise slowly from a supine position to a sitting position and remain in that position for a few minutes before standing.
- To make sure you're obtaining accurate blood pressure readings, use a cuff of the proper size for your patient. Using a cuff that's too small will cause a reading that's falsely elevated.

- If your patient has an intra-arterial line, frequently assess its integrity, observing carefully for signs of disconnection, dislodgment, and other complications.
- Be aware that hypertensive crisis may result from certain drug interactions—for example, MAO inhibitors given with tricyclic antidepressants, propranolol (Inderal), or meperidine (Demerol). If your patient takes an MAO inhibitor, warn him to avoid foods that contain the amino acid tyramine because the interaction could cause hypertensive crisis. Such foods include chicken liver, yeast, strong or aged cheeses, sour cream, coffee, wine, beer, raisins, chocolate, overripe bananas, avocados, and soy sauce.
- Discuss with your patient the importance of having his blood pressure checked regularly. Urge him not to skip appointments or stop taking prescribed antihypertensive medications without consulting his physician. Tell him the names, indications, dosages, schedules, and possible adverse effects of all medications he'll be taking at home.

HYPERTHERMIA

Normally, the hypothalamus regulates the body's temperature within a narrow range by balancing heat production, heat conservation, and heat loss. However, certain environmental and physical challenges (such as exogenous heat gain, increased endogenous heat production, and decreased heat dispersion) can result in a body temperature that rises too high. (See *Types of hyperthermia*.)

A persistently elevated body temperature can lead to excessive fluid loss and hypovolemic shock (heat exhaustion.) What's more, untreated hyperthermia can lead to failure of the patient's thermoregulatory mechanisms and heatstroke. If your patient develops hyperthermia, you'll need to assess her rapidly and intervene correctly to prevent life-threatening complications.

WHAT TO LOOK FOR
Clinical findings vary with the type of hyperthermia involved.

Heat cramps
- patient unaccustomed to heat
- strenuous activity in very warm climates
- severe, spasmodic cramps in abdomen and extremities
- prolonged sweating
- fever
- tachycardia
- elevated blood pressure.

Heat exhaustion
- exposure to high environmental temperatures
- prolonged elevation of core body temperature

TYPES OF HYPERTHERMIA

Types of hyperthermia include heat cramps, heat exhaustion, heatstroke, and malignant hyperthermia.

HEAT CRAMPS

Heat cramps usually occur in people who are not accustomed to heat and in those who perform strenuous activities in very warm climates. After prolonged sweating (and subsequent sodium loss), they experience severe, spasmodic cramps in the abdomen and extremities. Other findings may include fever, tachycardia, and elevated blood pressure.

HEAT EXHAUSTION

When a person is exposed to high environmental temperatures or experiences prolonged elevated core body temperatures—either of which causes profound vasodilation and profuse sweating—heat exhaustion may occur. This can lead to dehydration, decreased plasma volume, hypotension, decreased cardiac output, and tachycardia.

Typically, the person is alert and reports syncope or confusion. Other findings include normal, slightly elevated, or elevated temperature (up to 104° F [40° C]); pale, moist skin; weakness; dizziness; nausea; headache; and muscle cramping.

HEATSTROKE

The result of overstressed thermoregulatory activity within the body, heatstroke is usually caused by exposure to excessive heat or vigorous activity in warm weather. The brain's regulatory center stops functioning and, eventually, the sweat glands cease to function as well.

Usually, the patient exhibits bizarre behavior or irritability progressing to confusion, combativeness, delirium, and coma as well as tremors, seizures, and fixed and dilated pupils. Body temperature is greater than 105° F (40.6° C) with hypotension, rapid pulse (bounding or weak), tachypnea, and flushed, hot skin (in early heatstroke, skin may be moist, but as heatstroke progresses, the skin becomes dry because the sweat glands stop functioning). Death may result if treatment is not started immediately.

MALIGNANT HYPERTHERMIA

Characterized by life-threatening body temperature elevation and muscle rigidity, malignant hyperthermia is an autosomal dominant trait that typically occurs after a genetically predisposed patient receives a combination of a muscle relaxant, such as succinylcholine, and an inhalation general anesthetic, such as halothane.

Because of the muscle cell's faulty calcium channel regulator, an excessive amount of calcium enters the cell, causing sustained, uncoordinated skeletal muscle contraction. This increases oxygen consumption and raises the lactic acid level, causing acidosis. Acidosis leads to an increase in body temperature with tachycardia and arrhythmias, hypotension, decreased cardiac output, and cardiac arrest. General anesthesia diminishes heat loss.

The combination of heat production and inability to dissipate heat causes hyperthermia.

H

- profound vasodilation
- profuse sweating
- dehydration
- decreased plasma volume
- hypotension
- decreased cardiac output
- tachycardia
- syncope or confusion
- normal to elevated body temperature (up to 104° F [40° C])
- pale, moist skin
- weakness
- dizziness
- nausea
- headache
- muscle cramping.

Heatstroke

- body temperature above 105° F (40.6° C)
- reports of vigorous activity in high heat
- bizarre behavior or irritability progressing to confusion, combativeness, delirium, and coma
- tremors or seizures
- fixed, dilated pupils
- hypotension
- rapid pulse rate (bounding or weak)
- tachypnea
- flushed, hot skin (possibly moist at first but then dry when sweating ceases).

Malignant hyperthermia

- recent administration of a muscle relaxant, such as succinylcholine (Anectine), and an inhaled general anesthetic, such as halothane, to a genetically predisposed person
- life-threatening body temperature elevation
- muscle rigidity
- acidosis
- tachycardia and other arrhythmias
- hypotension
- decreased cardiac output
- cardiac arrest.

WHAT TO DO IMMEDIATELY

Successful treatment involves rapid reduction of core temperature. Notify the physician, and follow measures appropriate to your patient's condition.

For heat cramps

- Place the patient in a cool environment and give cool fluids.
- If she's too nauseated to drink cool fluids, establish I.V. access and administer I.V. fluids, as ordered. Anticipate the need for sodium replacement.
- Offer cool cloths and comfort measures.

For other hyperthermia types

- Assess the patient's airway, breathing, and circulation.
- Evaluate her oxygen saturation levels by way of pulse oximetry or arterial blood gas (ABG) analysis, as ordered; give supplemental oxygen as needed.
- Check the patient's vital signs and assess her core temperature every 15 to 30 minutes during early therapy.
- Place the patient in a cool environment (about 70° F [21.1° C]) and remove her clothes.

- Apply or spray tepid water on the patient's skin while fans blow over her to encourage evaporative heat loss.
- ➡ **NurseALERT** Avoid cold baths because of the increased risk for shivering, which increases metabolic rate and oxygen consumption. Watch for tensing or clenching of the patient's jaw muscles because it's an early indicator of shivering.
- Apply ice packs to the patient's groin, neck, axillary, and scalp areas. Alternatively, apply wet sheets or towels. Continue to have fans blowing over the patient to increase heat loss.
- Place the patient on a hypothermia blanket.
- If her temperature doesn't decline, anticipate the need for internal cooling measures, such as iced saline lavage, cool-fluid peritoneal dialysis, and cool-fluid bladder or rectal irrigation.
- Obtain a baseline neurologic assessment. If the patient has a reduced level of consciousness, take safety and seizure precautions.
- Begin continuous cardiac monitoring, as ordered. If arrhythmias develop, prepare to treat possible hyperkalemia and acidosis.
- Administer antipyretic therapy and I.V. fluid therapy, as ordered. Also give fluids orally if the patient has an intact gag reflex.
- If the patient is receiving a neuroleptic agent, discontinue it, as ordered.
- Anticipate insertion of a pulmonary artery or central venous catheter to evaluate the patient's hemodynamic parameters.
- Obtain laboratory tests, as ordered, including complete blood count, coagulation studies, and serum electrolyte and liver enzyme levels.

WHAT TO DO NEXT
Once your patient's temperature begins to decline, take these steps:
- Anticipate insertion of an indwelling urinary catheter to assess her hourly urine output.
- Monitor cooling measures and core temperature continuously. Your goal is to reduce the patient's temperature to 102° F (38.9° C) as rapidly as possible without causing hypothermia.
- ➡ **NurseALERT** Keep in mind that hyperthermia may spontaneously recur within about 4 hours after the initial temperature reduction.
- Assess the patient's neurologic status every 30 to 60 minutes.
- Continue to assess her respiratory status and ABG values for changes. If her oxygen saturation and respiratory status deteriorate, anticipate endotracheal intubation and mechanical ventilation.
- Monitor her ECG continuously for changes that suggest ischemia or arrhythmias.
- Administer benzodiazepines and phenothiazines, as ordered, for shivering or anxiety.
- Follow her laboratory results, including complete blood count, clotting studies, and serum electrolyte, liver enzyme, and creatine kinase levels.

- Keep the patient on complete bed rest until her temperature returns to normal.
- If she has malignant hyperthermia, give I.V. dantrolene (Dantrium), as ordered.

FOLLOW-UP CARE
- Continue to monitor all physiologic parameters for changes.
- Continue cooling measures, as indicated. Discontinue active measures when her temperature reaches 102° F (38.9° C). Remember that her temperature will continue to fall even after cooling measures have stopped.
- Assess the patient's renal function to identify rhabdomyolysis as a possible complication.
- Monitor for the presence of a hematologic disorder because coagulopathy may occur. Monitor laboratory studies.

SPECIAL CONSIDERATIONS
- Teach patients at risk for heat exhaustion and heatstroke about preventive measures.
- If malignant hyperthermia is the cause, educate the patient and her family about the condition, what triggers it, and ways to avoid it.

HYPERVOLEMIA

An abnormal increase in extracellular fluid (ECF) volume, hypervolemia may involve the interstitial or intravascular space. Water balance profoundly influences the composition of both ECF and intracellular fluid. To maintain fluid balance, the distribution of electrolytes and other substances in the body's fluid compartments must remain fairly constant.

In hypervolemia, the normal balance of ECF is disrupted and expands. This expansion may result from the following conditions:
- excessive replacement of isotonic I.V. fluids
- excessive sodium and water intake
- excessive sodium and water retention (as in heart failure, cirrhosis, and corticosteroid therapy)
- reduced excretion of sodium and water (as in acute or chronic renal failure)
- shifting of fluid from the interstitial to the intravascular space (as in burn injuries and hypertonic I.V. fluid therapy)
- too-rapid infusion of blood or blood products.

Hypervolemia is rare in a patient with normal cardiac and renal function because his body can compensate for the excess fluid volume. However, with underlying cardiac or renal dysfunction, adequate compensation doesn't occur, and the patient may progress to heart failure and pulmonary edema.

Stay alert for characteristic signs and symptoms of this potentially life-threatening condition, and be prepared to intervene promptly. Your quick actions may prevent this condition from progressing to cardiopulmonary arrest.

WHAT TO LOOK FOR
Clinical findings in hypervolemia may include:
- weight gain
- restlessness and anxiety
- moist skin
- distended neck veins
- hypertension
- polyuria (in a patient with normal renal function)
- tachycardia
- bounding peripheral pulses
- dyspnea
- crackles and wheezes
- rapid respirations
- peripheral edema
- ascites (see *Assessing for ascites,* page 202).

Some patients also show signs and symptoms of pulmonary edema, including a persistent cough (with frothy, pink fluid when edma is severe), paroxysmal nocturnal dyspnea, orthopnea, labored and rapid breathing, and a decreased level of consciousness.

Diagnostic tests
Diagnostic indicators of hypervolemia include:
- decreased hematocrit and serum electrolyte and osmolarity levels
- increased blood urea nitrogen (BUN) and serum creatinine levels (in patients with renal failure)
- increased central venous pressure, pulmonary artery pressure, and pulmonary artery wedge pressure
- fluid in the chest (diffuse haziness of the lung field on X-ray).

WHAT TO DO IMMEDIATELY
If you suspect that your patient has hypervolemia, notify the physician. Then take the following measures:
- Obtain blood samples, as ordered, for repeat measurement of hematocrit as well as BUN and serum electrolyte, creatinine, and osmolarity levels.
- Place the patient on continuous cardiac monitoring, and observe his ECG for signs of heart failure.
- Measure the patient's blood pressure and pulse and respiratory rates every 5 to 15 minutes. Stay especially alert for tachycardia, which may indicate heart failure.

H

ASSESSING FOR ASCITES

In a patient with hypervolemia, abdominal distention may signal ascites—an abnormal accumulation of intraperitoneal fluid. To evaluate for ascites, check for shifting dullness and an abdominal fluid wave.

DETECTING SHIFTING DULLNESS

If your patient has ascites, the location at which his abdominal percussion note changes from tympany to dullness will shift with gravity when he changes position. By marking that shift, you can confirm ascites.

Start by percussing from the umbilicus outward toward the flank with the patient in a supine position. Mark the skin at the point where tympany changes to dullness. Now have the patient turn onto his side. Percuss again, marking the change from tympany to dullness. Any difference between the two lines may signal ascites.

EVALUATING FOR A FLUID WAVE

Another test for ascites involves assessing for a fluid wave. For this examination, have an assistant place a hand and forearm vertically against the patient's abdomen, as shown in the illustration. Doing so helps to block transmission of a wave through fat tissue.

Now place your hands on either side of the patient's abdomen. With one hand, strike one side of the abdomen sharply with your fingertips and, with the other hand resting lightly on the skin surface, note whether you feel a wavelike reaction to the blow on the opposite side of the abdomen. If you do, the patient may have ascites.

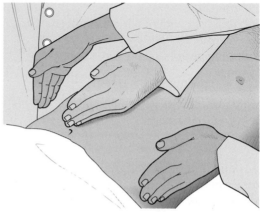

Assessing for a fluid wave

➡ **NurseALERT** To detect pulmonary edema early, evaluate the patient's respiratory status closely. Check for cough, dyspnea, and labored, rapid breathing. Auscultate his lungs for breath sounds, and check for distended neck veins.

• Prepare to assist with insertion of a central venous or pulmonary artery catheter to track the patient's hemodynamic status.

• Establish I.V. access. As prescribed, administer diuretics, such as furosemide (Lasix) and bumetanide (Bumex).

➡ **NurseALERT** Remember that these diuretics increase potassium excretion. When administering them, watch closely for signs and symptoms of hypokalemia, including fatigue, muscle cramps or weakness, paralysis, and such ECG changes as depressed ST segments, broad or inverted T waves, and enlarging U waves.

• Monitor the patient's fluid output and urine specific gravity, and report significant changes. Anticipate the need for an indwelling urinary catheter to ensure accurate output measurement.

• Prepare the patient for chest X-rays, as indicated.

• Monitor oxygen saturation using pulse oximetry or arterial blood gas analysis. Administer supplemental oxygen, as prescribed. Anticipate the need for endotracheal intubation and mechanical ventilation if respiratory distress occurs.

WHAT TO DO NEXT
Once your patient is stable, carry out the following interventions:
- Monitor laboratory studies, including hematocrit; BUN levels; serum electrolyte, osmolarity, and creatinine levels; and urine osmolarity level, every 4 hours, as ordered. Report significant changes immediately.
- Monitor the patient's vital signs every hour, and report changes that suggest cardiac or respiratory insufficiency. Especially watch for changes in respiratory rate, rhythm, and depth; breath sounds; and oxygen saturation.
- Restrict the patient's fluid and sodium intake, as ordered. To help prevent circulatory overload and cardiopulmonary complications, the physician may want to restrict all fluids, including I.V., oral, and enteral.
- If the patient has new-onset ascites of unexplained origin, assist with paracentesis to help identify the cause. Before this procedure, measure abdominal girth to establish a baseline. Then remeasure his girth at least daily. Report increases to the physician. (See *Assisting with paracentesis,* page 204.)
- Weigh the patient to establish a baseline, and then weigh him daily, watching for changes in fluid balance. Report weight gains.
- Be aware that your patient will need additional treatment if he experiences renal insufficiency.
- If the physician orders dialysis to remove excess fluid, prepare the patient for the procedure.
- As prescribed, administer total parenteral nutrition with concentrated nutrients to decrease fluid intake while ensuring adequate nutrition.
- Monitor for progression of peripheral edema, and check for pitting edema.

FOLLOW-UP CARE
- Continue to monitor the patient's laboratory results throughout therapy.
- Closely monitor the patient's fluid intake and output and urine specific gravity. Assess renal function indicators continually to detect signs of renal insufficiency or the need for dialysis.
- Keep the patient's head elevated to promote optimal ventilation and relieve dyspnea.

SPECIAL CONSIDERATIONS
- Teach the patient about the importance of maintaining fluid and electrolyte balance, such as by restricting his fluid or sodium intake or both.

H

ASSISTING WITH PARACENTESIS

A patient with ascites may require paracentesis to remove excess fluid from his abdomen and help determine the cause. When assisting with this procedure, use standard infection-control precautions and follow these steps.

BEFORE THE PROCEDURE
- Explain the procedure to the patient.
- Bring necessary supplies to the patient's bedside.
- Help the patient into an upright position on the edge of the bed, with his feet supported on a footstool or chair.
- Begin monitoring the patient's blood pressure.

DURING THE PROCEDURE
- Support the patient and urge him to stay still and upright.
- After injecting a local anesthetic, the physician inserts a trocar through a puncture wound in the abdomen, midline and below the umbilicus. The fluid drains slowly from the peritoneal cavity into a vacuum bottle or syringe.

- Monitor the patient's vital signs throughout the procedure, watching for signs of vascular collapse, such as pallor, decreased blood pressure, and an increased pulse rate.
- After fluid removal is completed and the physician removes the trocar, apply a dressing over the incision site.

AFTERCARE
- Help the patient to a comfortable sitting or lying position.
- Measure and document the amount of fluid withdrawn, including the number of specimens collected.
- Send the specimens to the laboratory for analysis.
- Monitor the patient's vital signs every 15 minutes for the first hour, every 30 minutes for the second hour, every hour for the next 4 hours, and then every 4 hours for 24 hours.
- Regularly inspect the dressing over the incision. If you note fluid leakage around the site, alert the physician.

- Also teach the patient to weigh himself daily at the same time of day, wearing clothing of similar weight. Tell him to report a sudden weight gain of 3 lb (1.4 kg) or more.
- Teach the patient about the underlying condition or disease process responsible for his hypervolemic state.

HYPOCALCEMIA

Hypocalcemia is defined as a total serum calcium level below 8.5 mg/dl or an ionized calcium level below 4.0 mg/dl. When acute, this electrolyte imbalance is a medical emergency because it increases neuromuscular excitability, causes laryngeal spasm, and impairs respiratory function. Hypocalcemia also may alter cardiac conduction, possibly triggering ventricular arrhythmias and heart failure. (See *About calcium,* page 172.)

Hypocalcemia usually occurs secondary to such medical conditions as:
- acute pancreatitis
- alkalosis
- hyperphosphatemia
- hypomagnesemia
- hypoparathyroidism

- malabsorption syndrome
- renal insufficiency
- severe burns, diarrhea, or infection
- vitamin D deficiency
- massive blood transfusions
- drugs, such as loop diuretics, aluminum-containing antacids, phosphates, plicamycin (Mithracin), or calcitonin.

If your patient develops hypocalcemia, her well-being may hinge on your expert and rapid response. Make sure you can identify the signs and symptoms of this disorder and know how to intervene appropriately.

WHAT TO LOOK FOR
Signs and symptoms vary with the severity of hypocalcemia, speed of onset, and the underlying cause. Acute hypocalcemia causes more severe signs and symptoms than chronic hypocalcemia, to which the body may adapt over time.

Neurologic signs and symptoms may include:
- anxiety
- irritability
- personality changes
- altered mental status
- tingling sensations around the mouth, hands, and feet
- increased deep tendon reflexes
- tetany, characterized by muscle twitching and cramps, carpopedal spasm, and (with severe hypocalcemia) laryngospasm and seizures (see *Identifying hypocalcemic tetany,* page 206)
- painful tonic muscle spasms.

Cardiac signs and symptoms may include:
- prolonged QT intervals on the ECG
- ventricular arrhythmias
- cardiac arrest.

GI signs and symptoms may include:
- nausea and vomiting
- diarrhea.

WHAT TO DO IMMEDIATELY
If your patient exhibits signs and symptoms of hypocalcemia, notify the physician. (Keep in mind that normal serum electrolyte values may differ among health-care facilities.) Then take these actions:
- Obtain blood samples for repeat measurement of total and ionized serum calcium and other serum electrolytes.
- Place the patient on continuous cardiac monitoring. Monitor her ECG for such changes as prolonged QT intervals and arrhythmias.

H

DANGER SIGNS AND SYMPTOMS

IDENTIFYING HYPOCALCEMIC TETANY

A life-threatening condition caused by hypocalcemia (low serum calcium levels), tetany is characterized by muscle twitching, cramps, seizures, and sharp wrist and ankle flexion. To detect hypocalcemic tetany, evaluate your patient for its classic signs.

TESTING FOR TROUSSEAU'S SIGN
Place a blood pressure cuff on your patient's upper arm and inflate the cuff to a point above her systolic pressure. Then watch her hand. If a carpopedal spasm—ventral contraction of the thumb and fingers—appears within 4 minutes, this is a positive Trousseau's sign.

TESTING FOR CHVOSTEK'S SIGN
Tap the patient's cheek over the facial nerve just in front of her ear, as shown in the illustration. As you do, watch for a positive response: abnormal contraction of the facial muscles, twitching of the lip, or, possibly, contraction of all muscles on one side of the face.

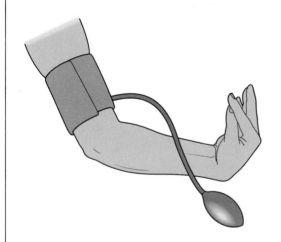

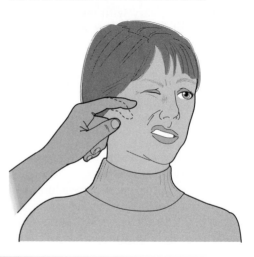

- Establish I.V. access. If prescribed, administer I.V. calcium (gluconate, chloride, or gluceptate solution). Be sure to note the amount of calcium administered and the amount of fluid infused. (See *Administering calcium safely*.)
- ➡ **NurseALERT** Before giving a calcium preparation, find out if the patient takes digoxin (Lanoxicaps). Calcium administration can result in hypercalemia, which enhances digoxin effects, placing the patient at greater risk for digitalis toxicity. When administering calcium, watch for evidence of digitalis toxicity, including arrhythmias, nausea, visual changes, and fatigue.
- Check the patient's blood pressure, pulse and respiratory rates, and mental status every 5 to 15 minutes.
- Observe for signs of neuromuscular irritability.
- Watch closely for signs of laryngeal obstruction, and frequently assess the patient's airway, breathing, and circulation. Keep a tracheostomy tray and manual resuscitation bag readily available in case of laryngospasm.

ADMINISTERING CALCIUM SAFELY

When administering calcium gluconate, chloride, or gluceptate solution to treat hypocalcemia, use standard precautions and follow the steps outlined below.
- Start an I.V. line if one isn't already in place. Remember that inserting a small needle into a large vein minimizes the risk of irritating the vein wall.
- When giving calcium as an infusion, use a volume-control device to ensure a consistent, accurate flow rate.
- If possible, warm the solution before administering it to prevent crystallization.
- As ordered, administer 7 to 14 mEq calcium—the usual adult dose for treatment of hypocalcemia.

IMPORTANT PRECAUTIONS
- To avoid incompatibilities, don't mix calcium with solutions containing carbonates, phosphates, or sulfates.
- Remember that giving calcium concomitantly with

digoxin enhances digoxin's effects and puts your patient at greater risk for toxicity. Watch closely for signs and symptoms of digitalis toxicity, including arrhythmias, nausea, visual changes, and fatigue.
- Monitor the patient's vital signs frequently during calcium therapy. Report bradycardia, hypotension, and syncope—signs of too-rapid calcium infusion. In addition, closely monitor the patient's fluid intake and output, which will also help prevent infusing calcium too rapidly.
- Anticipate the need for continuous cardiac monitoring to detect cardiac changes. If the patient complains of chest discomfort, stop the calcium infusion immediately and notify the physician.
- After calcium administration, keep the patient recumbent for about 15 minutes to prevent hypotension.

H

- If your patient has severe hypocalcemia, initiate seizure precautions, such as padding and raising the side rails, and bring emergency airway equipment to the bedside. If she has a seizure, protect her from injury, and notify the physician.
- As indicated, keep other emergency equipment (including intubation equipment, a defibrillator, and emergency medications) readily available in case of respiratory distress or heart failure.

WHAT TO DO NEXT
Once the patient is stable, take the following steps:
- Obtain a complete patient history to help identify the underlying cause of hypocalcemia and guide long-term treatment. Be sure to check for evidence of hypomagnesemia (a possible cause of hypocalcemia). Signs and symptoms of this magnesium imbalance include confusion, delusions, seizures, arrhythmias, hypotension, neuromuscular irritability, and leg and foot cramps.
- Continue to monitor her ionized or total serum calcium level and other electrolyte levels every 4 hours, as ordered. Report abnormalities at once.
- Monitor your patient's vital signs every hour for the duration of I.V. calcium therapy.
- Maintain continuous ECG monitoring, checking for prolonged QT intervals and ST segments, bradycardia, ventricular fibrillation, and other arrhythmias.

- Regularly assess the patient's neurologic status, including level of consciousness and personality changes.
- Insert an indwelling urinary catheter, as indicated, and monitor hourly fluid intake and output.

FOLLOW-UP CARE
- Continue to monitor your patient's laboratory test results.
- Be aware that treating hypocalcemia can lead to hypercalcemia. Monitor your patient for signs and symptoms of hypercalcemia, such as muscle weakness, decreased deep tendon reflexes, and confusion.
- Continue to document your patient's fluid intake and output to help prevent fluid overload from rapid I.V. fluid infusion.
- Frequently evaluate her respiratory status, including breath sounds and respiratory rate, rhythm, and depth.
- Continue to monitor the patient's neuromuscular status, assessing for Trousseau's and Chvostek's signs and muscle cramps and twitching.
- Frequently evaluate the patient's mental status for changes.
- Because calcium can irritate veins and cause tissue necrosis, monitor the I.V. site for signs of infiltration, such as redness, swelling, warmth, and pain. If infiltration occurs, discontinue I.V. therapy, apply warm compresses, and restart therapy at a new I.V. site.
- Maintain seizure precautions. Be aware that as your patient's serum calcium level returns to normal, her seizure risk decreases.

SPECIAL CONSIDERATIONS
- Don't combine supplemental calcium with bicarbonate or phosphate solutions; the interaction instantly produces a white precipitate.
- ➡ **NurseALERT** Rapid calcium infusion may cause bradycardia, which may trigger cardiac arrest. To prevent too-rapid infusion, use a volume-control device and monitor the infusion closely.
- Calcium chloride is more likely than other I.V. calcium preparations to increase the serum ionized calcium level.

HYPOGLYCEMIA

An acute, potentially fatal metabolic disorder, hypoglycemia refers to a blood glucose level of less than 60 mg/dl. Because brain cells require glucose to function, a glucose deficit rapidly can lead to brain damage and death. Hypoglycemia usually arises as a complication of treatment for diabetes mellitus. However, some people may experience it as a primary disorder or as a complication of another condition, such as adrenal insufficiency, myxedema, pancreatic cancer, and salicylate intoxication.

How hypoglycemia progresses
The sympathetic nervous system reacts to a low blood glucose level by releasing counterregulatory hormones (glucagon, epinephrine, cor-

tisol, and growth hormone) into the bloodstream. These hormones in turn stimulate the liver to release glucose and block insulin release from the pancreas—actions that account for early signs and symptoms of hypoglycemia.

In a diabetic patient, these compensatory mechanisms may not take place, and hypoglycemia quickly becomes life-threatening. Even in other patients, these mechanisms may not completely restore blood glucose to a normal level. As hypoglycemia progresses, late signs and symptoms arise, reflecting central nervous system involvement. Without treatment, permanent brain damage and, eventually, death are likely.

Your familiarity with the signs and symptoms of hypoglycemia and appropriate treatment is critical. You'll need to respond quickly to raise your patient's blood glucose level before devastating effects occur.

WHAT TO LOOK FOR

Early clinical findings in hypoglycemia may include:
- hunger
- weakness
- shakiness
- nervousness or anxiety
- palpitations
- tachycardia
- diaphoresis
- tingling of the lips, tongue, and fingers
- pallor around the nose and mouth.

Late findings involve the central nervous system and may include:
- dizziness
- drowsiness
- headache
- inability to concentrate
- confusion
- extreme fatigue
- slurred speech
- irritability
- anger or aggressive behavior
- blurred or double vision
- seizures
- incoordination
- coma
- decreased response time.

Be aware that the point at which hypoglycemia triggers obvious signs and symptoms varies greatly among individuals. One person may be asymptomatic, whereas another person with the identical blood glucose level shows classic signs and symptoms of hypoglycemia. Also, patients with long-standing, uncontrolled diabetes typically lose their ability to respond to sympathetic nervous stimulation and don't exhibit early (adrenergic) signs and symptoms.

WHAT TO DO IMMEDIATELY

If your patient's clinical findings or blood glucose level indicates hypoglycemia, notify the physician. Then take these steps:

- Rapidly assess the patient's airway, breathing, and circulation. If necessary, begin cardiopulmonary resuscitation at once.
- Quickly obtain a blood glucose reading.
- Administer 15 g of a simple carbohydrate. If the patient is conscious and able to swallow, give her a food or beverage. If she's unconscious or unable to swallow, quickly establish I.V. access and administer 25 g of dextrose 50%, as prescribed. If rapid insertion of an I.V. line isn't possible, give 1 mg of glucagon (0.5 mg for a child) by subcutaneous or intramuscular injection.
- Turn the patient onto her side so she won't aspirate vomitus. If she's unconscious, keep her on her side until she regains consciousness and is able to swallow.
- Institute seizure precautions, such as padding and raising the side rails and bringing an artificial airway to the bedside.

WHAT TO DO NEXT

After taking initial steps, follow these guidelines:

- Recheck the patient's blood glucose level 15 minutes after the initial treatment and every 15 minutes thereafter until it returns to normal.
- Assess the patient's vital signs and her response to the initial treatment.
- If her blood glucose level remains below normal, repeat the initial treatment measures every 15 minutes, as ordered, until her glucose rises to a normal level.
- Continue to maintain seizure precautions.

FOLLOW-UP CARE

- Try to determine the underlying cause of hypoglycemia.
- If the patient's next meal is more than 1 hour away or if she received glucagon, give her a snack consisting of one bread product and one meat product—for example, six crackers and 1 oz of cheese or half of a meat sandwich, consisting of 1 oz of meat and one slice of bread.
- Check the patient's blood glucose level every hour for several hours after a severe hypoglycemic reaction.

SPECIAL CONSIDERATIONS

- Teach the patient and family ways to avoid hypoglycemic recurrences and how to recognize signs and symptoms of hypoglycemia. Provide instructions on treating a hypoglycemic episode, including which foods or beverages to give and how to administer glucagon.

Instruct family members to call 911 if the patient doesn't respond within 15 minutes after glucagon administration.
- Advise the patient or family to call the physician if she has a severe hypoglycemic reaction (indicated by loss of consciousness or a blood glucose level below 40 mg/dl), if she has more than two unexplained reactions in 1 week, or if the reactions become more frequent or severe.

HYPOKALEMIA

When severe and untreated, hypokalemia can progress to cardiac or respiratory arrest and death. Although typically defined as a serum potassium level below 3.5 mEq/L, this electrolyte imbalance seldom causes clinically detectable signs until the potassium level drops below 3 mEq/L. (See *About potassium*, page 185.)

Hypokalemia can result from:
- anorexia, malnutrition (decreased potassium intake)
- antibiotics (such as carbenicillin and aminoglycosides)
- diarrhea
- excessive renal potassium losses as can occur with high mineralocorticoid secretion and distal (type I) or proximal (type II) renal tubular acidosis
- extreme diaphoresis
- glucocorticoid excess (for instance, Cushing's syndrome or excess steroid administration)
- liver disease
- hyperaldosteronism
- laxative or enema abuse
- magnesium deficiency
- malabsorption syndrome
- metabolic alkalosis
- nasogastric suctioning
- osmotic diuresis
- potassium-depleting diuretics (such as thiazide and loop diuretics)
- villous adenoma of the colon (rare)
- vomiting.

To help prevent the disastrous consequences of hypokalemia, make sure you're familiar with its clinical features and ready to respond with the proper treatment.

WHAT TO LOOK FOR
Clinical findings in hypokalemia may include:
- malaise, fatigue, generalized weakness
- decreased level of consciousness, lethargy, confusion
- muscle cramps, muscle twitches

- muscle weakness
- decreased deep tendon reflexes
- flaccid paralysis (starting in the legs and progressing to the trunk, arms, and facial and respiratory muscles)
- paresthesias
- ECG changes, such as depressed ST segments; broad or inverted T waves that flatten progressively; enlarging U waves that may hide the T wave, producing what resembles a prolonged QT interval; increased P-wave amplitude; prolonged PR interval; widened QRS complex; and atrial and ventricular arrhythmias (see *ECG changes in hypokalemia*)
- tachyarrhythmias
- orthostatic hypotension
- anorexia
- nausea and vomiting
- gaseous abdominal distention
- constipation
- decreased bowel sounds
- paralytic ileus
- dilute urine
- polyuria, nocturia, and polydipsia.

WHAT TO DO IMMEDIATELY

If your patient has suggestive signs or symptoms or a serum potassium level below 3.5 mEq/L, notify the physician. (Keep in mind that normal serum electrolyte values may differ somewhat among health-care facilities.) Then take the following actions:

- Place the patient on continuous cardiac monitoring, and watch for the telltale ECG changes described above.
- Draw a blood sample for repeat measurement of serum potassium and other electrolytes.
- Establish I.V. access. As prescribed, administer oral potassium replacement or I.V. potassium chloride solution (to treat potassium depletion when chloride depletion accounts for hypokalemia) by slow infusion. Dilute the potassium chloride solution first, according to manufacturer's instructions, to prevent pain and vein irritation (which could lead to sclerosis and postinfusion phlebitis). Administer with a volume-control device, monitoring closely to prevent rapid infusion, which could lead to arrhythmias or cardiac arrest.
- ➡ **NurseALERT** Always give potassium chloride slowly as a dilute solution, never by I.V. push or intramuscularly. Bolus I.V. administration can trigger cardiac arrest.
- Administer potassium acetate or potassium phosphate solution, if prescribed. Typically, the physician prescribes potassium acetate to treat hypokalemia accompanied by metabolic acidosis, and potassium phosphate to treat hypokalemia accompanied by hypophosphatemia.
- Hypokalemia predisposes a patient to digitalis toxicity, even if he is receiving relatively low doses of digoxin (Lanoxicaps). To help detect

E.C.G. CHANGES IN HYPOKALEMIA

If your patient has hypokalemia, expect his ECG to reveal the changes shown below.

Normal ECG waveform

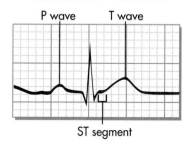

Hypokalemia

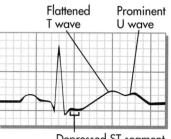

digitalis toxicity early, find out if the patient takes digoxin or digitoxin (Crystodigin) and watch for indications of toxicity, such as arrhythmias, nausea, visual changes, and fatigue.
- Carefully monitor your patient's hourly fluid intake and output.
- Check his blood pressure and pulse and respiratory rates every 5 to 15 minutes, noting tachycardia or a decreased respiratory rate.
- Check neuromuscular function every 5 to 15 minutes by assessing his leg and trunk muscles for paralysis and paresthesias. If paralysis progresses to affect respiratory muscles, respiratory arrest may occur.
- Prepare to assist with emergency cardiopulmonary resuscitation if the patient's heart or respiratory muscles fail. Keep emergency equipment, such as a manual resuscitation bag, endotracheal intubation set, defibrillator, and emergency medications, on hand.
- Administer oxygen, as prescribed.
- Prepare to assist with endotracheal intubation and mechanical ventilation in case of respiratory distress.

WHAT TO DO NEXT
Once the immediate crisis eases, carry out these interventions:
- Obtain a complete medical history to help identify the underlying cause of hypokalemia and guide long-term treatment.
- Continue to monitor the rate of I.V. potassium infusion to make sure it's not too rapid.
- Monitor serial serum electrolyte levels and report significant changes.
- Continue to monitor the patient's ECG for changes in heart rate and cardiac function and for atrial and ventricular arrhythmias.
- Assess the patient's vital signs every hour.
- Continue to monitor the patient's hourly fluid intake and output to

evaluate renal function and help detect signs of overly rapid potassium infusion.
- Regularly assess the patient's neuromuscular function, noting improvement of paralysis or paresthesias.
- Observe the I.V. site for signs and symptoms of infiltration, such as redness, swelling, warmth, and pain. If infiltration occurs, discontinue I.V. therapy, apply warm soaks, and restart therapy at a new I.V. site. Extensive subcutaneous damage from drug extravasation may require skin grafting.

FOLLOW-UP CARE
- Continue to monitor the patient's laboratory test results.
- Regularly assess his respiratory rate, rhythm, and depth and auscultate his lungs to assess breath sounds.
- Continue to monitor the patient's fluid intake and output.
- Enforce bed rest until the patient's serum electrolyte values return to normal. Assist him with ambulation because he's at risk for orthostatic hypotension.

SPECIAL CONSIDERATIONS
- When adding potassium chloride to the infusion solution, be sure to mix it thoroughly by inverting and agitating the bottle.
- ➡ **NurseALERT** Don't add potassium chloride to a hanging container of I.V. solution. It will pool at the bottom and infuse as a bolus, possibly inducing cardiac arrest.

HYPONATREMIA

Hyponatremia refers to a decreased sodium concentration in the extracellular fluid (ECF). This electrolyte imbalance can occur with normal, decreased, or increased total body sodium, provided a relative water excess is present. (See *Types of hyponatremia.*)

Hyponatremia may result from any condition that triggers sodium loss or water gain. Causes of *sodium loss* leading to hyponatremia include:
- adrenal insufficiency
- extreme sweating
- GI losses (as from severe vomiting or diarrhea)
- salt-depleting nephritis
- thiazide diuretics.

Causes of *water gain* leading to hyponatremia include:
- adrenal hypofunction (Addison's disease)
- heart failure
- hyperglycemia

- hyperlipidemia
- hypothyroidism
- liver cirrhosis
- renal failure or insufficiency
- psychogenic polydypsia
- syndrome of inappropriate antidiuretic hormone secretion (SIADH, which may occur with such conditions as bronchogenic carcinoma, brain tumor or abscess, or meningitis or as an adverse effect of certain drugs.

As the patient's serum sodium level decreases, water shifts from the ECF to the intracellular spaces. Without treatment, the sodium deficit eventually may produce generalized cellular edema, which in turn causes neurologic damage and death. If your patient is at risk for hyponatremia, you'll need to stay alert for signs and symptoms of this life-threatening disorder—and then respond rapidly and effectively.

WHAT TO LOOK FOR
Clinical findings associated with hyponatremia may include:
- irritability and restlessness
- agitation, disorientation, and confusion
- decreased level of consciousness, ranging from drowsiness and lethargy to coma
- severe headache
- seizures
- muscle cramps
- weakness
- gait disturbances
- nausea and vomiting
- abdominal cramps
- hyperactive bowel sounds
- tachycardia
- weak pulse
- hypotension
- serum sodium level below 135 mEq/L
- urine sodium level below 15 mEq/L.

When hyponatremia stems from SIADH, clinical findings also include:
- generalized weight gain
- serum sodium level below 125 mEq/L
- urine sodium level above 20 mEq/L
- urine specific gravity above 1.012
- below-normal serum osmolality level
- decreased blood urea nitrogen (BUN) and serum creatinine levels.

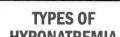

TYPES OF HYPONATREMIA

Depending on the pathophysiologic process involved, your patient may have one of three types of hyponatremia:
- *Hypervolemic hyponatremia.* In this situation, both total body sodium and water volume increase, but water volume increases more.
- *Hypovolemic hyponatremia.* Here, both total body sodium and water decrease, but sodium decreases more.
- *Euvolemic hyponatremia.* Serum sodium drops, but the extracellular fluid volume remains normal.

H

WHAT TO DO IMMEDIATELY

If you suspect that your patient has hyponatremia, notify the physician. Then intervene as follows:

- Obtain blood samples for repeat measurement of BUN and serum electrolyte, osmolality, and creatinine levels.
- Obtain samples for measuring urine sodium level and urine specific gravity.
- Establish I.V. access, and administer hypertonic saline solution (3% or 5%), as prescribed. To prevent overly rapid infusion, use a volume-control device.
- ➡ **NurseALERT** A rapid rise in serum sodium level may lead to pulmonary edema, cerebral swelling, neurologic deterioration, and death. Make sure to monitor the infusion carefully and watch your patient's serum sodium level closely; it should increase no more than 2 mEq/L/hour (unless the physician specifies otherwise). Because of the dangerous consequences of a rapid serum sodium rise, this therapy usually is administered in the intensive care unit.
- Monitor the patient's blood pressure and pulse and respiratory rates every 5 to 15 minutes, especially noting hypotension and tachycardia.
- Place the patient on continuous cardiac monitoring. Watch for ECG changes that suggest shock, such as heart rate changes and tachycardia or other arrhythmias.
- If your patient has severe hyponatremia, initiate seizure precautions, such as raising and padding the side rails, administering anticonvulsants if prescribed, and keeping an emergency airway on hand. If a seizure occurs, maintain a patent airway, protect the patient from injury and accidental removal of the I.V. line, and notify the physician. After the seizure, assess the patient and obtain blood samples to measure serum electrolyte levels.
- If your patient is receiving an anticonvulsant, monitor him for signs and symptoms of anticonvulsant toxicity.
- Record the patient's hourly fluid intake and output to detect signs of fluid overload and pulmonary edema.
- As prescribed, administer furosemide (Lasix) to promote water excretion and prevent pulmonary edema. During this therapy, monitor the patient for urinary sodium and potassium losses; anticipate further electrolyte replacement therapy if these losses become excessive.

WHAT TO DO NEXT

Once your patient has been stabilized, take these actions:

- Continue to monitor BUN level; serum electrolyte, osmolality, and creatinine levels; urine sodium level; and urine specific gravity. Alert the physician immediately if serum sodium rises too quickly.
- Assess the patient's vital signs and mental status every 15 minutes during the infusion of hypertonic saline solution and every 30 minutes for several hours afterward.
- Continue to monitor the patient's hourly fluid intake and output.

➡ **NurseALERT** Reduced output may signal pulmonary or cerebral edema.

- Maintain seizure precautions.
- Obtain a complete patient history to help identify the underlying cause of hyponatremia and guide long-term treatment.

FOLLOW-UP CARE

- Continue to monitor serum electrolyte and other laboratory test results; report significant changes immediately.
- Continue to record the patient's hourly fluid intake and output, and check his urine specific gravity.
- Continue to assess his mental status for signs of improvement or deterioration.
- Maintain seizure precautions. As therapy corrects his hyponatremia, the risk of seizures decreases.
- Observe the I.V. site for signs and symptoms of infiltration, such as redness, swelling, warmth, and pain. If any occur, discontinue I.V. therapy, apply warm soaks, and restart therapy at a new I.V. site.
- Provide a quiet environment to minimize confusion and agitation.
- Restrict the patient to bed rest until his serum electrolyte values return to normal. Because hyponatremia can cause gait disturbances, provide assistance during ambulation.

SPECIAL CONSIDERATIONS

- Closely monitor the patient for signs and symptoms of circulatory overload—respiratory changes, dyspnea, crackles, agitation, and anxiety. Keep emergency airway equipment, a defibrillator, and emergency medications on hand at all times.
- If your patient has SIADH, monitor his fluid intake and output especially closely. Intracellular water retention may be fatal. Patients with SIADH may be treated by fluid restriction (500 to 800 ml/24 hours) for 3 to 5 days. If hypertonic sodium infusions are prescribed, it is essential to administer the fluid slowly.

HYPOTENSION

Hypotension usually refers to a systolic blood pressure below 90 mm Hg—a level that for many patients is too low for adequate tissue perfusion. If the pressure decrease significantly impairs tissue perfusion and oxygenation, signs and symptoms of hypotension arise. Markedly decreased blood pressure may indicate that your patient is in shock—an emergency that calls for rapid intervention to avert death.

Causes

Hypotension may result from a cardiovascular, respiratory, neurologic, or metabolic disorder; use of certain drugs; stress; or even a change of position (orthostatic hypotension). In fact, any clinical condition that al-

H

ters the heart rate, myocardial pumping ability, or fluid volume can cause hypotension.

- *Heart rate alterations* that commonly cause hypotension include sinus bradycardia, second- and third-degree heart block, and pacemaker malfunction. These conditions can be detected by checking the patient's pulse rate or ECG.
- *Pump-related* hypotension may result from myocardial infarction, cardiomyopathy, acute papillary muscle dysfunction, acute aortic insufficiency, prosthetic valve dysfunction, ruptured intraventricular septum, or myocarditis.
- *Fluid volume problems* leading to hypotension may be absolute or relative. An absolute volume problem results from actual loss of fluid, as from hemorrhage, prolonged vomiting or diarrhea, polyuria, dehydration, and insensible water losses. A relative volume problem occurs when reduced systemic vascular resistance leads to vasodilation (as in anaphylactic shock, for example), and blood volume is inadequate to fill the vascular system. Fluid redistribution from the vascular space into the interstitial spaces also may lead to a relative volume problem.

WHAT TO LOOK FOR

Besides a systolic blood pressure below 90 mm Hg, hypotension may cause signs and symptoms that stem from compensatory mechanisms that attempt to keep vital organs perfused. For example, sympathetic stimulation may lead to:

- tachycardia
- cool, pale, mottled skin
- reduced urine output
- hypoactive bowel sounds.

If these compensatory mechanisms become ineffective, the patient also may develop:

- myocardial ischemia
- reduced level of consciousness
- dizziness, faintness, syncope.

WHAT TO DO IMMEDIATELY

If your patient has clinically significant hypotension, notify the physician. Then take these measures:

- Begin continuous blood pressure monitoring with a noninvasive system or through direct intra-arterial measurement, as ordered.
- Obtain a 12-lead ECG and begin continuous ECG monitoring.
- Measure the patient's oxygen saturation using pulse oximetry. Administer supplemental oxygen, as prescribed. (See *Understanding pulse oximetry.*)
- Insert a peripheral I.V. line.

UNDERSTANDING PULSE OXIMETRY

A noninvasive technique, pulse oximetry allows continuous monitoring of your patient's oxygen saturation—specifically, the percentage of oxygen-bound hemoglobin. When measured by pulse oximetry, the result is called SpO_2; when measured by arterial blood gas (ABG) analysis, it's called SaO_2. In a healthy adult, SpO_2 should be at least 95%.

Pulse oximetry works on the principle that well-oxygenated blood and poorly oxygenated blood absorb light differently. The degree of blood oxygenation determines how much light is transmitted through the vascular bed to the photodetector of the pulse oximetry system.

TWO COMPONENTS

A pulse oximeter has two main components:
- a probe, which shines red and infrared light through one of the patient's vascular beds (in a finger, ear, nose, or toe) to a photodetector
- a microprocessor, which displays a digital reading of the patient's SpO_2, possibly along with her pulse, as shown in the illustration.

INFLUENCING FACTORS

Pulse oximetry reliably measures oxygen saturation as long as your patient's SpO_2 is 70% or above. Several physiologic and technical factors can affect the accuracy of measurements.

Physiologic factors that can affect measurements include:
- abnormal hemoglobin, such as carboxyhemoglobin or methemoglobin
- intravascular dyes, such as fluorescein
- poor blood flow in the area selected for measurement
- anemia
- dark skin color
- fingernail or toenail polish inadequately removed before starting oximetry.

Technical factors that can influence SpO_2 include:
- too much motion
- bright lights around the probe
- improper probe placement
- use of the wrong probe (a finger probe used on a toe, for example)
- inadequate knowledge about how to use the device.

If you're not sure whether pulse oximetry results are accurate or if your patient's SpO_2 reading doesn't match her clinical condition, obtain ABG values for verification.

H

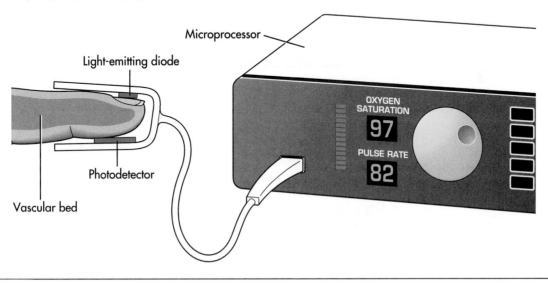

Microprocessor

Light-emitting diode

Photodetector

Vascular bed

OXYGEN SATURATION
97
PULSE RATE
82

Managing an altered heart rate

If your patient's hypotension stems from an altered heart rate, follow these guidelines:

- Determine the nature of the heart rate disorder (bradycardia, tachycardia, pacemaker dysfunction) and implement treatment as prescribed.
- If your patient has bradycardia with serious signs and symptoms (such as chest pain, dyspnea, decreased level of consciousness, pulmonary congestion, and heart failure), prepare to give atropine, 0.5 to 1.0 mg in repeated doses every 3 to 5 minutes, to a total of 0.04 mg/kg, as prescribed. Also expect to give dopamine or epinephrine and, if ordered, to begin transcutaneous pacing.
- If your patient has tachycardia accompanied by chest pain, dyspnea, decreased level of consciousness, pulmonary congestion, or heart failure, expect to administer medications, as prescribed, to treat the specific tachyarrhythmias.

Coping with a pump problem

If your patient's hypotension stems from a pump problem, take these actions:

- Assist in treating the underlying cause. For example, prepare your patient for emergency surgery if her intraventricular septum has ruptured.
- Unless she has pulmonary edema, quickly infuse 250 to 500 ml of normal saline solution, as prescribed.
- If fluids don't boost her blood pressure, give a combination of norepinephrine (Levophed), dopamine (Intropin), and dobutamine (Dobutrex), as prescribed, to support it.

Dealing with a fluid volume problem

If your patient's hypotension stems from a fluid volume problem, follow these steps:

- Anticipate insertion of a central venous or pulmonary artery catheter to continually assess hemodynamic status.
- Based on the patient's hemodynamic status, administer I.V. fluid replacement, as prescribed.
- Implement ordered treatments to correct the underlying cause of the volume problem.
- Once the patient's fluid volume has been restored, give vasopressors (such as norepinephrine or dopamine), as prescribed, to increase her systemic vascular resistance.
- ➡ **NurseALERT** When giving vasopressors, monitor the I.V. site carefully for signs of extravasation, such as blanching. Notify the physician if these occur, and prepare to give phentolamine (Regitine) to help avoid tissue necrosis and sloughing.

WHAT TO DO NEXT

Once the cause of hypotension is determined and treatments have begun, take these steps:
- Continue to monitor the patient's blood pressure closely.
- Watch for adverse drug effects, such as arrhythmias.
- Continue to assess the patient's cardiovascular status, including vital signs, heart rate and rhythm, heart and breath sounds, peripheral pulses, capillary refill, and skin color and temperature.
- Weigh the patient, and assess her mucous membranes, skin turgor, and fluid intake and output to help evaluate her fluid volume status.
- Assess her oxygenation status using pulse oximetry; limit any activities that decrease arterial saturation (SpO_2). Continue giving supplemental oxygen, as prescribed and necessary, and call the physician if SpO_2 falls below 95%.
- Take safety precautions to minimize the patient's risk of injury.

FOLLOW-UP CARE

- Continue to monitor your patient's blood pressure, cardiovascular status, and fluid status. Watch for changes in level of consciousness.
- Instruct the patient to change positions slowly; help her rise slowly to a sitting position before standing up. Sitting or standing too rapidly could result in orthostatic hypotension, causing dizziness and syncope.

SPECIAL CONSIDERATIONS

- As appropriate, teach your patient about the underlying condition that caused her hypotension (such as an arrhythmia). Discuss the disease process and treatments, and tell her which signs and symptoms she should report to the physician.

HYPOTHERMIA

Defined as a core body temperature below 95° F (35° C), hypothermia occurs when the body loses more heat than it produces. Although hypothermia is most common among neonates, trauma patients, elderly people, and homeless people, it also affects patients who have certain medical conditions or receive certain drugs. (See *Gauging your patient's hypothermia risk,* page 222.)

Because early signs and symptoms tend to be nonspecific, hypothermia is easily overlooked. In more than half of those affected, in fact, hypothermia is fatal. However, it can be reversed fully—even in patients with severe hypothermia—if detected and treated in time.

WHAT TO LOOK FOR

Clinical findings vary with the patient's degree of hypothermia, ranging from apathy and increased heart and respiratory rates in mild hypothermia to absence of brain waves, asystole, and apnea in deep hypothermia.

H

GAUGING YOUR PATIENT'S HYPOTHERMIA RISK

A patient who is affected by any the following conditions or circumstances may be at increased risk for hypothermia.

Central nervous system disorders
- Decreased level of consciousness
- Dementia, Alzheimer's disease
- Hypothalamic lesion
- Cerebrovascular accident
- Spinal cord injury

Metabolic disorders
- Hypoadrenalism
- Hypoglycemia
- Hypopituitarism
- Hypothyroidism
- Malnutrition
- Myxedema
- Wernicke's encephalopathy

Drug and substance use
- Alcohol
- Barbiturates
- Benzodiazepines
- Cyclic antidepressants
- General anesthetics
- Parasympatholytic agents
- Phenothiazines
- Narcotics

Other conditions and factors
- Burn injury
- Environmental exposure
- Erythroderma
- Exfoliate dermatitis
- Hepatic failure
- Renal failure
- Sepsis
- Severe trauma
- Extremes of age: neonates and elderly people

WHAT TO DO IMMEDIATELY

If you suspect that your patient is hypothermic, notify the physician. Then take these measures:

- Assess his airway, breathing, and circulation. If he has no pulse or respirations, begin cardiopulmonary resuscitation.
- Prepare to assist with defibrillation and endotracheal intubation, if indicated. Be aware that defribrillation may not be effective unless the patient's temperature is at least 86° F (30° C).
- Measure the patient's core body temperature. For greatest accuracy, use a continuous-reading thermistor probe with a scale range of 68° to 107.6° F (20° to 42° C). Insert the probe at least 5 cm into the patient's rectum. If the patient requires endotracheal intubation, expect to assist with insertion of an esophageal temperature probe, which correlates most closely with cardiac temperature. (Although an indwelling urinary catheter with a thermometer may be used to obtain bladder temperature, few hospitals routinely stock this item.)
- Administer warmed and humidified oxygen, as prescribed.
- Remove any wet clothing from the patient. Cover him with blankets and turn up the heat, if possible, to prevent further heat loss. If a reflective blanket (a space blanket) is available, place it over him and shine a heat lamp on it. Make sure you position the lamp at a safe distance; it should warm the patient gently without burning him.
  ➡ **NurseALERT** Keep the patient covered at all times—especially his head.

- Start an I.V. line and administer warm I.V. fluids, as prescribed.
- Institute continuous cardiac monitoring and obtain a baseline ECG, as ordered. Remember that arrhythmias pose an immediate threat to the patient's life.
- ➡ Nurse**ALERT**   Stay alert for an "Osborne" (J) wave on the ECG. This slow, positive deflection in the latter part of the QRS complex is characteristic of hypothermia. The appearance of J waves may warn of impending ventricular fibrillation. (See *Detecting a J wave*, page 224.)

WHAT TO DO NEXT
After taking initial steps, follow these guidelines:
- Begin rewarming the patient, as ordered and indicated by his temperature. For mild hypothermia (93.2° to 95° F [34° to 35° C]) and moderate hypothermia (86° to 93.2° F [30° to 34° C]), anticipate using passive and active external rewarming techniques. Passive external rewarming allows the patient's body to generate heat, whereas active external rewarming usually involves immersing the patient in warm water or covering him with an air- or a fluid-filled heating blanket.
- For severe hypothermia (below 86° F [30° C]), use active internal rewarming, which may include administration of warm oxygen, infusion of warm I.V. fluids, lavage of the peritoneum with warm dialysis solution (potassium-free), or other measures.
- Expect to assist with insertion of an arterial line, central venous catheter, and pulmonary artery catheter.
- Continue to administer warmed I.V. fluids, as ordered.
- Administer transfusions of warmed blood, if indicated and prescribed.
- ➡ Nurse**ALERT**   Be sure to warm donor blood at least to body temperature before transfusing it.
- If the patient is on a mechanical ventilator, maintain humidifier temperature on the ventilator at 120° F (48.9° C).
- Monitor your patient's laboratory test results, including complete blood count, serum electrolyte level, blood urea nitrogen level, blood glucose level, coagulation screen, arterial blood gas (ABG) values, and blood alcohol and drug levels, as indicated.
- ➡ Nurse**ALERT**   When sending arterial blood samples for ABG analysis to the laboratory, always write the patient's core temperature on the tube. Hypothermia affects the oxyhemoglobin dissociation curves, increasing affinity of hemoglobin for oxygen.
- Prepare the patient for a chest X-ray (to check for aspiration pneumonia and pulmonary edema) and an abdominal X-ray (to rule out free air if the patient will undergo heated peritoneal dialysis).

FOLLOW-UP CARE
- Continuously monitor all the patient's physiologic parameters, including core temperature and cardiopulmonary status.
- Assess him for afterdrop, a condition that causes core body temperature to drop. Afterdrop may occur during rewarming as blood that

H

DETECTING A J WAVE

The illustrations below compare a normal ECG waveform with that of a patient with hypothermia. In the normal ECG waveform, note the J point where the QRS complex meets the ST segment.

In hypothermia, the patient develops a characteristic wave—called a J wave—at the J point, making it difficult to determine where the QRS complex ends and the ST segment begins.

Normal ECG waveform

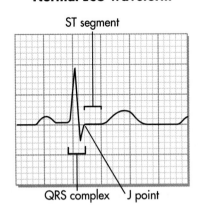

ST segment

QRS complex   J point

ECG waveform with J wave

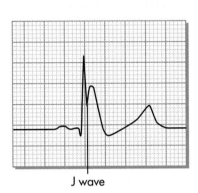

J wave

has flowed through cold peripheral tissues returns to the central circulation. By chilling the heart further, afterdrop may induce heart failure, decreased cardiac output, and reduced systemic blood pressure (rewarming shock). Myocardial cooling also may increase the risk of ventricular fibrillation.

- Watch the cardiac monitor to detect arrhythmias. Be aware that atrial fibrillation and other arrhythmias are common when body temperature falls below 93.4° F (34° C).
- Closely monitor your patient for metabolic acidosis during rewarming. Because insulin release and glucose metabolism are impaired by hypothermia, hyperglycemia may occur.
- Be aware that electrical cardioversion of the hypothermic heart is difficult—sometimes impossible—especially when core body temperature is below 86° F (30° C).
- If the patient has had severe or prolonged hypothermia, assess for evidence of noncardiogenic pulmonary edema, gastric submucosal hemorrhage, pancreatic necrosis, cerebrovascular accident, and myocardial infarction.
- ➡ **NurseALERT** Watch closely for signs and symptoms of pneumonia.

SPECIAL CONSIDERATIONS
- Be aware that no single rewarming method is best for all patients in all situations. The physician will choose the method or combination of methods that best suits your patient's individual needs.

HYPOVOLEMIC SHOCK

In hypovolemic shock, inadequate intravascular volume causes stroke volume to diminish. As a result, cardiac output and blood pressure decrease and blood flow through the capillaries dwindles, reducing perfusion to the tissues and vital organs.

Hypovolemic shock results from acute loss of intravascular fluid volume (in the absence of adequate fluid replacement) brought about by external fluid losses or internal fluid shifts.

External fluid losses that may cause hypovolemic shock include:
- blood loss due to hemorrhage, GI bleeding, severe hemoptysis, ruptured esophageal varices
- plasma loss due to burns, draining wounds or skin ulcers, fistulas
- GI fluid loss due to prolonged vomiting or diarrhea
- renal fluid loss due to diabetic ketoacidosis, hyperglycemic hyperosmolar nonketotic syndrome, diabetes insipidus, adrenal insufficiency, high-output renal failure, or overly aggressive diuretic therapy
- cutaneous fluid loss due to excessive sweating from heatstroke.

Internal fluid shifts that may lead to hypovolemic shock include:
- internal bleeding, such as from dissecting aortic aneurysm, fractured long bones, hemothorax, ruptured spleen, retroperitoneal hemorrhage, hemorrhagic pancreatitis
- third-spacing of fluid, in which fluids move out of the intravascular space and collect in a body cavity, such as ascites secondary to cirrhosis or large pleural effusions or chylothorax secondary to cancer
- movement of fluid out of the cell and into the interstitial spaces, which causes edema and may result from burns, severe allergic reactions, or the body's response to bacterial endotoxins.

The severity of hypovolemic shock depends on how much intravascular volume the patient loses, how quickly the loss occurs, and how effectively compensatory mechanisms respond. In an otherwise healthy person, sudden loss of 25% or more of total intravascular volume can cause extreme circulatory failure by overwhelming the body's compensatory mechanisms and causing severe hypotension. If the same amount of volume loss occurs over several days rather than several hours, the body may be able to compensate more effectively, improving the patient's prognosis.

A patient in hypovolemic shock is at risk for developing acute respiratory distress syndrome, renal failure, and multisystem organ failure. Clearly, she'll survive only if her condition is detected early and treated effectively.

H

WHAT TO LOOK FOR
Clinical findings in hypovolemic shock may include:
- decreased blood pressure
- hypotension
- tachycardia
- rapid and thready pulse, diminished pulse, or nonpalpable periph-eral pulses
- pale, clammy, or mottled skin
- delayed capillary refill
- cool extremities
- restlessness, anxiety
- decreased level of consciousness
- rapid, shallow respirations
- dyspnea
- cyanosis
- decreased urine output
- fever
- obvious bleeding
- elevated serum potassium, serum lactate, and blood urea nitrogen (BUN) levels
- decreased hematocrit and serum hemoglobin level
- arterial blood gas (ABG) abnormalities, including decreased blood pH, reduced partial pressure of arterial oxygen, and increased partial pressure of arterial carbon dioxide.

WHAT TO DO IMMEDIATELY
If you suspect that your patient is in hypovolemic shock, notify the physician. Then follow these guidelines:
- Obtain blood samples to measure or recheck hematocrit, red blood cell and platelet counts, ABG values, BUN level, and serum electro-lyte, hemoglobin, and creatinine levels.
- Establish I.V. access, using the largest-diameter I.V. device available. As prescribed, administer I.V. fluid resuscitation therapy. Use a vol-ume-control device, and monitor the amount and rate of fluid in-fused. (See *Fluids used to treat hypovolemic shock*.)
- ➡ **NurseALERT** Keep in mind that rapid infusion of cold I.V. fluids may induce hypothermia and arrhythmias. If your patient requires mas-sive infusions, warm the fluids before administering them.
- Begin to keep a meticulous record of the patient's intake and output. As indicated, insert an indwelling urinary catheter to ensure an ac-curate output measurement. Monitor the patient's urine output every 30 to 60 minutes. If output drops below 30 ml/hour, notify the physician.
- As indicated, place the patient on continuous cardiac monitoring, and watch her ECG for arrhythmias and ischemia.
- Check the patient's blood pressure, heart rate, and mental status every 5 minutes; report any changes.

TREATMENT OF CHOICE

FLUIDS USED TO TREAT HYPOVOLEMIC SHOCK

Fluid resuscitation serves as the cornerstone of treatment for hypovolemic shock. Familiarize yourself with the fluids typically administered in this emergency.

HYPERTONIC FLUIDS

Hypertonic fluids, which have an osmotic pressure higher than that of serum and interstitial fluid, are used to increase serum osmolality. By increasing the osmolality of fluid in the intravascular space, they draw fluid out of the intracellular and interstitial spaces, thus expanding intravascular volume. Examples of hypertonic fluids include 3% and 5% sodium chloride.

Be aware that administering hypertonic fluids too quickly can cause fluid volume overload, possibly leading to pulmonary edema and even death.

HYPOTONIC FLUIDS

Hypotonic fluids, which have a lower osmotic pressure than serum, draw water out of the vessels and into the intracellular and interstitial spaces. They are used to replenish fluids lost from tissues. An example of a hypotonic fluid is half-normal saline solution.

ISOTONIC FLUIDS

Isotonic fluids have the same osmotic pressure as serum and are used to increase intravascular volume. They include normal saline solution as well as lactated Ringer's solution, which provides more balanced electrolyte replacement.

Keep in mind that infusing large amounts of normal saline solution may lead to metabolic acidosis by increasing the serum chloride level and decreasing the serum bicarbonate concentration.

ALBUMIN

A plasma volume expander, human serum albumin may be indicated for a patient with a low serum albumin level and low plasma oncotic pressure (usually from blood or plasma loss). Albumin increases serum osmolality, thus drawing fluid out of the extracellular space and into the intravascular space.

Avoid administering albumin too rapidly because it could result in fluid volume overload. Monitor the patient for signs of vascular overload, such as crackles and dyspnea.

BLOOD PRODUCTS

Blood replacement therapy may be necessary in a patient who has lost more than 20% of total blood volume. Whole blood may be given to patients suffering from severe hemorrhage who require rapid replacement of a large volume of blood (more than 3 units). Packed red blood cells are generally preferred because of the decreased risk of adverse reactions.

Remember that administering blood products exposes the patient to the risks of transfusion reaction, transmission of bloodborne diseases (such as hepatitis and acquired immunodeficiency syndrome), and circulatory overload.

COLLOIDS

Colloids, such as hetastarch and dextran, are plasma volume expanders. Hetastarch, a hydroxyethal starch, is nonallergenic and has colloidal properties much like albumin. The glucose polymer dextran also acts as a colloidal plasma volume expander. But dextran can produce serious adverse effects, such as anaphylactic reactions, bleeding disorders (from interference with platelet and coagulation function), and renal dysfunction.

H

➡ **NurseALERT** Suspect worsening of hypovolemic shock if you detect decreasing blood pressure, an increased heart rate, and a decrease in level of consciousness.

• Perform a baseline neurologic assessment, and monitor for changes that signal decreased cerebral perfusion, such as a change in level of consciousness and increasing restlessness or confusion.

• Assess your patient's peripheral skin for color, warmth, and capillary refill. Evaluate the rate, strength, and regularity of her radial, brachial, pedal, and popliteal pulses every 5 to 15 minutes. Hard-to-detect peripheral pulses may mean that your patient's condition is deteriorating.

- Monitor the patient's respiratory status every 5 minutes, including respiratory rate, depth, and character and ease of breathing. Ask her if she's having trouble breathing.
- Auscultate her lungs every 15 minutes to check for signs of pulmonary edema. Prepare for possible endotracheal intubation and mechanical ventilation if she experiences respiratory distress.
- Administer supplemental oxygen, as indicated and prescribed. Monitor oxygen saturation by way of pulse oximetry.
- Prepare to assist with insertion of a central venous or pulmonary artery catheter to evaluate the patient's hemodynamic status and track the effectiveness of fluid resuscitation.
- Monitor the patient's mean arterial pressure (MAP).
- ➡ **NurseALERT** A MAP below 60 mm Hg adversely affects cerebral perfusion.
- Monitor the patient closely for signs and symptoms of circulatory overload: crackles, dyspnea, agitation, and anxiety. Keep emergency airway equipment available. If ordered, prepare the patient for dialysis.

WHAT TO DO NEXT
Once your patient has stabilized, take these steps:
- Monitor laboratory test results and report abnormalities immediately.
- Continue cardiac monitoring, noting changes in cardiac function, tachycardia or other arrhythmias, and hypotension.
- Monitor the patient's neurologic status, including level of consciousness, and personality changes.
- Assess her vital signs every 5 to 15 minutes during I.V. fluid therapy. Remember that I.V. fluids can cause circulatory overload and lead to cardiac arrest and respiratory insufficiency.
- Monitor the patient's fluid output every hour. Keep in mind that an output below 30 ml/hour may signal decreased renal perfusion and, possibly, renal failure. Notify the physician immediately.
- Continue to monitor the patient's renal function through urine specific gravity, BUN level, serum creatinine level, and other test results as appropriate. Report abnormal values.
- Administer ordered treatments to correct the underlying cause of hypovolemic shock. If indicated, prepare the patient for surgery.

FOLLOW-UP CARE
- Continue to monitor laboratory results and report abnormalities.
- Record the patient's fluid intake and output every 2 to 4 hours. Monitor urine specific gravity, assessing for normal, concentrated, or dilute urine.

SPECIAL CONSIDERATIONS
- As indicated, keep emergency equipment (defibrillator, emergency medications, endotracheal or tracheal intubation set, and mechanical ventilator) on hand in case of respiratory or cardiac arrest.

- Teach the patient about the importance of maintaining normal hydration. Encourage adequate fluid intake.

HYPOXEMIA

A state of deficient oxygen in arterial blood, hypoxemia typically is further defined as a partial pressure of arterial oxygen (PaO_2) below 60 mm Hg at sea level in an adult (younger than age 60) who is breathing room air. The condition causes inadequate tissue perfusion with varying degrees of cyanosis.

Many medical conditions and certain drugs can lead to hypoxemia. Because it may lead to respiratory failure, you'll need to stay alert for signs, symptoms, and diagnostic markers in any patient at risk. If you detect hypoxemia, you'll need to act fast to prevent your patient's condition from deteriorating. (See *Conditions that cause hypoxemia*, page 230.)

WHAT TO LOOK FOR
Clinical findings in hypoxemia may include—
- *Neurologic*: restlessness, drowsiness, confusion, and hallucinations
- ➡ **NurseALERT** Changes in level of consciousness are the earliest signs of hypoxemia.
- *Cardiovascular:* tachycardia, elevated blood pressure, elevated pulmonary artery pressure; with severe hypoxemia, possible hypotension and bradycardia
- *Respiratory:* tachypnea, dyspnea
- *Integumentary:* mottled skin, periorbital and peripheral cyanosis
- *Hepatic:* hepatic dysfunction; elevated serum bilirubin, alkaline phosphatase, and transaminase levels (late signs indicative of severe hypoxemia)
- *Hematologic:* prolonged prothrombin and partial thromboplastin times
- *GI:* severe abdominal pain (late sign indicative of bowel ischemia)
- *Renal*: decreased glomerular filtration rate and increased secretion of antidiuretic hormone (late sign)
- *Metabolic:* serum sodium deficit (hyponatremia).

WHAT TO DO IMMEDIATELY
If your patient's PaO_2 drops below normal or he shows signs and symptoms of hypoxemia, notify the physician. Then take these measures:
- Obtain the patient's vital signs and assess his level of consciousness for subtle changes.
- Institute pulse oximetry to assess oxygen saturation, and draw blood for baseline arterial blood gas (ABG) values. (See *Performing Allen's test*, page 231.)
- Provide supplemental oxygen, as prescribed. Expect to give the least amount of oxygen needed to improve oxygenation and then titrate

H

TREATMENT OF CHOICE

CONDITIONS THAT CAUSE HYPOXEMIA

The conditions that may produce hypoxemia fall into four general categories.

HYPOVENTILATION ABNORMALITIES
Always accompanied by hypercapnia (increased carbon dioxide content of the blood), hypoventilation abnormalities commonly result from damage to the brain's respiratory center, such as from head trauma, cerebrovascular accident, or drugs that depress the central nervous system (for instance, narcotics). Less often, they're caused by emphysema, asthma, and bronchitis.

DIFFUSION ABNORMALITIES
These conditions result from the inability of alveolar gases to move across the alveolocapillary membrane to the pulmonary capillary bed and from the pulmonary bed across the membrane to the atmosphere. They may stem from fluid accumulation (as in heart failure and pulmonary edema), collagen accumulation (as in pulmonary fibrosis and sarcoidosis), or a decreased diffusion area (as in lung resection and emphysema).

$\dot{V}/\dot{Q}$ MISMATCH
An abnormal relationship between the oxygen volume reaching the alveoli and perfusion through pulmonary capillaries, a ventilation-perfusion ($\dot{V}/\dot{Q}$) mismatch may take the form of inadequate ventilation with normal perfusion or inadequate perfusion with normal ventilation. Mismatches are common in chronic obstructive pulmonary disease, restrictive lung disorders caused by obesity, kyphoscoliosis, and interstitial lung disease.

BLOOD SHUNTING
When blood passes through portions of the lungs that don't participate in gas exchange (for example, when alveoli are filled with fluid or have collapsed), it's shunted—meaning that blood can't receive oxygen or release carbon dioxide. This results in decreased systemic arterial oxygenation and, consequently, hypoxemia.

Blood shunting occurs in acute respiratory distress syndrome, atelectasis, pneumonia, pulmonary edema, pulmonary embolism, and lung tumors.

---

upward as indicated. If necessary, be prepared to administer 1.0 fraction of inspired oxygen by manual resuscitation bag.
- Auscultate the patient's lungs for adventitious sounds, which may indicate pulmonary edema or obstruction.
- Instruct the patient to take deep breaths, but don't let him hyperventilate.
- ➡ **NurseALERT** Hyperventilation puts the hypoxemic patient at risk for respiratory alkalosis.
- Prepare for possible endotracheal intubation and mechanical ventilation if your patient's PaO_2 continues to fall.
- Elevate the head of the bed to semi-Fowler's or high Fowler's position to promote lung expansion.
- Begin continuous cardiac monitoring to detect myocardial ischemia and arrhythmias.
- Anticipate assisting with insertion of a pulmonary artery catheter to evaluate the patient's hemodynamic status.

WHAT TO DO NEXT
Once your patient is stable, follow these guidelines:
- Prepare him for diagnostic tests, as ordered, including chest X-ray, pulmonary function tests, and ventilation-perfusion ($\dot{V}/\dot{Q}$) scanning, to find the underlying cause of hypoxemia.

PERFORMING ALLEN'S TEST

Before drawing an arterial blood sample, perform Allen's test to make sure the patient has adequate collateral circulation and arterial function in his hand. Follow these steps:

- Rest the patient's arm on a bedside table, palm up. Support his wrist on a rolled towel.
- Instruct him to clench his fist.
- Apply pressure over the radial and ulnar arteries with the middle and index fingers of both your hands.

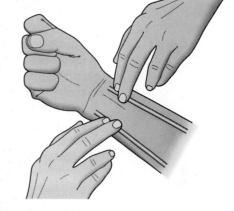

- With your fingers still pressing on the arteries, ask the patient to unclench his fist. His palm should look blanched because you're occluding the arteries.

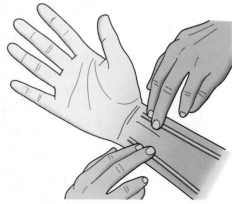

- Now release pressure on the ulnar artery. If it has normal blood flow, his palm will turn pink within a few seconds, even though you're still occluding the radial artery.
- If his palm takes longer than a few seconds to turn pink, suspect an inadequate blood supply from the ulnar artery and find another puncture site.

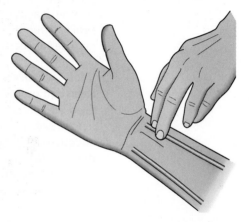

H

- Continue to monitor the patient's vital signs, cardiopulmonary status, level of consciousness, pulse oximetry readings, and ABG values; report significant changes.

➡ **NurseALERT** Stay alert for respiratory acidosis, indicated by increased partial pressure of arterial carbon dioxide with decreased blood pH.

- Assess serial serum lactate levels. Keep in mind that inadequate oxygenation causes cells to shift to anaerobic metabolism, resulting in lactic acidosis.
- Enforce bed rest to minimize oxygen demands until the patient's condition improves.
- Continue to give supplemental oxygen, as prescribed. However, remember that oxygen won't correct hypoxemia caused by shunting.
- Administer antibiotics, diuretics, and vasoactive medications, as prescribed and indicated.
- If your patient's hypoxemia results from a diffusion abnormality, expect to give diuretics, as prescribed, and provide frequent oral hygiene. Monitor his urine output often to track diuretic effectiveness.
- If his hypoxemia results from a $\dot{V}/\dot{Q}$ mismatch, expect to give bronchodilators, antibiotics, and other medications, as prescribed and necessary, to improve gas exchange.

FOLLOW-UP CARE

- Continue to monitor the patient's vital signs, level of consciousness, and ABG and pulse oximetry values; report significant changes.
- Encourage frequent coughing, deep breathing, and incentive spirometry to improve ventilation and optimize gas exchange.
- Keep the head of the patient's bed elevated 45 degrees or higher to promote adequate lung expansion.
- Change the patient's position frequently to mobilize secretions and prevent them from pooling.
- Have him ambulate as soon as tolerated to prevent respiratory complications related to immobility. Perform passive range-of-motion exercises to help prevent venous stasis. Assess his oxygen saturation by pulse oximetry (SpO_2) in response to activity; report any decrease and adjust his activity level as indicated.
- Provide frequent oral hygiene to minimize dry mouth because oxygen therapy can cause mucous membrane dryness.

SPECIAL CONSIDERATIONS

- Keep in mind that although the terms *hypoxemia* and *hypoxia* often are used interchangeably, their meanings differ. Hypoxemia refers to an inadequate oxygen partial pressure in arterial blood; hypoxia, to inadequate oxygenation of body tissues. However, hypoxemia may precipitate hypoxia, as may certain blood cell disorders, cardiovascular disorders, and cellular poisoning. Unlike hypoxemia, hypoxia can't be measured directly.

I, L, M

ILEUS

A general term for intestinal obstruction, ileus also specifically denotes a type of functional obstruction called paralytic, or adynamic, ileus. In this condition, intestinal peristalsis decreases or stops because of a disturbance or interruption of the bowel's intrinsic nervous system.

Ileus most often results from abdominal surgery. Other causes include peritoneal injury and conditions that induce severe physiologic stress, such as burns, peritonitis, blunt trauma to the abdomen, intra-abdominal vascular occlusion, severe electrolyte imbalance, myocardial infarction, severe pyelonephritis, rib fracture, and extensive GI ulceration.

Because GI secretions continue despite the intestine's impaired motility, fluid accumulates in the bowel lumen. If the fluid isn't reabsorbed or if it's lost through vomiting or mechanical suction, the patient may become dehydrated and develop potentially life-threatening electrolyte imbalances.

Indeed, the patient with ileus is particularly vulnerable to potassium deficit (hypokalemia) and metabolic alkalosis from hydrogen loss. Without fluid and electrolyte replacement, he'll suffer dehydration, hypovolemic shock, and renal failure.

WHAT TO LOOK FOR
Clinical findings for a patient with ileus may include:
- decreased or absent bowel sounds
- absence of flatus or bowel movements
- abdominal distention
- sensation of abdominal fullness
- abdominal pain (described as gas pains)
- vomiting
- increased drainage from a nasogastric (NG) tube
- signs and symptoms of dehydration, such as oliguria, tachycardia, poor skin turgor, and dry mucous membranes
- distention of the intestinal lumen, shown by plain abdominal X-ray films.

I

ASSESSING BOWEL SOUNDS

Evaluating a patient for ileus requires expertise in auscultating the abdomen and interpreting bowel sounds. Follow the guidelines below to sharpen your technique.

PREPARING FOR THE EXAMINATION
- Warm your hands and stethoscope before you touch the patient. Otherwise, contact with your cold hand or stethoscope may cause his abdominal muscles to contract. Also, to prevent chilling, make sure the room is warm and the patient isn't unnecessarily exposed.
- If your patient has a nasogastric tube attached to suction, turn off the suction or clamp the tube temporarily while you auscultate. The suction device could produce misleading sounds or interfere with your hearing.

STEPS TO FOLLOW
- Always auscultate the abdomen *before* percussing or palpating it. Otherwise, your manipulation may exaggerate bowel sounds or produce sounds not usually heard.
- Mentally divide your patient's abdomen into quadrants. Using the diaphragm of your stethoscope, start at one quadrant and listen for 1 to 2 minutes for air and fluid moving through the intestines. Keep in mind that bowel sounds normally are high-pitched gurgling or bubbling noises with an irregular pattern. They occur roughly every 5 to 15 seconds.
- If you don't hear bowel sounds after auscultating for 1 to 2 minutes, try gently flicking the patient's abdomen with your finger or pressing on it gently. Then listen again for up to 5 minutes before you decide that the patient has no bowel sounds in that quadrant.
- After auscultating in one quadrant, move to another and listen there. Do this until you've listened in all four quadrants. Try to develop a routine pattern for auscultation so you don't skip a quadrant.
- Be aware that abdominal wall thickness can affect what you hear. Consequently, expect to have more difficulty hearing bowel sounds in obese patients. A full bladder can obscure bowel sounds as well.
- Avoid dragging your stethoscope across the patient's abdominal wall. Doing so could increase irritation and cause muscle spasm.

WHAT TO DO IMMEDIATELY

If you suspect that your patient has ileus, notify the physician. Then take these steps:
- Auscultate the patient's abdomen for bowel sounds in all quadrants. (See *Assessing bowel sounds*.)
- If you don't detect any bowel sounds, withhold oral intake, expect to insert an NG tube, as ordered, and attach it to low intermittent suction.
- Ask the patient about his recent bowel elimination pattern, including the last time he moved his bowels or passed flatus.
- Establish I.V. access and administer I.V. fluids, as prescribed.
- Monitor the patient's fluid intake and output carefully, making sure to include any drainage from the NG tube.
- Assess his skin and mucous membranes for signs of dehydration.
- Ask him to describe his abdominal pain; then regularly evaluate for changes in the nature of the pain.
- Measure the patient's abdominal girth to obtain a baseline. To ensure accurate repeat measurements, mark the area where you measured with an indelible pen.
- Assess for vomiting or increased drainage from the NG tube.

WHAT TO DO NEXT

After taking those initial steps, follow these guidelines:
- Obtain blood samples for measurement of complete blood count, hemoglobin level, and hematocrit.
- Maintain NG tube decompression and suction, as ordered. Anticipate the need for tube irrigation to maintain patency.
- As tolerated by the patient, encourage ambulation to stimulate bowel activity.
- Administer cholinergic drugs, such as bethanechol (Duvoid), if prescribed, to stimulate bowel motility. Monitor for therapeutic and adverse effects.
- Every 4 to 8 hours, assess your patient's bowel sounds and abdominal girth, and ask him about the passage of flatus or stool.

FOLLOW-UP CARE

- If ileus resulted from abdominal surgery, realize that your patient may not understand why his bowels aren't working. Also, be aware that he's likely to be hungry despite ileus. Explain to him what ileus is, stressing that it's common after abdominal surgery. Reassure him that normal intestinal function usually returns spontaneously within 3 days. Emphasize the importance of frequent ambulation to stimulate bowel activity.
- As the patient's condition resolves, introduce liquids gradually and advance his diet as tolerated.
- Continue to assess his bowel sounds, abdominal girth, and bowel elimination frequently.
- Assess his nasal area often for irritation from the NG tube. Apply water-soluble soothing ointment as needed.

SPECIAL CONSIDERATIONS

- Remember that many patients are embarrassed by questions about their bowel movements. Maintain a professional, straightforward approach to help put your patient at ease.

INTESTINAL OBSTRUCTION

Intestinal obstruction refers to a complete or partial blockage of the lumen of the small or large intestine that impedes passage of intestinal contents. An intestinal obstruction may be mechanical or functional. (See *Mechanical intestinal obstruction,* pages 236 and 237; and *Functional obstruction,* page 238.)

In an obstructed intestine, normal absorption of the intestinal contents diminishes but intestinal secretions continue and may even increase. As a result, fluid and gas accumulate in the intestinal lumen behind the blockage. The bowel proximal to the obstruction dilates and intraluminal pressure rises.

MECHANICAL INTESTINAL OBSTRUCTION

A mechanical obstruction results from a problem outside or inside the intestinal walls or within the intestinal lumen. The following illustrations show common causes of mechanical obstruction.

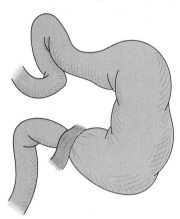

Adhesions

Adhesions (scar tissue from previous surgery) can obstruct the intestinal lumen and block the flow of intestinal contents.

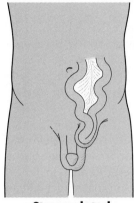

Strangulated inguinal hernia

A hernia in the inguinal area constricts intestinal blood flow and may lead to gangrene if circulation is not restored.

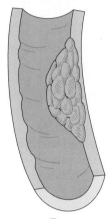

Tumor

Abnormal tumor growth from adjacent organs or within the intestinal wall (as shown here) or lumen can obstruct the flow of intestinal contents.

Ultimately, the bowel mucosa becomes ischemic and necrotic and the intestinal wall grows more permeable, allowing bacteria to move into the abdominal cavity. Without treatment, the bowel may perforate and the spilled intestinal contents may cause peritonitis. Seepage of plasma into the peritoneal cavity causes dehydration; the patient may progress to shock, vascular collapse, and death within hours.

An obstruction high in the bowel causes severe vomiting with moderate abdominal distention. An obstruction low in the bowel causes pronounced distention but less vomiting until later in the disorder. Prolonged vomiting may induce serious fluid and electrolyte imbalances, reflective of the level of obstruction. Obstruction high in the intestinal tract results in hypokalemia and hypochloremia with metabolic alkalosis from loss of acidic gastric fluids. Obstruction below the distal duodenum causes loss of alkaline digestive fluids, leading to metabolic acidosis.

Clearly, you need to be able to recognize clues to intestinal obstruction because its effects—peritonitis, dehydration, electrolyte imbalances, and shock—jeopardize your patient's life.

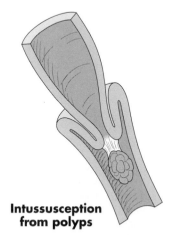

**Intussusception
from polyps**

Polyps on the intestinal wall may
cause one segment of the intestinal lumen to prolapse into another segment.

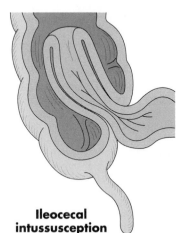

**Ileocecal
intussusception**

A prolapse of the valve between the
small intestine and the cecum of
the large intestine, ileocecal intussusception can cause intestinal obstruction.

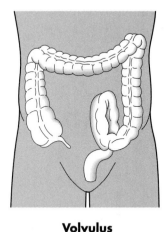

Volvulus

Volvulus, a twisting of the intestine at
least 180 degrees on its mesentery,
can cause an obstruction of the flow
of intestinal contents.

WHAT TO LOOK FOR
Clinical findings in intestinal obstruction may include:
- intermittent or continuous abdominal pain and cramping (pain typically is poorly localized)
- abdominal distention
- vomiting (if obstruction is in the large intestine, vomiting of fecal
  matter)
- passage of watery, mucoid stools (in incomplete obstruction)
- high-pitched hyperactive bowel sounds (reflects intestinal attempts
  to force contents past the obstruction)
- failure to pass stools or flatus
- absence of bowel sounds
- signs and symptoms of dehydration (oliguria, tachycardia, poor skin
  turgor, and dry mucous membranes)
- decreased urine output
- increased hematocrit and hemoglobin level from dehydration
- air or fluid in the GI tract, visible on abdominal X-rays.

FUNCTIONAL OBSTRUCTION

A functional obstruction results from a physiologic or neurologic condition that depresses or stops peristalsis or from vascular compromise that leads to bowel ischemia.

One of the most common neurologic causes of functional obstruction is surgical manipulation of the intestines. Other conditions that affect the neuromuscular activity of the intestines include peritonitis, pancreatitis, and disorders that cause overstimulation (shock, trauma, and critical illness). Vascular compromise leading to functional obstruction may stem from embolism or thrombosis of the mesenteric vessels.

Mesenteric occlusion

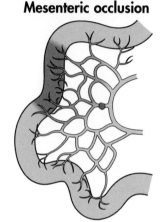

This illustration shows an occlusion in the area of the mesenteric artery that normally provides blood flow to the intestines. Here, however, the occlusion has blocked the blood flow, causing a functional obstruction.

WHAT TO DO IMMEDIATELY

If you suspect that your patient has an intestinal obstruction, notify the physician. Then carry out these interventions:

- Assess the patient's vital signs, especially noting an increased temperature; rapid, weak pulse; rapid respirations; and hypotension.
- Withhold oral intake. Monitor the patient's intake and output hourly.
- Insert a nasogastric (NG) or an intestinal tube, as ordered. As appropriate, assist with the insertion of an intestinal tube, such as a Cantor or Miller-Abbott tube.
- Evaluate vomitus or NG drainage for amount, color, odor, and consistency.
- Palpate the patient's abdomen gently, checking for rigidity and rebound tenderness. (See *Eliciting rebound tenderness*, page 3.)
- ➡ **NurseALERT** Know that a rigid, distended abdomen with rebound tenderness signals peritonitis—an emergency that calls for immediate intervention.
- Assess bowel sounds in all quadrants. (See *Assessing bowel sounds*, page 234.)
- Ask the patient when she had her last bowel movement or passed flatus.

- Check for abdominal distention by measuring the patient's abdominal girth. To ensure accurate future measurements, use an indelible pen to mark the spot where you took the baseline measurement.
- Establish I.V. access, and administer I.V. fluids and electrolytes, as prescribed.
- Assess the patient's hydration status by checking her skin turgor and inspecting her oral mucous membranes for dryness.
- Assess the patient's pain status and administer analgesics, as needed and prescribed.
- Obtain blood samples for complete blood count, hematocrit, and serum electrolyte and hemoglobin levels.

WHAT TO DO NEXT
After taking initial actions, follow these guidelines:
- Monitor the patient's vital signs closely for changes that suggest dehydration or hypovolemia.
- Continue to give I.V. fluids and electrolytes, as prescribed.
- If the patient is hemodynamically unstable, anticipate instituting hemodynamic monitoring, such as central venous pressure monitoring or pulmonary artery pressure monitoring. Once the monitoring system is in place, assess the patient's central venous pressure every 2 to 4 hours.
- Administer antibiotics, as prescribed, for peritonitis or other abdominal infection.
- Assess the functional status of the NG or intestinal tube. Irrigate the tube with normal saline solution, as ordered, to keep it patent. Monitor all drainage for amount, color, and consistency.
- Continue to assess the patient's bowel sounds every 4 hours and measure her abdominal girth at least every 8 hours and more often if indicated. Regularly ask her about passage of flatus or feces.
- If indicated, obtain arterial blood gas values and monitor the results for metabolic alkalosis.
- Monitor repeat laboratory test results.
- Provide frequent oral hygiene.
- ➡ Nurse**ALERT** To help prevent electrolyte washout, limit the number of ice chips you give the patient to moisten her mouth while NG suction is being used to drain her GI contents.
- Inspect the patient's nares for signs of irritation from the tube. If necessary, apply a water-soluble lubricant to soothe the nasal area.

FOLLOW-UP CARE
- Continue to monitor the patient's bowel sounds, abdominal girth, and bowel elimination.
- If the patient requires surgery to relieve the obstruction, prepare her, as ordered, and provide preoperative teaching.
- Once the intestinal obstruction has been resolved and bowel sounds return, introduce oral fluids gradually, as ordered, and assess the patient's tolerance of oral intake.

SPECIAL CONSIDERATIONS

- Provide discharge teaching as indicated. Be sure to stress the importance of eating a high-fiber diet, drinking plenty of fluids, and getting sufficient exercise to help ensure normal bowel function.
- Teach the patient about signs and symptoms of recurrent intestinal obstruction, such as vomiting, constipation, and abdominal distention. Instruct her to report these at once.

INTRACRANIAL PRESSURE, INCREASED

Intracranial pressure (ICP) refers to the pressure exerted by the intracranial contents—brain, cerebrospinal fluid (CSF), and blood—against the inside of the skull. The rigid skull can't expand to accommodate an increase in intracranial volume. Thus a change in the volume of the brain, CSF, or intracranial blood demands a reciprocal change in one or both of the other components to keep pressure stable.

An ominous sign rather than a primary condition in itself, increased ICP can result from any condition that alters the normal balance of brain, intracranial blood, and CSF volume. (See *Understanding the normal balance of intracranial contents.*)

- *Increased brain volume* may result from cerebral edema (as occurs after trauma) or a space-occupying lesion (such as a tumor or an abscess).
- *Increased blood volume* occurs with conditions that increase cerebral blood flow (such as hypercapnia), intracranial hemorrhage or hematoma, and conditions that obstruct venous outflow.
- *Increased CSF volume* results from increased CSF production (as in choroid plexus disease), decreased CSF absorption (as in communicating hydrocephalus, which may occur after subarachnoid hemorrhage or bacterial meningitis), and obstructed CSF flow (as in noncommunicating hydrocephalus).

This sequence of events leads to neurologic deterioration:

- As ICP rises, blood flow to the brain decreases and perfusion pressure falls.
- Cellular hypoxia triggers vasodilation, which boosts cerebral blood-flow and causes ICP to rise even higher.
- Further compression of brain tissue and blood vessels causes dwindling blood flow to the brain.
- As ICP continues to increase, the brain begins to shift under pressure and, ultimately, may herniate through the foramen magnum, killing the patient.

Clearly, the results of increased ICP can be disastrous without prompt detection and a rapid, expert response.

UNDERSTANDING THE NORMAL BALANCE OF INTRACRANIAL CONTENTS

The skull houses three main components: brain tissue (80%), blood (10%), and cerebrospinal fluid (10%). In a normal human being, the total volume of intracranial contents is estimated to be between 1700 and 1900 ml.

Typically, this intracranial volume—and the percentages of the intracranial components in relation to each other—remains relatively constant. And even if small changes occur in the volume and relative percentages of the intracranial contents, the body can usually compensate—for example, by increasing cerebrospinal fluid absorption or the flow of venous blood out of the cerebral circulation and into the jugular vein. This natural compensation helps maintain normal intracranial pressure.

Sometimes, however, these natural compensation mechanisms fail. And if a volume increase in one or more components develops, and there is no compensation from another component, intracranial pressure will continue to rise, and the patient will develop neurologic deterioration.

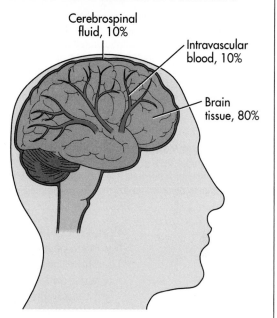

Cerebrospinal fluid, 10%

Intravascular blood, 10%

Brain tissue, 80%

I

WHAT TO LOOK FOR

Clinical findings in increased ICP may include:
- altered level of consciousness, including irritability, restlessness, lethargy, confusion, and stupor
- papilledema
- pupillary changes, including unequal pupils, altered responsiveness to light (sluggish to nonreactive), and change in size or shape
- cranial nerve palsies, including ptosis (eyelid drooping) and dysfunctions in extraocular movements
- headache (an inconsistent sign)
- focal neurologic deficit
- seizures.

Ominous clinical findings, which reflect pressure on the brain stem, include:
- altered vital signs, including elevated blood pressure, widened pulse pressure, and bradycardia
- decorticate or decerebrate posturing in response to stimulation
- impaired brain stem reflexes, such as corneal and gag reflexes
- projectile vomiting (seen mostly in young children).

REDUCING I.C.P. THROUGH OSMOTIC DIURESIS

Because increased intracranial pressure (ICP) often stems from or is complicated by cerebral edema, the physician may order hyperosmotic diuretics to draw water out of the brain's interstitial spaces, thereby decreasing brain mass and ICP. The patient's blood-brain barrier must be intact for osmotic diuresis to be effective. Otherwise, the hyperosmotic agent may pass into the brain, worsening cerebral edema and increasing brain mass.

ADMINISTERING MANNITOL
Mannitol (Osmitrol, 20% or 25% solution) is the hyperosmotic agent of choice because it reduces ICP rapidly. Typically, its effects peak within 15 minutes of administra-

tion; the duration of action is approximately 2 to 6 hours.

Expect to give mannitol 20% I.V. initially at a dosage of 1.5 to 2.0 g/kg of body weight over 15 to 30 minutes for maximal effect. You may repeat the dose every 1 to 4 hours, if needed.

To maintain adequate blood pressure and avoid a marked decrease in intravascular volume, most physicians order albumin (50 ml of a 25% solution) concomitantly with mannitol. Albumin enhances cerebral perfusion and minimizes mannitol's rebound effect.

Keep in mind that mannitol can cause severe dehydration and electrolyte imbalances. For the duration of therapy, monitor your patient's serum electrolyte levels and serum osmolality closely.

WHAT TO DO IMMEDIATELY

If you suspect that your patient has increased ICP, notify the physician. Then take these measures:

- Ensure and maintain an adequate airway. Prepare for endotracheal intubation if the patient's level of consciousness is severely decreased and she can't maintain a patent airway.
- Administer supplemental oxygen, as prescribed, to maintain her partial pressure of arterial oxygen (PaO_2) above 90 mm Hg. Monitor the patient's oxygen saturation level by pulse oximetry or arterial blood gas analysis, as indicated.
- Carefully assess and monitor the patient's level of consciousness. Changes in level of consciousness are the earliest indicators of increasing ICP.
- Assess the patient's vital signs, but keep in mind that vital sign changes are late findings in increased ICP.
- Prepare her for an immediate computed tomographic scan, as ordered.
- Establish I.V. access, and begin administering osmotic diuretics, if prescribed, to help reduce ICP. (See *Reducing ICP through osmotic diuresis.*)
- Perform frequent neurologic assessments and report significant changes.
- Elevate the head of the bed 15 to 30 degrees to promote venous outflow. Keep the patient in a neutral position, avoiding extreme neck or hip flexion (which increase ICP).
- Obtain baseline serum electrolyte and osmolarity levels, as ordered, to help guide drug therapy.
- Insert an indwelling urinary catheter, as ordered, to monitor urine output.
- Monitor intake and output closely (as often as every hour).

- Assist with the insertion of an ICP monitoring device if the patient requires continuous monitoring.

WHAT TO DO NEXT

Once your patient has been initially stabilized, carry out the following interventions:

- Continue to monitor her neurologic status, correlating the findings with ICP monitor readings (if an ICP monitoring device has been inserted).
- ➡ **NurseALERT** Stimulation, such as from physical care, repositioning, and treatment, can cause the patient's ICP to temporarily increase. To prevent serious elevations in ICP, space the patient's activities to allow her ICP to return to baseline. Be especially alert for a transient decrease in her neurologic status, which can warn of impending decompensation.
- Assess the patient for adequate ventilation; maintain mechanical ventilation, if ordered. Continuously assess her oxygen saturation level, and provide supplemental oxygen, as indicated and ordered, to maintain adequate PaO_2.
- Suction the patient if necessary, but not routinely. Only perform this procedure when needed, and limit the suctioning time to the briefest time possible.
- ➡ **NurseALERT** Before suctioning, preoxygenate the patient for 30 to 60 seconds.
- Monitor the patient's vital signs, watching closely for hypotension (a possible effect of diuretic therapy).
- ➡ **NurseALERT** In the presence of increased ICP, systolic blood pressure must be sufficient to deliver blood to the brain despite increased resistance in cerebral vasculature. The goal of treatment is to keep the patient mildly hypertensive (140 mm Hg systolic). Hypotension can lead to a dangerous decrease in cerebral perfusion pressure, resulting in cerebral hypoxia.
- Monitor her fluid intake and output closely to avoid hypovolemia (from osmotic diuresis).
- To prevent hyperthermia, provide antipyretic drugs, as prescribed, and hypothermia blankets as necessary. Remember—hyperthermia increases the metabolic rate and therefore can raise ICP.
- Maintain a quiet environment and avoid excessive environmental stimulation.
- Administer stool-softening agents, as prescribed, and implement other measures to prevent constipation and the need for straining at stool (which increases ICP).
- Carefully maintain the ICP monitoring device according to your facility's guidelines, using strict aseptic technique. Take measures to ensure accurate readings and avoid infection. If an intraventricular catheter is in place, take precautions to avoid inadvertent loss of CSF.

I

- Monitor the patient's serum electrolyte and osmolarity levels for the duration of diuretic therapy.

FOLLOW-UP CARE
- To help prevent complications of immobility, turn and reposition the patient every 2 hours and provide meticulous skin care to prevent breakdown. Perform passive range-of-motion exercises on all extremities, and maintain joints in their functional positions.
- Using aseptic technique, provide care for the insertion site of the ICP monitoring device; monitor the site closely for signs of infection.
- As the patient's ICP stabilizes, prepare for removal of the ICP monitoring device.
- Continue to monitor the patient's neurologic status to detect any changes.

SPECIAL CONSIDERATIONS
- If a fiber-optic ICP monitoring system is used, prevent the catheter from kinking or bending to avoid interfering with accurate readouts or breaking the catheter.
- Be sure to keep a fluid-filled ICP monitoring system correctly positioned, balanced, and free of air. Calibrate it as indicated to ensure accurate readouts. Check your facility's policy for flushing the system.
- Assess the patient's rehabilitation needs and make appropriate referrals early during her hospital stay.

I.V. CATHETER PROBLEMS

Usually, careful management and assessment can keep your patient's I.V. catheter intact and his infusion running smoothly. However, occasionally a catheter may become occluded or a piece of it may be severed. (See *Assessing the I.V. catheter site.*)

An occluded catheter can create problems by blocking your patient's infusion. A severed catheter can imperil your patient's life if a piece of the catheter tip floats into his systemic circulation; the piece may lodge near the original site or may advance to the heart or even to the pulmonary vascular bed.

If you suspect that your patient has an I.V. catheter problem, your quick action could improve his outcome—even save his life.

WHAT TO LOOK FOR
Clinical findings depend on whether the catheter is severed or occluded.

Indications of a severed catheter
Clinical findings in a patient with a severed catheter may include:
- an obvious break or fracture in the catheter lumen

- leakage of I.V. fluid from the catheter shaft
- a missing internal catheter tip, discovered when you remove the venous access device
- visibly reduced catheter length on removal of the venous access device
- pain along the vein used for an existing catheter or at the site of a previous catheter entry site
- findings that correspond to the location of a migrating catheter tip, including chest pain, dyspnea, cyanosis, tachycardia, and hypotension.

Indications of an occluded catheter
Clinical findings produced by an occluded catheter may include:
- backflow of blood into the catheter, administration tubing, or both
- a reduced flow rate or cessation of flow
- lack of change in the flow rate when you raise the solution container
- inability to flush the catheter.

WHAT TO DO IMMEDIATELY
Tailor your response to the suspected problem—a severed catheter or an occluded one.

For a severed catheter
- If the severed portion of the catheter is visible, try to retrieve it.
- If you can't retrieve it or it isn't visible, apply pressure or wrap a tourniquet above the I.V. site to try to stop the catheter fragment from migrating into the central venous system, heart, and lungs.
- Notify the physician, and obtain an order for X-rays to locate the catheter in the patient's body.
- ➡ **NurseALERT** Continue to apply pressure or keep the tourniquet in place until you've obtained radiographic confirmation of the catheter's location.
- Support the patient as needed if he develops circulatory or pulmonary symptoms.

For an occluded catheter
- Check the tubing for kinks or a closed roller clamp, and adjust as necessary.
- Attempt to aspirate the clot with a syringe. If you're successful, flush the catheter with a mild flush solution, such as heparin flush solution or normal saline for injection.
- ➡ **NurseALERT** Don't force the flush solution because you could dislodge an embolus, which would enter the patient's systemic circulation. Also, be aware that if your patient complains of sharp pain when you flush the catheter, you might have dislodged a thrombus and caused intimal damage. If so, assess the site closely for signs of phlebitis.
- If you can't remove the occlusion by aspiration, you'll have to remove the catheter and start a new I.V. line at another site.

ASSESSING THE I.V. CATHETER SITE

Careful assessment and sound site management will help you avoid most problems with I.V. catheters. Your assessment of the insertion site should reveal:
- no tenderness or discomfort
- no discoloration or redness
- no swelling
- no induration
- no moisture accumulation under the dressing
- a secure and intact dressing.

I

WHAT TO DO NEXT
After the initial problem has been identified, take these steps:
- If the catheter is severed, stay with the patient until the fragment is located and removed. A catheter fragment usually can be removed by performing a radiologic snare procedure. If not, the patient may need surgery. Prepare him as needed.
- Start a new I.V. line at another site and resume I.V. therapy, as ordered.
- Care for the I.V. site and maintain the infusion according to your facility's policy. As appropriate, use an I.V. pump or controller to maintain the proper rate.
- If a snare retrieval procedure was performed, assess and care for the puncture site. Inspect the area routinely for signs and symptoms of infection.

FOLLOW-UP CARE
- Continue to monitor the patient's vital signs, cardiopulmonary status, and related symptoms, such as dyspnea and chest pain.

SPECIAL CONSIDERATIONS
To prevent a catheter from becoming severed or occluded, follow these measures:
- Keep fluid moving through the catheter to prevent clotting or occlusion. For example, don't allow the I.V. infusion container to run dry before replacing it. Also make sure to flush all I.V. lines (including heparin locks and other intermittent infusion devices) before and after each use, according to your facility's policy.
- The cannula tip of an over-the-needle I.V. device should never be moved past the bevel tip until the catheter is threaded into the vein lumen. By moving an I.V. cannula past a stylet bevel tip and reseating it onto the metal stylet, you risk causing a catheter emboli or sheering the I.V. catheter material.
- Never retract an over-the-needle I.V. catheter against the needle's bevel tip.
- Secure all I.V. catheters properly to avoid excessive tension on the catheter lumen.
- When irrigating a Silastic catheter, use a 5-ml syringe or larger (to decrease pounds per square inch) and avoid using excessive force.
- Don't apply pressure over the I.V. site when withdrawing the catheter.
- After removing the catheter, inspect its internal tip to make sure it's complete and intact.

LATEX HYPERSENSITIVITY REACTION

The increasing use of latex gloves and condoms to prevent transmission of acquired immunodeficiency syndrome and hepatitis has had an unexpected result: increased latex hypersensitivity. Health-care workers are at high risk for hypersensitivity because they wear latex gloves and work with or around other latex-containing medical products every day. With thousands of latex-containing products in common use—from clothing and toys to adhesives—latex hypersensitivity is a potential threat to virtually anyone. (See *How latex hypersensitivity arises,* page 248.)

Latex hypersensitivity may present as a type I (immediate) reaction, a type IV (delayed) reaction, or chemical irritation dermatitis.

- A type I reaction, the most dangerous, may arise within minutes or up to 1 hour after contact with latex. Type I reactions are subdivided according to severity, with localized urticaria being the least severe and anaphylaxis the most severe.
- A type IV reaction remains localized to the skin or mucous membranes.

In a severe hypersensitivity reaction, the victim may die of acute respiratory failure and vascular collapse if she doesn't receive immediate, effective treatment. To make matters worse, even as she's being treated for anaphylaxis, her latex exposure is likely to continue—unless you and other members of the health-care team recognize this emergency and remove all latex items immediately.

Stay alert for possible latex hypersensitivity in any patient who has suggestive signs and symptoms. And make sure to keep appropriate equipment, such as a latex-free emergency cart, readily available to ensure that you and your colleagues render safe care.

WHAT TO LOOK FOR

Clinical findings in anaphylaxis caused by latex hypersensitivity may include:

- angioedema (swelling of the face, neck, lips, larynx, hands, feet, and genitalia)
- dyspnea
- wheezing
- stridor (from laryngeal edema or bronchoconstriction)
- tachycardia
- urticaria
- hypotension.

WHAT TO DO IMMEDIATELY

If you suspect that your patient's having an anaphylactic reaction to latex, establish and maintain a patent airway, ensure that the patient has

HOW LATEX HYPERSENSITIVITY ARISES

Composed of the milky sap from the rubber tree *Hevea brasiliensis*, latex contains proteins, lipids, nucleotides, and cofactors. After processing, it consists of 2% to 3% protein and more than 200 polypeptides. Latex hypersensitivity occurs after a person has been sensitized to the proteins in natural latex rubber or once the barrier protection of the skin has broken down from the additives used to manufacture latex.

On the first exposure to latex—whether direct, as from wearing latex gloves, or indirect, as from inhaling the airborne powder released from another person's glove—a person may become sensitized. Although her body forms antibodies to the latex proteins at this time, symptoms don't arise until a subsequent exposure. With each successive exposure, her symptoms may worsen.

CROSSEXPOSURE THREAT

Many of the polypeptides found in latex also exist in plants (such as poinsettia) and tropical fruits (including papayas, avocados, kiwifruit, and bananas). Therefore, a latex-sensitive person may experience a crossreaction from ingesting or coming into contact with one of these plants or foods.

IDENTIFYING THOSE AT RISK

The following people are at risk for latex hypersensitivity:

- health-care providers, from daily exposure to latex examination gloves and many other medical products that contain latex
- people with a history of allergy or asthma
- people with spina bifida because of their frequent exposure to latex-containing items during medical care
- patients who've had multiple genitourinary or intra-abdominal surgeries, from direct exposure of body cavities to latex
- patients who undergo frequent or continuous catheterization
- rubber industry workers and other people with occupational exposure to latex, such as food service workers.

effective respiration and circulation, and notify the physician. Then follow these guidelines:

- Administer epinephrine 1:1,000 by subcutaneous injection, 0.01 ml/kg to a maximum of 0.3 ml every 10 to 15 minutes, as prescribed, to halt anaphylaxis.

  ➡ **Nurse ALERT** A patient who is experiencing anaphylaxis must receive epinephrine as soon as possible to stay alive.

- Establish and maintain a patent airway using latex-free supplies, such as a latex-free endotracheal tube. If the patient has oral or laryngeal edema (making oral intubation impossible), gather latex-free cricothyrotomy supplies and assist with the procedure, as ordered.

- Establish an I.V. line. Be sure to use I.V. tubing without latex injection ports. Remember to use latex-free gloves when caring for a patient with known or suspected latex hypersensitivity.

- Monitor the patient's blood pressure every 5 to 15 minutes for hypotension, but make sure to use a latex-free blood pressure cuff and tubing. Or place Webril (a stretchable cotton material used to prevent irritation from plaster casts) between the patient and the blood pressure cuff so the latex won't touch her skin.

- Auscultate the patient's chest for wheezing or decreased air movement.

- Assess her oxygen saturation continuously by way of pulse oximetry. As prescribed, provide high-flow supplemental oxygen and aerosolized bronchodilators.

➡ **NurseALERT** Keep in mind that the straps on some oxygen face masks contain latex; if in doubt, remove the strap and have the patient hold the mask in place or tie the mask with cloth straps.

- Using latex-free leads, begin continuous cardiac monitoring; monitor the patient's ECG for tachycardia and cardiac response to epinephrine.
- Give secondary I.V. medications, such as diphenhydramine (Benadryl), steroids, and fluids, as prescribed. Depending on the patient's response to epinephrine, the physician also may prescribe I.V. vasopressors.
- Remove all latex-containing items from the room and from possible contact with the patient. In a health-care setting, such items may include gloves, drug vials with latex stoppers, I.V. tubing with latex injection ports, latex hand-held resuscitation bags, anesthesia ventilator bellows, plastic syringes with latex-tipped plungers, and some nasopharyngeal tubes.

WHAT TO DO NEXT
Once your patient is stable, take these measures:
- Continue to monitor her vital signs.
- Stay alert for another episode of anaphylaxis, which may result from inadvertent latex exposure during treatment or from epinephrine's short half-life. (Some patients need more than one epinephrine injection, depending on the type and duration of latex exposure.)
- If possible, arrange for a private room to minimize potential latex exposure near the patient.
- Place a sign on the patient's door informing staff members and visitors of her latex hypersensitivity. Don't allow the use of latex gloves or other latex items in the room.
- Keep a cart stocked with latex-free products at the patient's bedside in case she needs further interventions.

FOLLOW-UP CARE
- Continue to guard the patient against latex exposure throughout her hospital stay.
- Enforce bed rest to keep her oxygen demands down and slow her heart rate (epinephrine speeds the heart rate).
- Regularly auscultate the patient's chest for wheezing.
- Maintain I.V. fluid therapy, as prescribed, to support blood pressure.
- To help determine which latex item might have triggered the hypersensitivity reaction, ask the patient about her activities just before anaphylaxis began.
- Find out if an allergist previously diagnosed the latex hypersensitivity and provided follow-up treatment. If not, provide referrals according to facility policy.

SPECIAL CONSIDERATIONS
- Keep in mind that caring for a patient with latex hypersensitivity requires a knowledgeable health-care team.

L

- Remember—you never know when a latex-sensitive person may enter your area. Even a patient with no history of latex hypersensitivity may experience anaphylaxis while receiving care for another medical problem. Staff members and visitors are at risk too. Stock an emergency kit with crucial supplies for treating latex-hypersensitivity anaphylaxis: epinephrine, latex-free (vinyl or neoprene) gloves, latex-free I.V. equipment (such as tubing with latex-free ports), latex-free tape, and latex-free electrodes.
- Make sure your facility also has larger carts stocked with additional latex-free items, such as urinary catheters, endotracheal tubes, blood pressure cuffs, and dressings.
- Provide the patient with written materials about latex hypersensitivity and a list of items she must avoid to prevent another life-threatening reaction.
- To guard yourself and your colleagues from latex hypersensitivity reactions, ask your supervisor to obtain latex-free product substitutes.
- Urge your administrator to conduct latex hypersensitivity training during orientation for new employees and during yearly in-service classes.

METABOLIC ACIDOSIS

A primary bicarbonate deficit, metabolic acidosis is characterized by excess acid or deficient base (bicarbonate) in response to an underlying pathologic condition. As a result, the patient's pH—which buffering systems normally maintain at about 7.35—may drop below its normal level. (See *Understanding blood pH and acid-base balance*.)

Conditions that may cause *acid accumulation* include:
- lactic acidosis
- renal failure
- tissue hypoxia
- ketoacidosis from diabetes or starvation
- salicylate, paraldehyde, or ethanol toxicity.

Conditions that may lead to *bicarbonate loss* include:
- severe, prolonged diarrhea
- drainage of the small intestine or pancreas
- pancreatic fistulas
- ureterosigmoidostomy or jejunal loop
- rapid administration of saline solution.

Clinical effects of metabolic acidosis reflect the body's efforts to correct the acidosis through renal, respiratory, and cellular compensation. For instance, decreased blood pH causes the brain's respiratory center to increase respiratory rate and depth in an attempt to eliminate excess carbon dioxide (an acid) and return blood to its normal (neutral) pH. The

UNDERSTANDING BLOOD pH AND ACID-BASE BALANCE

A normal pH (hydrogen ion concentration) in arterial blood is essential to survival. In a healthy person, compensatory mechanisms and chemical buffering systems maintain blood pH between 7.35 and 7.45.

In uncompensated or partially compensated *metabolic acidosis*, arterial pH typically drops below 7.35 and the serum bicarbonate level measures less than 22 mEq/L. However, a patient with chronic, compensated metabolic acidosis may have a normal pH.

DIAGNOSING ACID-BASE DISORDERS

All acid-base disorders must be evaluated through arterial blood gas (ABG) values. ABG analysis measures the partial pressures of oxygen and carbon dioxide and the pH of an arterial sample as well as the bicarbonate concentration and oxygen saturation.

WHAT THE ANION GAP SHOWS

Calculating the anion gap—the difference between cation and anion concentrations in the blood—can help identify the underlying cause of metabolic acidosis. Normally, the gap measures between 8 and 18 mEq/L.

In metabolic acidosis stemming from bicarbonate loss, the anion gap is normal. In metabolic acidosis resulting from acid accumulation, the gap rises above normal.

---

kidneys respond to falling pH by secreting more hydrogen, chloride, and ammonia ions while retaining bicarbonate and sodium.

Severe or untreated metabolic acidosis can deteriorate quickly to cardiac and respiratory arrest and, ultimately, death. Be alert for telltale signs and symptoms, especially when caring for a patient with a predisposing condition, such as diabetes, anorexia, and shock.

WHAT TO LOOK FOR

Clinical findings in metabolic acidosis may include:
- decreased level of consciousness (possibly stupor or coma)
- disorientation, confusion
- headache
- increased respiratory rate and depth
- Kussmaul's respirations (abnormally slow, deep respirations)
- acetone breath (if the patient has ketoacidosis)
- fever
- evidence of dehydration, such as increased thirst and decreased skin turgor
- signs and symptoms of shock (such as distended neck veins, hypotension, diminished or thready peripheral pulse, tachycardia, pallor, poor capillary refill, and decreased skin temperature)
- cardiac changes, such as arrhythmias (tachycardia or bradycardia) and decreased cardiac output
- arterial blood gas (ABG) values showing blood pH below 7.35, bicarbonate below 22 mEq/L, and partial pressure of carbon dioxide in arterial blood below 35 mm Hg (see *Interpreting ABG values*, page 253).

WHAT TO DO IMMEDIATELY

If you suspect that your patient has metabolic acidosis, notify the physician. Then follow these guidelines:

M

- Obtain blood samples for repeat ABG analysis. Monitor ABG values, anion gap, and serum electrolyte levels throughout therapy.
- As indicated, place the patient on continuous cardiac monitoring, and monitor for disturbances of rate and rhythm on his ECG.
- Establish I.V. access and administer medications prescribed to correct the underlying cause of metabolic acidosis and restore fluid and electrolyte balance. For metabolic acidosis that stems from diabetic ketoacidosis, expect to give I.V. insulin and fluids. For lactic acidosis, anticipate administering I.V. sodium bicarbonate to neutralize blood acidity.
- ➡ **NurseALERT** Be aware of the potential risks of sodium bicarbonate infusion, including hypernatremia, metabolic alkalosis, fluid volume overload, and acute hypokalemia. Also, monitor the patient closely for signs and symptoms of cardiac and respiratory arrest.
- Use a volume-control device to prevent overly rapid infusion of I.V. medications and fluids. Monitor the infusion closely.
- Check the patient's blood pressure; pulse rate; respiratory rate, rhythm, and depth; and level of consciousness every 5 to 15 minutes; report significant changes. Auscultate breath sounds every 15 minutes.
- As indicated, monitor the patient's oxygen saturation levels continuously by way of pulse oximetry; as needed and prescribed, administer supplemental oxygen.
- Anticipate the need for endotracheal intubation and mechanical ventilation if the patient develops respiratory insufficiency leading to respiratory arrest.
- For metabolic acidosis caused by renal failure, expect to prepare the patient for peritoneal dialysis or hemodialysis. Assist during the procedure, as ordered.
- If metabolic acidosis is severe, initiate seizure precautions, such as padding and raising the side rails. Keep emergency airway equipment on hand and give anticonvulsants, if prescribed.

WHAT TO DO NEXT
Once your patient has been stabilized, take these steps:
- Continue to monitor his ABG and serum electrolyte values. Report significant changes immediately.
- Continue to watch his ECG for arrhythmias and other abnormalities.
- Frequently assess his vital signs, especially observing for cardiac and respiratory changes.
- Monitor the patient's hourly fluid intake and output. Remember that diminished output may lead to circulatory overload. Monitor closely for evidence of overload, such as respiratory changes, dyspnea, crackles, agitation, and anxiety. Anticipate dialysis to remove excess fluid.
- Continue seizure precautions. If a seizure occurs, ensure a patent airway, protect the patient from injury and accidental removal of the I.V. catheter, and notify the physician at once. After the seizure, assess the

INTERPRETING A.B.G. VALUES

If you suspect that your patient has an acid-base disturbance, you'll need to analyze his arterial blood gas (ABG) values closely to determine which disturbance is present and whether his body is compensating for it. Review the following information to help sharpen your ABG interpretation skills.

THREE CRUCIAL VALUES

When assessing for an acid-base disturbance, focus on your patient's pH, partial pressure of arterial carbon dioxide ($Paco_2$), and HCO_3^- values.

Blood pH

Blood pH indicates whether the patient's blood is neutral (pH of 7.35 to 7.45), alkaline (higher than 7.45), or acidic (lower than 7.35).

$Paco_2$

The $Paco_2$ value indicates the partial pressure of carbon dioxide in the blood. The normal range for $Paco_2$ is 35 to 45 mm Hg. $Paco_2$ relates inversely to pH: As $Paco_2$ rises, pH decreases.

$Paco_2$ is considered the respiratory component in acid-base determination because the lungs exert primary control over it. However, metabolic disturbances also can alter the $Paco_2$ level because the lungs compensate for primary metabolic acid-base disorders. For instance, in metabolic acidosis, the lungs "blow off" carbon dioxide in an effort to raise the pH; in metabolic alkalosis, they retain carbon dioxide in an attempt to lower the pH.

HCO_3^-

HCO_3^- refers to blood bicarbonate. An index of the alkali reserve, HCO_3^- is the metabolic component of the acid-base equilibrium. The normal bicarbonate range is 22 to 26 mEq/L.

HCO_3^- and pH are directly related: as one rises, so does the other. HCO_3^- increases in metabolic alkalosis and decreases in metabolic acidosis.

PUTTING THE VALUES IN PERSPECTIVE

To determine which acid-base imbalance your patient has, start by looking at pH. If it's below 7.35, suspect acidosis; if it's above 7.45, suspect alkalosis. If pH is normal, don't assume that nothing is wrong until you've checked to see that the $Paco_2$ and HCO_3^- are normal. A normal pH may reflect that the body has compensated for an acid-base imbalance.

Metabolic or respiratory disturbance?

Next, determine whether the primary disturbance is metabolic or respiratory by checking to see how the HCO_3^- and $Paco_2$ values relate to the pH value.
- If both HCO_3^- and pH are abnormal but $Paco_2$ is normal, the primary disturbance is metabolic.
- If both $Paco_2$ and pH are abnormal but HCO_3^- is normal, the primary disturbance is respiratory.

Alkalosis or acidosis?

Now put all three values together to find out which type of metabolic or respiratory disturbance your patient has.
- Increased HCO_3^- and pH, normal $Paco_2$: metabolic alkalosis
- Decreased HCO_3^- and pH, normal $Paco_2$: metabolic acidosis
- Normal HCO_3^-, increased $Paco_2$, decreased pH: respiratory acidosis
- Normal HCO_3^-, decreased $Paco_2$, increased pH: respiratory alkaosis.

Clues to compensation

Finally, determine whether compensation is occurring by looking at the value that represents that *nonprimary* disorder. For example, if your patient's primary disorder is metabolic, look at the $Paco_2$ value. If his primary disorder is respiratory, look at the HCO_3^- value.

Suspect compensation if the nonprimary component is moving in the same direction as the primary component; this reflects the body's attempt to bring the pH into a normal range. The following scenarios indicate probable compensation:
- $Paco_2$ is decreased slightly in a patient with metabolic acidosis (primary problem is decreased HCO_3^-).
- $Paco_2$ is slightly increased in a patient with metabolic alkalosis (primary problem is increased HCO_3^-).
- HCO_3^- is slightly increased in a patient with respiratory acidosis (primary problem is increased $Paco_2$).
- HCO_3^- is slightly decreased in a patient with respiratory alkalosis (primary problem is decreased $Paco_2$).

M

patient and obtain a blood sample to evaluate his fluid and electrolyte status.
- Continue to monitor the patient's oxygen saturation level.

FOLLOW-UP CARE
- Continue to monitor laboratory results; report significant changes.
- Continue to record the patient's fluid intake and output.
- Assess his level of consciousness, including orientation, regularly.
- Maintain seizure precautions. As therapy corrects metabolic acidosis, the risk of seizures decreases.
- Obtain a complete patient history to help identify the underlying cause of metabolic acidosis and guide long-term treatment.

SPECIAL CONSIDERATIONS
- As indicated, keep emergency equipment such as a defibrillator and emergency medications on hand in case of cardiopulmonary arrest.

METABOLIC ALKALOSIS

Metabolic alkalosis is characterized either by excess bicarbonate (base) or by decreased hydrogen ions (acid). It's commonly accompanied by deficits in serum potassium and chloride.

Conditions that may cause a *loss of hydrogen ions* include:
- prolonged vomiting or gastric suctioning
- severe diarrhea
- electrolyte imbalances, such as hypercalcemia, hypomagnesemia, and hypokalemia
- diuretic use (except carbonic anhydrase inhibitors)
- renal insufficiency
- laxative abuse
- excess aldosterone secreted by adrenal glands (as in Cushing's syndrome, hyperadrenocorticism, and primary hyperaldosteronism).

Conditions that may cause a *gain in bicarbonate* include:
- milk-alkali syndrome
- excessive ingestion of alkalis (such as baking soda and antacids)
- administration of I.V. sodium bicarbonate, calcium carbonate, or parenteral nutrition solutions
- excessive or rapid administration of stored blood.

The lungs try to compensate for metabolic alkalosis through hypoventilation, which retains carbon dioxide and lowers serum pH. The kidneys compensate by retaining hydrogen ions and excreting bicarbonate ions. Without treatment, these compensatory mechanisms eventually fail, and the patient lapses into a coma.

Early detection and prompt treatment of metabolic alkalosis usually ensure a good prognosis. To safeguard your patient's well-being, make sure you're thoroughly familiar with the clinical and laboratory indicators of metabolic alkalosis and the rapid interventions you must take.

WHAT TO LOOK FOR
Clinical findings in metabolic alkalosis may include:
- nervousness, anxiety, and shakiness
- irritability, agitation , and confusion
- decreased level of consciousness
- tingling of the fingers and toes
- muscle weakness or twitching
- hyperactive reflexes (see *Evaluating deep tendon reflexes,* page 256)
- Chvostek's and Trousseau's signs (if hypocalcemia is present)
- tetany
- seizures
- arrhythmias, such as atrial tachycardia
- other ECG changes, such as decreased T-wave amplitude and, in later stages, prolonged QT intervals and T waves merging with P waves
- arterial blood gas (ABG) values revealing blood pH above 7.45, bicarbonate above 26 mEq/L, and partial pressure of arterial carbon dioxide above 40 mm Hg.

WHAT TO DO IMMEDIATELY
If you suspect that your patient has metabolic alkalosis, notify the physician. Then take these steps:
- Obtain blood samples for repeat ABG analysis and serum electrolyte measurement. Monitor these levels throughout therapy.
- Evaluate the patient's blood pressure, pulse and respiratory rates, and level of consciousness every 5 to 15 minutes; report significant changes.
- Begin continuous cardiac monitoring, and observe the ECG for low T waves, atrioventricular arrhythmias, and, in later stages, merging of T and P waves.
- Establish I.V. access. As prescribed, in severe metabolic alkalosis, administer I.V. ammonium chloride to increase hydrogen ion concentration and raise the serum chloride level. Use an infusion-control device to prevent too-rapid an infusion. Monitor the infusion closely throughout therapy.
- ➡ **NurseALERT** Be aware that I.V. ammonium chloride may cause hyperchloremic metabolic acidosis in a patient with renal or hepatic impairment. Use extreme caution when administering this agent to such a patient.
- Implement other ordered treatments to correct the underlying cause of metabolic alkalosis and restore fluid and electrolyte balance. For

M

EVALUATING DEEP TENDON REFLEXES

Deep tendon (muscle stretch) reflexes are brief, involuntary muscle contractions in response to sudden stretching. In a number of conditions, including electrolyte imbalances, acidosis, and alkalosis, deep tendon reflexes may become hypoactive or hyperactive.

ASSESSMENT STEPS
Follow these steps to evaluate your patient's biceps, triceps, patellar, Achilles, and bracheoradialis reflexes:
- Ask the patient to relax.
- Position the arm or leg to be tested so that it's stretched slightly.
- Distract the patient's attention from this area to decrease cognitive inhibition of the reflex. For example, before testing a reflex in the arm, instruct her to clench her teeth; before testing a reflex in her leg, ask her to grasp her hands and pull.
- Hold your thumb firmly against the tendon and tap it briskly with a reflex hammer, or strike the tendon with the reflex hammer directly.
- Observe the muscle's response to the tapping; normally, it extends and contracts rapidly. In a hyperactive response, muscle movement is jerky and exaggerated. In a markedly hyperactive response, you may even note clonus—involuntary, rapidly alternating muscle contraction and relaxation.

- Compare the reflex response on the opposite side of the patient's body, using the same amount of force. Bilateral responses should be equal.

GRADING REFLEX RESPONSES
Grade your patient's reflex responses on a scale of 0 to 4+ as follows:
- 4+: Hyperactive with sustained clonus
- 3+: Hyperactive
- 2+: Normal
- 1+: Hypoactive
- 0: Absent

You may want to transfer the patient's scores to a stick figure like the one shown below.

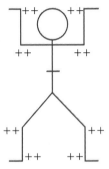

instance, if gastric losses led to metabolic alkalosis, anticipate giving normal saline solution and I.V. potassium chloride to restore normal electrolyte levels. Use a volume-control device to ensure the proper infusion rate.
- If administering I.V. solutions with potassium chloride, monitor the patient closely for arrhythmias. Because potassium is primarily excreted by the kidneys, monitor her urine output to check for normal renal function. Make sure to dilute the I.V. solution as directed by the manufacturer to prevent pain and irritation of the vein. Keep in mind that too-rapid an infusion of potassium may lead to cardiac arrest.
- If the patient has hypocalcemia, expect to give I.V. calcium (gluconate, chloride, or gluceptate), as prescribed.
- ➡ **Nurse**ALERT Infuse I.V. calcium *slowly* to prevent bradycardia, which may trigger cardiac arrest. Before starting calcium therapy, check the patient's medication history for digoxin use; calcium enhances the effects of this drug and puts the patient at increased risk for digitalis toxicity. During calcium therapy, watch closely for evidence of toxicity, including nausea, fatigue, vision changes, and arrhythmias.

- Prepare to assist with cardiopulmonary resuscitation if the patient's heart stops or respiratory muscles fail.
- As indicated, initiate seizure precautions, such as raising and padding the side rails, administering anticonvulsants, if prescribed, and bringing an emergency airway to the bedside.

WHAT TO DO NEXT
Once your patient has been stabilized, take these steps:
- Monitor her vital signs, ABG values, and serum electrolyte levels every hour during electrolyte replacement therapy and every 4 hours thereafter. Report significant changes immediately.
- Continue to monitor her ECG for signs of altered heart function, T-wave changes, tachycardia, and other arrhythmias.
- Continue to monitor the patient's level of consciousness closely.
- Record her hourly fluid intake and output. Be sure to take into account any I.V. fluids that have been infused.
- Continue to maintain seizure precautions, as indicated. If a seizure occurs, protect the patient from injury and accidental removal of the I.V. catheter, ensure a patent airway, and notify the physician. After a seizure, assess the patient and draw blood samples to evaluate her fluid and electrolyte status.

FOLLOW-UP CARE
- Continue to keep a close watch on the patient's ABG values and serum electrolyte levels; report significant changes at once.
- Assess her level of consciousness often for changes.
- Continue to record her hourly fluid intake and output, and measure urine specific gravity.
- Maintain seizure precautions. Remember that as therapy relieves your patient's acid-base imbalance, her risk for seizures declines.
- Restrict the patient to bed rest until her ABG and electrolyte levels return to normal. Assist with ambulation when she gets out of bed because she's at risk for muscle weakness.
- Obtain a complete patient history to help identify the underlying cause of metabolic alkalosis and guide long-term treatment.

SPECIAL CONSIDERATIONS
- As indicated, keep emergency equipment (such as a resuscitation bag, endotracheal intubation set, defibrillator, and emergency medications) on hand at all times in case of cardiopulmonary arrest.

M

MURMUR, ACUTE-ONSET

Heart murmurs don't always indicate life-threatening events. However, after an acute myocardial infarction (MI), the sudden onset of a new murmur may signal a ventricular septal defect (VSD) or papillary muscle rupture—both potentially fatal complications of MI.

Murmur caused by VSD

Occasionally, a patient with an anterior, an inferior, or a septal MI develops a perforation in the interventricular septum. When this happens, some amount of blood from the left ventricle passes through the perforation to the right ventricle, forcing the heart's right side to work harder. Right ventricular preload rises and, eventually, the right ventricle fails. The patient's prognosis depends on the perforation's size and the extent of decompensation from acute heart failure and shock.

Murmur caused by papillary muscle rupture

If an infarct develops in or near a papillary muscle, the muscle may become ischemic or rupture; the chordae tendineae may rupture as well. As a result, papillary muscles can't keep the mitral valve tightly closed against the backflow of blood from the high-pressure left ventricle, which may allow severe mitral regurgitation into the left atrium and pulmonary vasculature during contractions. The patient then may suffer massive pulmonary edema and shock; without immediate valve replacement surgery, he may die.

WHAT TO LOOK FOR

Clinical findings in acute murmur depend on whether the patient has a VSD or a papillary muscle rupture. (See *New murmur after MI*.)

Findings in VSD

A patient with a VSD may have the following signs and symptoms:
- loud, harsh holosystolic murmur
- hypotension
- elevated left ventricular end-diastolic pressure
- palpable precordial thrill
- dyspnea
- chest pain
- syncope.

Findings in papillary muscle rupture

With papillary muscle rupture, expect signs and symptoms of acute mitral regurgitation, such as:
- loud, blowing systolic murmur
- crackles on auscultation
- tachycardia
- severe dyspnea
- V waves on pulmonary artery wedge pressure tracings
- third and fourth heart sounds (S_3 and S_4)
- thready peripheral pulses
- cool, clammy skin.

DANGER SIGNS AND SYMPTOMS

NEW MURMUR AFTER M.I.

If your patient suddenly develops a new murmur after a myocardial infarction (MI), his life could be in danger. That's because the murmur may signal development of a ventricular septal defect (VSD) or papillary muscle rupture. In either case, you'll hear variable—usually high-pitched—blowing, musical, or harsh sounds through the diaphragm of your stethoscope.

RECOGNIZING VSD MURMURS

A VSD produces a murmur when blood flows from the higher-pressure left ventricle to the lower-pressure right ventricle (see illustration at left).

With a VSD, expect to hear a high-pitched holosystolic murmur throughout ventricular systole. It is loud-est along the left sternal border and may intensify with inspiration.

RECOGNIZING PAPILLARY MUSCLE RUPTURE MURMURS

With a papillary muscle rupture, the murmur results from backward flow of blood from the high-pressure ventricle through an incompetent mitral valve to the lower-pressure atrium (see illustration at right).

Expect to hear a high-pitched systolic murmur that's loudest at the apex of the heart and that may radiate to the axilla. With dysfunction of the chordae tendineae, you may hear a midsystolic click.

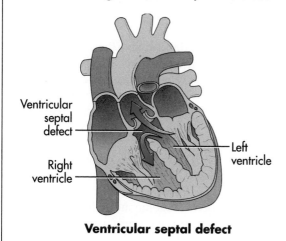

Ventricular septal defect

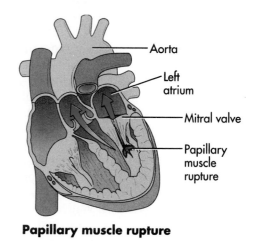

Papillary muscle rupture

M

WHAT TO DO IMMEDIATELY

If your patient has an acute murmur and you suspect VSD or papillary muscle rupture, notify the physician. Then take these steps:

- Begin continuous cardiac and blood pressure monitoring.
- Assist with insertion of a pulmonary artery catheter for hemodynamic monitoring.
- Insert and maintain an I.V. line. Administer I.V. medications, as prescribed.
- Obtain arterial blood gas measurements, and monitor the patient's oxygen saturation by way of pulse oximetry. Provide supplemental oxygen, if prescribed and needed.
- To confirm suspected VSD, collect blood samples from the distal and proximal ports of the patient's pulmonary artery catheter. The oxy-

gen level in these samples reveals whether oxygenated blood is being shunted from the left to the right ventricle.

- As prescribed, give medications to reduce afterload, such as nitroprusside sodium (Nitropress).
- As ordered, prepare your patient for insertion of a balloon catheter for intra-aortic balloon counterpulsation (IABP) therapy to reduce left-to-right shunting and promote forward blood flow.
- Withhold food and oral fluids in anticipation of emergency surgery to repair the septal defect (in VSD) or replace the mitral valve (in papillary muscle rupture).
- If mitral regurgitation results from ischemia, prepare the patient for revascularization. He may undergo thrombolysis, angioplasty, or bypass grafting to restore valvular competence by improving coronary artery flow.
- If the patient develops severe pulmonary edema, anticipate treatment with IABP therapy, oxygen, and such medications as diuretics, I.V. nitroglycerin, nitroprusside, morphine sulfate, and bronchodilators.

WHAT TO DO NEXT
Once your patient is out of immediate danger, take these steps:
- Assess his cardiovascular status frequently, including vital signs, skin color and temperature, peripheral pulses, capillary refill, urine output, level of consciousness, and heart and breath sounds.
- Monitor the murmur frequently for duration and timing in the cardiac cycle, auscultatory location, loudness, configuration, pitch, and quality. Notify the physician of any changes.
- To limit the patient's myocardial oxygen demands and improve his oxygen supply, keep him on bed rest, restrict his activities, and provide supplemental oxygen and sedatives, as prescribed.
- Watch for signs and symptoms of cardiogenic shock. If they develop, provide supplemental oxygen, as prescribed, and prepare for endotracheal intubation and mechanical ventilation if the patient's respiratory status deteriorates. Administer morphine sulfate, inotropic agents, and vasopressors, as prescribed.
- Watch the patient's ECG for arrhythmias and ischemic changes.
- Monitor hemodynamic parameters if he has a pulmonary artery catheter in place. Anticipate inserting an indwelling urinary catheter to assess hourly urine output.
- If the patient is receiving IABP therapy, observe for complications, such as improper balloon placement or inflation timing, catheter migration, thromboemboli, infection, or bleeding.
- Prepare the patient for surgery, as ordered. Afterward, provide appropriate postoperative care.

FOLLOW-UP CARE
- Increase your patient's activity level, as tolerated.
- If he received a prosthetic heart valve, give anticoagulants, as pre-

scribed, to reduce the risk of thrombus formation. Adjust the dose to keep his prothrombin time at 1½ to 2 times the control, as prescribed. Take measures to prevent hemorrhage, and watch for signs and symptoms of bleeding.
- Continue to assess his cardiovascular status. Report new or changing murmurs; they could signal a defective prosthetic valve.

SPECIAL CONSIDERATIONS
- If your patient received I.V. nitroprusside, monitor his serum thiocyanate and cyanide levels and watch for signs and symptoms of toxicity, such as hypotension, metabolic acidosis, dyspnea, headache, loss of consciousness, and vomiting.
- Teach your patient how to take prescribed anticoagulants correctly, how to prevent injuries and bleeding, and what symptoms to report to the physician. Emphasize the importance of keeping follow-up medical appointments.
- If he has a new valve, explain that he's at increased risk for endocarditis. Urge him to tell all health-care providers about the valve because he may need to take antibiotics before certain procedures, especially invasive ones.

MYOCARDIAL INFARCTION

In an acute myocardial infarction (MI), blood flow to certain areas of the myocardium decreases or stops; myocardial cells become ischemic, develop hypoxic damage, and, eventually, may die. Depending on the extent and location of the myocardial damage, the patient may face permanent functional deficits and even death.

Your immediate, effective response to this emergency may avert disaster. That's because it takes 4 to 6 hours for necrosis to affect the full myocardial thickness; prompt treatment during this interval can restore blood flow to ischemic areas, limiting the size of the infarcted area and, possibly, saving the patient's life.

Deprivation and damage
Most MIs arise when a thrombus forms in an area of a coronary artery already narrowed by atherosclerosis. Within about 20 minutes, myocardial cells deprived of oxygen-rich blood begin to die; this triggers an inflammatory response that causes release of certain enzymes. By the second or third day after an MI, neutrophils and macrophages begin to remove dead tissue; within about 2 weeks of the initial event, the myocardium has become thin and vulnerable. By 6 weeks post-MI, the infarcted area has been replaced by scar tissue that's strong but doesn't contract the way normal heart muscle does.

M

WHAT TO LOOK FOR
Clinical findings in MI may include:
- crushing chest pain that lasts for 20 or more minutes and doesn't abate with rest or nitroglycerin
- pain described as squeezing, crushing, viselike, stabbing, burning, or a heaviness or tightness in the chest; it may radiate to the neck, shoulders, jaws, arms, epigastrium, and back
- diaphoresis
- pallor
- nausea and vomiting
- anxiety
- a feeling of impending doom
- arrhythmias
- palpitations
- characteristic ECG changes (see *How MI alters ECG waveforms*)
- tachypnea
- weakness
- low-grade fever
- elevated leukocyte counts and an increased erythrocyte sedimentation rate
- pericardial friction rub.

With a left ventricular infarct, clinical findings may also include:
- third and fourth heart sounds (S_3 and S_4)
- a new murmur
- crackles on auscultation
- dyspnea.

With a right ventricular infarct, clinical findings may also include:
- Kussmaul's sign (jugular vein distention on inspiration)
- hypotension
- heart block
- peripheral edema.

WHAT TO DO IMMEDIATELY
If you suspect that your patient is experiencing an MI, notify the physician. Then follow these guidelines:
- Obtain the patient's vital signs to establish a baseline before therapy begins.
- Ask your patient to quantify his chest pain, using a scale from 0 to 10, with 0 being no pain and 10 being the worst pain possible. Also ask him to describe the pain's characteristics, such as pressure or sharpness, and its location.
- Give supplemental oxygen, as prescribed.
- As prescribed, administer one sublingual nitroglycerin tablet every 5 minutes to a maximum of three tablets, as needed.

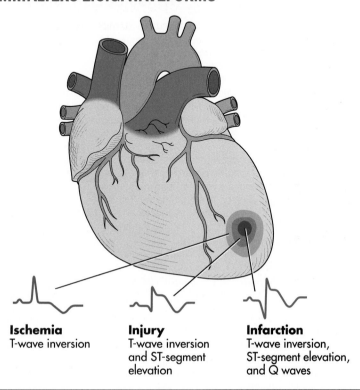

HOW M.I. ALTERS E.C.G. WAVEFORMS

Myocardial infarction (MI) causes three distinct zones of myocardial tissue damage:
- an inner zone of infarcted (necrotic) tissue
- a middle zone of injured tissue
- an outer zone of ischemic tissue.

Although infarcted tissue can never function again, ischemic and injured tissue might regain function if the patient receives prompt and effective treatment.

An ECG can help determine the size and location of the three zones. Although T waves and ST segments return to baseline as the heart heals, Q waves remain long after the MI occurs.

Ischemia
T-wave inversion

Injury
T-wave inversion and ST-segment elevation

Infarction
T-wave inversion, ST-segment elevation, and Q waves

- Give analgesics for pain relief, as prescribed. Know that morphine is often preferred because it dilates coronary arteries and improves blood flow while relieving pain.
- ➡ **NurseALERT** Monitor your patient's respiratory rate and depth because morphine may cause respiratory depression.
- Obtain a 12-lead ECG (if you haven't done so already), and begin continuous cardiac monitoring. Watch for ECG changes characteristic of MI. If you see elevated ST segments, prepare the patient for reperfusion with thrombolytic therapy or percutaneous transluminal coronary angioplasty (PTCA). (See *Thrombolytic therapy*, page 264.)
- Give aspirin, 160 to 325 mg orally, as prescribed.

After admission
Once your patient's MI has been confirmed and he's been admitted, take these steps:
- Monitor serial cardiac enzymes (such as creatine kinase [CK] and its isoenzyme CK-MB) and levels of troponin T and I. (See *Tests used to evaluate chest pain*, page 265.)

THROMBOLYTIC THERAPY

Has your patient had chest pain for more than 30 minutes but less than 6 hours? Does his ECG show elevated ST segments? If you can answer yes to both these questions, expect the physician to order thrombolytic therapy to lyse a newly formed clot in a coronary artery.

The ordered thrombolytic agent may be one that's clot-specific, such as alteplase (Activase). Or it may be one with general thrombolytic properties, such as streptokinase (Kabikinase), urokinase (Abbokinase), or anistreplase (Eminase).

Thrombolytic therapy is contraindicated in a patient with active bleeding, hemorrhagic stroke, severe hypertension, recent major surgery, trauma, head injury, a history of intracranial surgery, hemorrhagic retinopathy, aortic dissection, or previous allergic reactions.

If your patient is receiving thrombolytic therapy, focus your nursing care on the following.

PREPARING YOUR PATIENT
- Before thrombolytic therapy begins, make sure your patient has two—and preferably three—patent I.V. lines.
- Assess the patient's cardiovascular and neurologic status, and obtain a baseline ECG.
- Order laboratory tests, including hematocrit, white blood cell count, platelet count, prothrombin time, partial thromboplastin time (PTT), blood type and crossmatch, and hemoglobin, fibrinogen and fibrin split products, cardiac enzyme, blood urea nitrogen, and serum creatinine levels.
- Explain the purpose and risks of thrombolytic therapy to your patient and his family.

AFTERCARE
- Compare the patient's cardiovascular and neurologic status with baseline findings. Watch for hypotension if he received streptokinase.
- Assess his ECG for signs of successful thrombolytic therapy: return of ST segments and T waves to baseline, relief of chest pain, early peaking of CK-MB levels, and reperfusion arrhythmias.
- Intervene for symptomatic arrhythmias, as ordered.
- Report ischemic ECG changes and complaints of chest pain, which may indicate reocclusion. Anticipate immediate cardiac catheterization, percutaneous transluminal coronary angioplasty, or coronary artery bypass graft surgery.
- Give I.V. heparin, as prescribed, after your patient receives alteplase. Monitor his PTT level and titrate the heparin dose to keep it at 1½ to 2 times the control, as ordered.
- Assess for allergic reactions, such as fever, rash, itching, and chills, if your patient received streptokinase or anistreplase. Give antihistamines for mild reactions, as ordered.
- Check often for signs of bleeding, such as decreased hemoglobin level and hematocrit, tachycardia, hypotension, headache, flank pain, pale and cool skin, and restlessness. Test the patient's stools, urine, and emesis for blood. Monitor puncture sites for oozing blood and hematomas. Check all test results and report abnormal values that may indicate bleeding.
- Take measures to avoid trauma and injury to the patient's tissues. For instance, avoid intramuscular injections and urinary catheter insertion. (Preferably, a urinary catheter should be inserted before thrombolytic therapy begins.)

- Restrict the patient to bed rest with the use of a bedside commode until he's pain-free for 12 to 24 hours, as ordered.
- Administer antianxiety drugs, as prescribed and necessary.
- Assess for arrhythmias by way of continuous ECG monitoring. If arrhythmias develop, administer antiarrhythmic medications, as prescribed.
- ➡ **NurseALERT** Keep atropine, lidocaine, epinephrine, transcutaneous pacing patches, a transvenous pacemaker, and a defibrillator readily available to treat arrhythmias.
- Administer I.V. nitroglycerin for 24 to 48 hours, as prescribed, unless your patient experiences bradycardia, excessive tachycardia, or hypotension. Titrate the dose to the desired blood pressure and heart rate, as ordered.

DIAGNOSTIC TESTS

TESTS USED TO EVALUATE CHEST PAIN

If your patient with chest pain needs to be evaluated for myocardial ischemia or injury, expect to prepare him for one or more of the following diagnostic procedures.

CHEST X-RAY
A screening test for patients with chest pain, a chest X-ray demonstrates the size and shape of the heart, its chambers, and great vessels.

ECG
This test records electrical activity generated by the heart, as measured by skin electrodes connected to an amplifier and a strip-chart recorder. An ECG can evaluate and locate ischemic, injured, and infarcted myocardial tissue; identify arrhythmias, hypertrophy, and pericarditis; and evaluate pacemaker function.

EXERCISE STRESS TESTING
Also called exercise ECG, exercise stress testing provides indirect information about your patient's coronary arteries by evaluating his heart rate and blood pressure and revealing ST-segment changes on the ECG. The physician may order this test to detect cardiac abnormalities absent during rest and to evaluate the effectiveness of medical or surgical treatment.

STRESS ECHOCARDIOGRAPHY
This test uses ultrasound waves to record the size, shape, and movement of heart structures before and during exercise. It's especially helpful when ECG stress testing fails to yield definitive results.

THALLIUM SCAN
A nuclear imaging test, the thallium scan evaluates cardiac muscle perfusion. After an I.V. injection, the radioactive tracer thallium-201 accumulates in myocardial areas where blood flow is adequate. Areas of the myocardium that are underperfused (hence the myocardial cells that are injured or infarcted) show up as "cold spots" (areas of decreased thallium accumulation) on the scan.

POSITRON EMISSION TOMOGRAPHY
A positron emission tomographic (PET) scan evaluates cardiac metabolism and reveals the size of an MI resulting from coronary occlusion. By identifying viable heart tissue, a PET scan helps determine whether the patient is a good candidate for bypass surgery or angioplasty. A PET scan may be done in conjunction with exercise testing.

TECHNETIUM SCAN
This test uses a tracer isotope to show recently damaged areas of heart muscle. It also confirms the presence, size, and location of an acute MI and helps differentiate unstable angina from an acute MI.

CARDIAC CATHETERIZATION AND CORONARY ANGIOGRAPHY
These studies help determine the extent or severity of coronary artery disease, identify lesions and obstructions, and assess the extent of collateral circulation.

LIPOPROTEIN MEASUREMENT
Laboratory determinations of your patient's serum total cholesterol level, serum triglyceride levels, and lipoprotein-cholesterol fractionation help evaluate his fat metabolism and gauge his risk for coronary artery disease.

CARDIAC ENZYMES AND PROTEINS
In the hours and days after a myocardial infarction (MI), cardiac enzymes follow a characteristic pattern of rising, peaking, and returning to baseline. Key cardiac enzymes include creatine kinase (CK), lactate dehydrogenase (LD), and troponin, as shown in the graph below.

Because damage to other organs also may increase CK and LD levels, these tests focus on the isoenzymes CK-MB and LD_1 (which are specific to cardiac muscle) and the protein troponin (a contractile protein that serves as a more specific marker for acute MI). Troponin T levels rise for 3 hours to 10 days after an MI. Myoglobin levels also may aid early diagnosis of an MI.

M

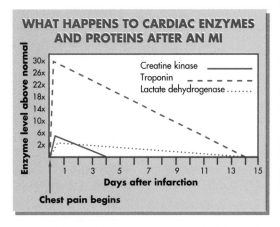

WHAT HAPPENS TO CARDIAC ENZYMES AND PROTEINS AFTER AN MI

- If your patient's acute MI continues to evolve, expect the physician to prescribe I.V. beta blockers.
- If your patient's ECG shows elevated ST segments or left bundle-branch block, give angiotensin-converting enzyme inhibitors, as prescribed. However, be aware that these agents may be contraindicated if he's hypotensive.
- If your patient has suffered a right ventricular infarct, administer I.V. fluids, as indicated and prescribed. Anticipate giving inotropic medications as well.

WHAT TO DO NEXT

- Continue to monitor the patient's ECG for evolution of the MI, arrhythmias, and signs of further ischemia.
- If the patient received thrombolytic therapy, assess for signs and symptoms of reperfusion, such as relief of chest pain, ST-segment resolution, early peaking of CK-MB levels, and reperfusion arrhythmias.
- Monitor the patient's vital signs, heart and breath sounds, urine output, level of consciousness, skin color and temperature, edema, capillary refill, and peripheral pulses. Immediately report abnormal findings, such as a new murmur or restlessness.
- Assess reports of chest pain using the PQRST approach. (See *PQRST approach to assessing chest pain*, page 22.)
- After your patient has been without chest pain for 12 hours, begin to increase his activity level. Help him to the bathroom and take him for short walks, as tolerated.
- Continue to administer beta blockers, as prescribed. Monitor your patient's heart rate and blood pressure during therapy, and report bradycardia or hypotension to the physician.
- Continue to administer aspirin, as prescribed.
- Within 48 hours, wean your patient off I.V. nitroglycerin and begin oral, transdermal, or other nitrate therapy, as ordered. Closely monitor his ECG, heart rate, and blood pressure and stay alert for complaints of chest pain.
- Administer magnesium sulfate, as prescribed, if the patient has hypomagnesemia.
- Anticipate giving I.V. heparin if the patient had a large anterior MI or a left ventricular thrombus or if he underwent PTCA. Monitor activated partial thromboplastin time (APTT) to keep the heparin dose within the prescribed therapeutic range. Watch carefully for signs and symptoms of embolic stroke, such as a sudden change in level of consciousness or the sudden onset of focal neurologic deficits.
- Continue administering I.V. heparin for 48 hours, as prescribed, if your patient received alteplase.
- If your patient had an inferior or a posterior MI, a right-sided ECG may be performed to rule out a right ventricular infarct. Place leads on the right side of his chest in positions that mirror the left side. Watch for ST-segment elevation in lead V_4R, which indicates a right ventricular infarction.

- Assess the patient for signs and symptoms of pericarditis, such as a pericardial friction rub and pleuritic chest pain. Administer aspirin, as prescribed, and monitor for cardiac tamponade and other complications of pericarditis.
- If your patient has recurrent chest pain, expect to give I.V. nitroglycerin, analgesics, and antithrombotic medications (such as aspirin and heparin), as prescribed. If he has continued pain, prepare him, as ordered, for angiography and either coronary artery bypass grafting or PTCA.
- Watch for signs and symptoms of heart failure, such as dyspnea, crackles, S_3 or S_4 heart sounds, and orthopnea. Anticipate giving diuretics, vasodilators, and inotropic agents, as prescribed.
- Suspect cardiogenic shock if your patient develops tachycardia, hypotension, restlessness, S_3 heart sound, increased pulmonary pressures, crackles, and oliguria. Prepare for insertion of an intra-aortic balloon pump and for emergency coronary angiography, and expect the patient to undergo PTCA or bypass surgery.
- If your patient develops atrial fibrillation with hemodynamic compromise or ischemia, prepare him for electrical cardioversion, as ordered. (See *Caring for your patient during synchronized cardioversion*, page 39.) Otherwise, anticipate giving beta blockers, calcium channel blockers, or digoxin to slow the ventricular rate and I.V. heparin to reduce the risk of embolus formation. Keep in mind that arrhythmias may occur with reperfusion.
- If the patient has pulseless ventricular fibrillation or monomorphic ventricular tachycardia, prepare to treat him with immediate direct-current countershock, as ordered. Administer lidocaine (Lidocaine), procainamide (Pronestyl), or amiodarone (Cordarone), as prescribed, if monomorphic ventricular tachycardia isn't causing symptoms.
- Give atropine for symptomatic sinus bradycardia and atrioventricular block, as prescribed. Be aware that some arrhythmias, such as third-degree heart block and newly acquired bundle-branch block, may warrant temporary pacing. (See *Understanding temporary pacemakers*, page 45.)
- ➡ **NurseALERT** Prepare your patient for immediate surgery if PTCA was unsuccessful and he still has chest pain or hemodynamic instability; if he has persistent chest pain and contraindications to catheter therapies; if he has cardiogenic shock and coronary anatomy incompatible with PTCA; or if he has a complication, such as papillary muscle rupture or ventricular septal defect. Stay alert for sudden hemodynamic collapse, which may indicate ventricular wall rupture, ventricular septal rupture, papillary muscle rupture, or cardiac tamponade.
- Stay alert for other complications of acute MI, including heart failure, pulmonary edema, ventricular aneurysm, Dressler's syndrome (pericarditis with effusion 1 to 4 weeks after MI), cardiogenic shock, pericarditis, and sudden death.

M

FOLLOW-UP CARE

- Continue giving aspirin, as prescribed.
- Monitor the patient's APTT, lipid profile, hematocrit, blood urea nitrogen level, and serum creatinine, cardiac enzyme, and electrolyte levels. Report abnormal values.
- Monitor his blood glucose level. Within the first 3 days of MI, stay alert for hyperglycemia. Stress-induced catecholamine release, such as norepinephrine, causes blood glucose levels to rise by mediating the release of glycogen and glucose from body cells and by suppressing pancreatic beta cell activity, which reduces insulin secretion and elevates blood glucose even further.
- Prepare your patient for a submaximal or symptom-limited ECG stress test.

SPECIAL CONSIDERATIONS

- Warn your patient to avoid Valsalva's maneuver because it can cause sudden, marked changes in heart rate and blood pressure.
- Teach your patient and his family about the medications he'll be taking at home. Discuss their purpose, administration schedules, dosages, and adverse effects and what symptoms to report.
- Help your patient identify his MI risk factors and develop a plan to reduce them. As indicated, advise him to focus on achieving and maintaining an ideal weight, following a low-cholesterol diet, stopping smoking, getting regular exercise, reducing stress, controlling his blood glucose level, and managing hypertension.
- Explain the components of an aerobic exercise program and review guidelines for safe exercise. Discuss when the patient can resume sexual activity.
- Inform the patient about support groups, educational programs, and cardiac rehabilitation programs available in his community.
- Teach your patient what to do if he has chest pain, including how to take sublingual nitroglycerin and when to seek emergency care.

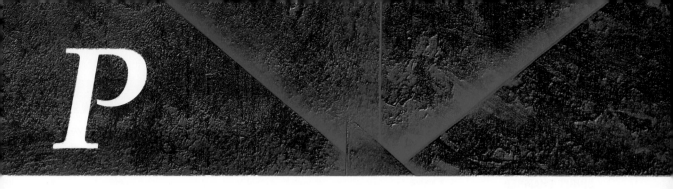

PACEMAKER MALFUNCTION

Implanted in a subcutaneous pocket in the chest or abdomen, a permanent pacemaker consists of a pulse generator and one or more pacing leads, each with an electrode at its tip. Electrodes are threaded transvenously to the patient's right atrium, right ventricle, or both. In a single-chamber pacemaker, the pacing lead usually is in the right ventricle. A dual-chamber, or atrioventricular-sequential, pacemaker has leads in both the atrium and the ventricle to mimic normal heart function more closely. (See *Viewing single- and dual-chamber pacemakers,* page 270.)

A pacemaker can save your patient's life, but a malfunctioning one could trigger life-threatening arrhythmias. What's more, pacemaker use can lead to such complications as infection, lead displacement, lead fracture and disconnection, ventricular perforation, and cardiac tamponade. Your prompt assessment and intervention for any one of these complications could mean the difference between life and death.

Pacemaker modes
Some pacemakers function only on demand; others, at a fixed rate. Demand pacemakers, the most common type, sense the heart's intrinsic rhythm. When the patient's heart rate falls below a predetermined rate set on the pacemaker, an electrical stimulus is sent through lead wires to the electrode. The stimulus causes the heart muscle to depolarize and contract.

Fixed-rate pacemakers, in contrast, fire at a predetermined rate, regardless of the patient's intrinsic cardiac activity. (See *Understanding pacemaker codes,* page 271.)

Common pacemaker problems
Pacemaker problems include failure to sense, oversensing, failure to capture, failure to pace, and pacing at an altered rate.

Failure to sense (undersensing). A pacemaker that fails to sense (recognize the heart's intrinsic electrical activity) fires inappropriately—for instance, causing pacemaker spikes to fall on the T wave (ventricular repolarization) of the ECG. This places the patient at risk for developing a life-threatening arrhythmia, such as ventricular tachycardia.

VIEWING SINGLE- AND DUAL-CHAMBER PACEMAKERS

Three types of permanent pacemakers, along with the ECG patterns they typically produce, are shown below.

SINGLE-CHAMBER ATRIAL PACEMAKER

In this pacemaker, the lead is positioned in the atrium. The ECG shows pacemaker spikes followed by a P wave.

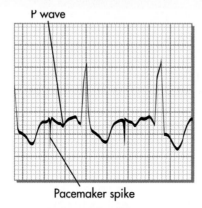

P wave

Pacemaker spike

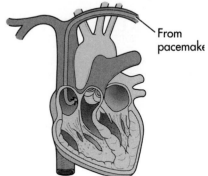

From pacemaker

SINGLE-CHAMBER VENTRICULAR PACEMAKER

The lead for this single-chamber ventricular pacemaker is positioned in the right ventricle. The ECG shows a spontaneous P wave followed by a pacemaker spike and a QRS complex.

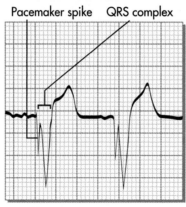

Pacemaker spike   QRS complex

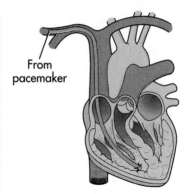

From pacemaker

DUAL-CHAMBER OR ATRIOVENTRICULAR SEQUENTIAL PACEMAKER

A dual-chamber pacemaker like the one shown here can pace both the atrium and the ventricle, providing the atrial contribution ("kick") to ventricular filling. The ECG shows both the atrial and the ventricular pacemaker spikes.

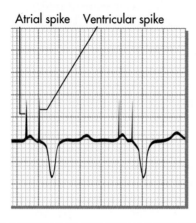

Atrial spike   Ventricular spike

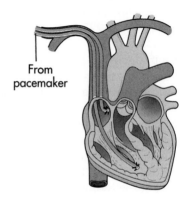

From pacemaker

UNDERSTANDING PACEMAKER CODES

A pacemaker's three-letter code indicates how the pacemaker has been programmed.
- The first letter signifies which heart chamber is being paced: A (atrium), V (ventricle), D (dual, or both chambers), or O (none, not applicable).
- The second letter tells which chamber the pacemaker senses: A (atrium), V (ventricle), D (dual), or O (none, not applicable).
- The third letter indicates how the pacemaker responds to the sensed event: I (inhibited), T (triggered), D (dual—atrial triggered and ventricular inhibited), or O (not applicable).

ADDITIONAL LETTERS

Some pacemaker codes have two additional letters.
- The fourth letter shows the number of available reprogrammable functions: P (programmable rate or output only), M (multiprogrammable), C (programmable with telemetry), R (rate responsive), or O (none).
- The fifth letter signifies how the pacemaker responds to tachycardia: P (pacing), S (shock), D (dual pacing and shock), or O (none).

Failure to sense may result from a fractured or displaced lead, a failing battery, a malpositioned electrode tip, an increased sensing threshold (as from edema or fibrosis at the electrode tip), incorrect pacemaker programming (such as inappropriate sensitivity or refractory periods), or electromagnetic interference (EMI, as from electrical generators and radio and television transmitters). Medical conditions that can cause failure to sense include myocardial infarction (MI) and electrolyte imbalances.

Oversensing. An oversensing pacemaker may pace at a rate slower than the set rate or fail to produce paced beats. Causes of oversensing include EMI, sensing of T waves or atrial activity, sensing of myopotentials (skeletal muscle contractions), and pacemaker sensitivity that's set too high.

Failure to capture. A pacemaker that doesn't capture produces ECG pacemaker spikes that aren't followed by QRS complexes (if the electrode is in the ventricle) or by P waves (if the electrode is in the atrium). A pacemaker may be misdiagnosed as failing to capture if it fires during the heart's refractory period, when the heart can't respond to a stimulus.

Most often, failure to capture results from a dislodged lead. Other causes include lead fracture, battery depletion, myocardial perforation by the lead wire, and improper lead insulation. Also, the stimulation threshold may increase from MI, medication, electrolyte abnormalities, and fibrosis at the electrode tip.

Failure to pace. Failure to pace may cause absence of apparent pacemaker activity on the ECG, and the patient's heart rate may fall below the pacemaker's set rate. If atrial stimulation is sensed by the ventricular amplifier in a dual-chamber pacemaker, ventricular stimulation may be inhibited. Sometimes, though, a normally functioning pacemaker is

RECOGNIZING R-ON-T PHENOMENON

If your patient's pacemaker fails to sense intrinsic QRS complexes, it may discharge during the heart's vulnerable period, causing pacemaker spikes to fall on or near T waves.

The rhythm strip shown here, for instance, reveals that the pacemaker isn't sensing the patient's spontaneous QRS complex and is firing on the T wave as a result, stimulating the heart during repolarization. This dangerous situation puts the patient at risk for ventricular tachycardia or fibrillation.

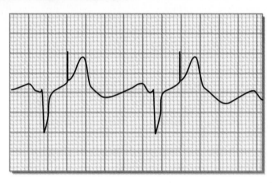

misdiagnosed with failure to pace because the patient's own heart rhythm is inhibiting it.

Usually, failure to pace results from circuitry or battery failure, lead displacement or fracture, or a broken or loose lead-generator connection.

Pacing at an altered rate. With an altered pacing rate, pacemaker spikes don't occur at the set rate, possibly triggering a dangerous condition called R-on-T phenomenon. (See *Recognizing R-on-T phenomenon.*) Causes of altered-rate pacing include oversensing of cardiac activity (leading to pacemaker inhibition), battery depletion, circuitry malfunction (resulting in a "runaway" pacemaker that fires at an excessive rate), sensing of myopotentials, and phantom reprogramming (such as by electrocautery or another unintentional source).

WHAT TO LOOK FOR

Clinical findings in a patient with pacemaker malfunction may include:
- dizziness
- syncope
- palpitations
- irregular pulse
- pulse rate below the pacemaker's programmed rate
- fatigue
- pallor
- hypotension
- chest pain
- dyspnea.

With a *dislodged* pacemaker electrode , the patient may also have:
- hiccups
- twitching of chest and abdominal muscles.

WHAT TO DO IMMEDIATELY

If you suspect that your patient's pacemaker is malfunctioning, notify the physician. Then follow these guidelines:

- Obtain a 12-lead ECG with a rhythm strip, and compare it with previous strips. However, keep in mind that a properly functioning pacemaker that's inhibited by the patient's own heart rhythm may not produce a pacemaker artifact.
- Begin continuous ECG monitoring.
- Bring an emergency cart with temporary pacing equipment to the bedside.
- Assess your patient's vital signs, level of consciousness, skin color and temperature, and capillary refill; auscultate his heart and breath sounds.
- Verify the type of pacemaker your patient has to help assess and correct the problem.
- ➡ Nurse**ALERT** To evaluate your patient's pacemaker function accurately, you'll need to know its mode and programmed rate and whether it's a single- or dual-chamber model.
- Obtain a chest X-ray, as ordered, to check lead position and identify any lead fracture or lead-generator disconnection. Compare findings with previous X-rays, noting any change in lead position.

WHAT TO DO NEXT

After taking initial steps, follow these guidelines:

- Place a magnet over the pacemaker, as ordered and if permitted by your facility. The magnet inhibits the pacemaker's sensing capability and causes it to pace at a fixed rate. This prevents the patient's own heart rate from inhibiting the pacemaker and allows you to evaluate whether or not the pacemaker is capturing appropriately. Also check for capture while the patient performs Valsalva's maneuver or while the physician performs carotid sinus massage to slow the patient's intrinsic heart rate and induce pacing.
- ➡ Nurse **ALERT** Use caution when placing a magnet over a pacemaker; be sure to observe the ECG for arrhythmias that may occur during asynchronous pacing.
- While watching your patient's ECG, determine if the pacemaker is functioning according to the set mode. For example, if it's programmed in the VVI mode, it should pace the ventricle whenever it doesn't sense a spontaneous ventricular depolarization. Spontaneous ventricular depolarization at a rate above the set rate, on the other hand, should inhibit pacing.
- If the pacemaker fails to sense the heart's intrinsic rhythm, expect to see pacing artifacts that compete with your patient's own rhythm. Be aware that R-on-T phenomenon may occur if the pacemaker fires too soon after a spontaneous QRS complex. Also, check the amplitude or height of the P or R wave on the patient's ECG. If the amplitude is low, the pacemaker's sensitivity may need to be increased to detect

P

them. The pacemaker senses the patient's P wave (with atrial pacing) or R wave (with ventricular pacing) to determine whether or not pacing impulses must be delivered. If this doesn't correct the problem, look for potential EMI sources and obtain a chest X-ray, as ordered, to check for lead displacement or fracture. If these problems are ruled out by the physician, he may replace the pulse generator because it may be defective.

- Observe for pacemaker capture. Assume that the pacemaker is capturing properly if the ECG shows a pacemaker artifact followed by a P wave when the atrium is being paced or followed by a QRS complex when the ventricle is being paced.
- Monitor your patient's heart rate; report a rate below the pacemaker's set rate. Be aware that a gradual rate decrease (rate drift) may indicate a failing battery.
- If pacing periods alternate with periods of failure to pace, suspect a fractured lead and report it to the physician.
- Check for EMI sources that may be interfering with your patient's pacemaker function. In the hospital, these include transcutaneous electrical nerve stimulation, radiation therapy, magnetic resonance imaging, and electrocautery. Immediately remove the patient from any EMI source.
- If indicated, prepare the patient for and assist with vector analysis or a noninvasive programmer to evaluate pacemaker function. For instance, the use of a noninvasive programmer may reveal the need to adjust the pacemaker's stimulus strength, sensitivity, rate, refractory periods, or pacing mode; it also allows measurement of lead impedance. Some programmers display such data as the number of paced and sensed events and the pacemaker's model and serial number.
- If these noninvasive methods fail to shed light on the cause of the pacemaker problem, prepare your patient for an invasive procedure, such as a pacing system analyzer. During this procedure, the physician can analyze pulse generator function, evaluate lead integrity and positioning, and provide electrophysiologic patient data.
- Monitor the patient's serum electrolyte levels and report any abnormalities. Expect to administer electrolyte replacement, as prescribed and needed, to correct electrolyte deficits.

FOLLOW-UP CARE

- After pacemaker insertion or lead reinsertion, repair, or repositioning, obtain a chest X-ray to verify lead placement and serve as a baseline for future comparison. Also obtain a baseline ECG.
- Maintain continuous ECG monitoring for the specified period after pacemaker adjustments have been made.

SPECIAL CONSIDERATIONS

- Teach your patient about the importance of keeping follow-up appointments with the physician or pacemaker clinic.

- Make sure the patient understands how to use telephone monitoring equipment to check pacemaker function between medical visits.
- Instruct the patient how to take his pulse and to report a high or low rate. Review symptoms of pacemaker malfunction—dizziness, fatigue, dyspnea, palpitations, irregular pulse, chest pain, hiccups, and twitching of chest and abdominal muscles. Tell him to report these at once.
- Advise the patient to stay away from EMI sources, such as power tools. Help him evaluate his home and workplace for equipment that may cause EMI. Tell him to move away immediately if a piece of equipment causes dizziness and not to go near it again.
- Instruct your patient to consult his cardiologist before undergoing a medical or surgical procedure that causes EMI emissions, such as magnetic resonance imaging and electrocautery.
- Caution him not to touch or move the pacemaker in its subcutaneous pocket because he may dislodge the leads.
- Keep a magnet available on your unit for troubleshooting pacemaker problems.
- When defibrillating a patient who has a permanent pacemaker, don't place the paddles directly over the pacemaker. Instead, place them at least 3" (7.5 cm) from the pulse generator to avoid electrical damage. After defibrillation, reassess pacemaker function.

PANCREATITIS

An inflammation of the pancreas, pancreatitis can take an acute or a chronic form. Acute pancreatitis, which carries significant mortality, typically comes on abruptly and has a short course. Resolution—or death—occurs within days.

Pathophysiologic features of acute pancreatitis include activation of pancreatic enzymes (especially trypsin before release into the duodenum), which triggers pancreatic autodigestion. This autodigestion in turn leads to diffuse pancreatic inflammation, cellular breakdown, and, eventually, necrosis. Elastic fibers of blood vessels begin to dissolve, triggering potentially massive blood loss.

Alcohol abuse and biliary disease together account for roughly 75% of cases of acute pancreatitis. Other precipitating conditions include infections (such as mumps and scarlet fever) and certain endocrine disorders. Human immunodeficiency virus infection has also been associated with acute pancreatitis.

Although sometimes mild and self-limiting, acute pancreatitis may present as a critical emergency. That's because systemic vasodilation and increased vascular permeability predispose the patient to hypovolemic shock, while fluid buildup in the peritoneal cavity and retroperitoneal space may cause respiratory distress. Under these conditions, the patient quickly may develop life-threatening acute respiratory distress syndrome (ARDS).

P

UNDERSTANDING CHRONIC PANCREATITIS

In chronic pancreatitis, tissue destruction is progressive and irreversible, even after the underlying cause is corrected. Protein plugs, some of which calcify, form in the pancreatic ducts. Acinar cells, which produce digestive enzymes, diminish in number, and pancreatic tissue becomes fibrotic.

These changes lead to malabsorption and nutritional deficiencies. Eventually, the insulin-producing pancreatic islet cells are affected and diabetes mellitus develops. Other complications may include pseudocysts, abscesses, and external fistulas.

Alcohol abuse is the most common cause of chronic pancreatitis, which has a gradual course with about 50% of those afflicted surviving 20 to 25 years after initial diagnosis.

TREATMENT OPTIONS

Treatment of chronic pancreatitis centers on preventing severe episodes by minimizing the work of the pancreas. Typically, the physician forbids alcohol and caffeine and prescribes a bland diet low in fat and high in carbohydrates and protein; a patient with inadequate enzyme production receives oral pancreatic enzymes. Anticholinergic drugs, antacids, and gastric acid inhibitors are given to decrease gastric acid (which stimu-lates pancreatic function).

If the patient has impaired vitamin B_{12} absorption, the physician may order parenteral administration of this vitamin. The hyperglycemic patient receives insulin or, if her islet cells can be stimulated, oral hypoglycemic agents.

Controlling pain

Pain control poses the greatest challenge in disease management. Usually, the physician prescribes a non-opioid narcotic, such as meperidine (Demerol). However, because the disease is chronic and may cause severe pain, the risk of drug tolerance is high. Nonnarcotic pain-control measures have had limited success.

Surgery

When pain becomes intractable or complications such as abscesses and fistulas compromise the patient's quality of life, surgery may be recommended to allow pancreatic secretions to drain into the intestine. Surgical options include pancreaticojejunostomy, revision of the sphincter of Oddi, and, sometimes, pancreatectomy. These procedures carry a high mortality risk, and symptoms commonly recur as the disease progresses.

An acute episode may resolve entirely, with no permanent organ damage. However, sometimes the disorder progresses to the chronic form. (See *Understanding chronic pancreatitis.*) Complications of acute pancreatitis include pancreatric abscess, peritonitis, respiratory disorders (atelectasis, hypoxemia, ARDS), impaired cardiac function, and hypocalcemia.

WHAT TO LOOK FOR

Clinical findings in acute pancreatitis may include:

- sudden onset of intense pain in the left upper abdominal quadrant, which may radiate to the middle of the back or to the left shoulder
- nausea and severe vomiting
- low-grade fever
- signs and symptoms of circulatory shock, including hypotension, tachycardia, tachypnea, and pallor
- abdominal rigidity and muscle guarding
- rebound tenderness
- periumbilical bruising (Cullen's sign)
- bruising of the flanks (Grey Turner's sign)
- respiratory distress

- decreased bowel sounds
- serum amylase level above 250 units/L
- decreased serum calcium level
- elevated serum lipase, serum glucose, blood urea nitrogen, lactate dehydrogenase, and urine amylase levels
- elevated white blood cell count.

In chronic pancreatitis, clinical findings may include:
- severe, unrelenting abdominal pain
- weight loss
- steatorrhea
- evidence of malnutrition, such as dry, flaky skin; dull, brittle hair; and a decreased serum albumin level
- hyperglycemia.

WHAT TO DO IMMEDIATELY
If your patient develops signs or symptoms of pancreatitis, notify the physician. Then follow these steps:
- Withhold all oral intake.
- Assess the patient's vital signs for indications of hypovolemic shock. Maintain a meticulous record of her intake and output.
- As ordered, insert a nasogastric tube and attach it to suction.
- Administer analgesics and anticholinergics, as prescribed, to relieve pain.
- ➡ **NurseALERT** Know that the patient with pancreatitis may require high-dose narcotic analgesia and may develop drug tolerance. However, keep in mind that she's *not* a drug addict; don't treat her as one. Monitor her response to the medication, and watch closely for signs of overdose. Commonly used analgesics include nonopioid narcotics, such as meperidine (Demerol) and pentazocine (Talwin), which don't cause spasm of the pancreatic sphincter of Oddi.
- Establish I.V. access, and administer I.V. fluids, as prescribed.
- Anticipate insertion of a central venous or pulmonary artery catheter to allow continuous monitoring of central venous or pulmonary artery wedge pressure. Assist with catheter insertion, as ordered, and obtain frequent readings.
- Insert an indwelling urinary catheter, as ordered, and monitor the patient's hourly urine output.
- Obtain blood samples for a complete blood count and to measure serum electrolyte and amylase levels. Also draw a sample for baseline arterial blood gas (ABG) analysis; monitor the patient's oxygen saturation through ABG values or pulse oximetry.
- Administer supplemental oxygen, as prescribed. Be prepared to assist with endotracheal intubation and mechanical ventilation if the patient's respiratory status deteriorates.

P

WHAT TO DO NEXT

Once the patient has been stabilized, follow these guidelines:

- Continue to monitor her vital signs and hemodynamic status frequently—as often as every hour if indicated.
- Administer antibiotic therapy, as prescribed.
- Assess the patient's abdomen for ascites and distention. Auscultate her bowel sounds at least every 4 hours.
- If indicated, prepare her for abdominal paracentesis to remove fluid.
- Monitor repeat serum glucose levels. Anticipate administering insulin if hyperglycemia develops.
- Observe for signs and symptoms of hypocalcemia (muscle twitching, tremors, and irritability). Keep I.V. calcium gluconate on hand, if needed, to prevent tetany.
- Assess the patient's respiratory status carefully for indications of developing respiratory complications.
- ➡ **NurseALERT** Because your patient is in severe pain, know that she's likely to have shallow, guarded respirations, which could make it difficult for you to assess for fluid accumulation in the lungs.
- Perform a nutritional assessment, including weighing the patient, measuring skin-fold thickness, and assessing her skin and mucous membranes.
- If indicated, prepare the patient for surgery to treat complications of pancreatitis, such as abscesses and fistula, or to resect necrotic tissue if pain becomes intractable. Surgical options range from simple abscess drainage (performed laparoscopically) to pancreaticojejunostomy (Whipple procedure, a major abdominal operation) to total pancreatectomy. After surgery, provide appropriate postoperative care.

FOLLOW-UP CARE

- Once the patient's bowel sounds return, resume oral feedings, as ordered. Expect to start with clear fluids and progress to high-carbohydrate foods and elemental protein feedings, which don't stimulate pancreatic secretions. Gradually introduce a bland, low-fat diet of six feedings per day. Consult the dietitian to assist with meal planning, as needed.
- ➡ **NurseALERT** Keep in mind that the physician usually restricts dietary carbohydrates if the patient has impaired glucose tolerance.

SPECIAL CONSIDERATIONS

- Make sure the patient and family understand the dietary plan for chronic pancreatitis. Stress that good nutrition is essential for healing, even though eating may be painful.
- Review the prescribed medication regimen, including the purpose and correct administration of pancreatic enzymes, histamine-2-receptor antagonists, and antacids.

• Teach the patient and family about the link between alcohol consumption and onset of acute pancreatitis or exacerbation of chronic pancreatitis. Urge the patient to avoid alcohol completely. Provide information on self-help groups and other community resources.

PERICARDITIS

Pericarditis refers to inflammation of the pericardial sac surrounding the heart. As part of the inflammatory response, neutrophils migrate to the pericardial sac, making it more vascular and causing fibrin to develop on the sac's visceral (inner) layer. (See *Inside view of the pericardial sac,* page 63.) The heart's epicardial layer and the pleura surrounding the lungs also may become inflamed.

Pericarditis most commonly results from viral infection. Other precipitating conditions include bacterial and fungal infections, tuberculosis, uremia, Dressler's syndrome (after myocardial infarction), neoplasms, trauma, connective tissue diseases (such as rheumatoid arthritis), cardiac surgery, and drug reactions.

Chronic constrictive pericarditis may develop when acute pericarditis results from neoplasm, radiation therapy, previous surgery, or tuberculosis. In this disease form, the pericardium thickens and a stiff membrane surrounds the heart, preventing it from stretching and filling during diastole. As right and left filling pressures increase, stroke volume and cardiac output decrease.

Sometimes pericarditis resolves on its own with symptomatic treatment, such as to relieve chest pain. However, a patient who develops pericardial effusions, cardiac tamponade, or other complications requires immediate treatment to correct those conditions.

WHAT TO LOOK FOR
In acute pericarditis, clinical findings may include:
• pericardial friction rub (see *Assessing for pericardial friction rub,* page 280.)
• severe, sharp chest pain over the left precordium, possibly radiating to the left shoulder, left trapezius ridge, neck, or abdomen (see *Identifying the origin of chest pain,* pages 20 and 21.)
• chest pain that worsens when the patient lies supine, takes a deep breath, coughs, or swallows and improves when he sits up and leans forward
• rapid, shallow respirations (an attempt to avoid chest pain)
• dyspnea
• low-grade fever
• characteristic ECG changes, including an elevated concave ST segment and upright T waves in most leads; a depressed ST segment in aVR and V_1; and a depressed PR interval that may appear with atrial inflammation.

ASSESSING FOR PERICARDIAL FRICTION RUB

The hallmark of acute pericarditis, a pericardial friction rub results from the friction created when the roughened pericardial and epicardial surfaces move against each other. To identify this dangerous sign, you'll need to auscultate your patient's heart.

WHERE TO LISTEN
To check for the high-pitched sound of a pericardial friction rub, press firmly against the patient's skin with the diaphragm of your stethoscope. A pericardial friction rub is loudest along the third intercostal space at the left sternal border, and it doesn't radiate widely.

Listen for the characteristic grating, scraping, or leathery sound, which may resemble the noise made by walking on dry snow. The rub may change each time you listen to it; it may even seem to disappear at times.

THREE COMPONENTS
Commonly, a pericardial friction rub has three components or sounds. The first component occurs as a result of ventricular systole, the second occurs early in diastole as the ventricles rapidly fill with blood, and the third occurs with atrial systole.

Pericardial effusion
With a large pericardial effusion, clinical findings may include:
- distant, muffled heart sounds
- cough
- dyspnea
- tachypnea
- hiccups (from phrenic nerve pressure)
- hoarseness (from laryngeal nerve damage)
- bell-shaped ("water-bottle") appearance of the heart on chest X-ray.

Constrictive pericarditis
With constrictive pericarditis, clinical findings may include:
- pericardial knock (a loud sound that reflects restricted ventricular filling, heard in early diastole along the left sternal border)
- dyspnea on exertion
- leg edema
- ascites
- fatigue
- anorexia
- weight loss
- elevated jugular venous pressure and vein distention.

WHAT TO DO IMMEDIATELY
If you suspect that your patient has acute pericarditis, notify the physician. Then take the following actions:
- Restrict the patient to bed rest and elevate the head of his bed 45 degrees. Assess his vital signs, including temperature.
- Obtain a 12-lead ECG; then begin continuous cardiac monitoring, reporting arrhythmias and other ECG changes .
- Expect to give antiarrhythmics, as prescribed, if your patient develops an arrhythmia.

- Insert an I.V. line and administer I.V. medications or fluids, as necessary and prescribed.
- Anticipate instituting hemodynamic monitoring if the patient has cardiac tamponade or constrictive pericarditis. Check readings frequently, especially right atrial and pulmonary artery pressures, cardiac output, and stroke volume.
- Administer supplemental oxygen, as prescribed and indicated.
- Assess your patient's oxygen saturation levels by way of pulse oximetry.
- To help rule out other causes of chest pain, ask the patient to describe his pain. Suspect ischemia as the cause of chest pain if he describes crushing, burning, tightness, or a sensation of pressure (possibly radiating to the arm or jaw). Suspect a pericardial source if he describes severe, sharp precordial pain, especially if it spreads to the left trapezius ridge, worsens on inspiration, and improves when he leans forward.
- Administer aspirin and nonsteroidal anti-inflammatory drugs (NSAIDs), such as ibuprofen (Motrin) and indomethacin (Indocin), as prescribed. To avoid GI upset, give them with food or milk.
- ➡ Nurse**ALERT** Indomethacin may cause sodium and fluid retention, which could trigger or aggravate heart failure. If this drug is prescribed, assess your patient often for signs and symptoms of heart failure, such as third and fourth heart sounds (S_3 and S_4), crackles, orthopnea, and dyspnea (including paroxysmal nocturnal dyspnea).
- Prepare the patient for an echocardiogram, as ordered, to confirm pericardial effusion or cardiac tamponade.
- As prescribed, administer antibiotics if pericarditis has a bacterial origin.
- Evaluate the patient for signs and symptoms of cardiac tamponade, such as pulsus paradoxus, narrowing pulse pressure, dyspnea, and hypotension. If you suspect cardiac tamponade, anticipate the need for pericardiocentesis or pericardiectomy. (See *Your role in pericardiocentesis*, page 282.) Administer inotropic and chronotropic drugs and volume expanders, as prescribed. Monitor for respiratory distress, and prepare for possible endotracheal intubation and mechanical ventilation.
- Auscultate heart sounds and inspect neck veins frequently. Call the physician if the patient's cardiovascular status deteriorates, as indicated by neck vein distention, pulsus paradoxus, muffled heart sounds, a new S_3 or S_4, or a murmur.

WHAT TO DO NEXT

Once the patient has been stabilized, carry out these interventions:
- Assess his respiratory status closely. Remember that because deep inspiration causes chest pain, he may take shallow, rapid breaths. Monitor his arterial blood gas and pulse oximetry values to evaluate his oxygenation status, and continue giving supplemental oxygen, as necessary and prescribed.

P

YOUR ROLE IN PERICARDIOCENTESIS

If your patient has pericarditis, you may need to assist with pericardiocentesis. This procedure removes excess fluid from the pericardial space, allowing the heart to expand during diastolic filling. It also allows removal of a pericardial fluid specimen to help identify the cause of pericarditis. Usually, pericardiocentesis is performed in a critical care unit, a cardiac catheterization laboratory, an operating room, or an emergency department.

PREPARING YOUR PATIENT

- Explain the procedure to the patient. Tell him that he'll receive a local anesthetic and will be asked to lie on his back without moving. Reassure him that he shouldn't feel pain but may feel pressure as the pericardial needle enters the pericardial space.
- Unless the procedure will be done on an emergency basis, instruct your patient not to eat or drink for 4 to 6 hours before the procedure.
- Start an I.V. line in case your patient requires fluid or medications.
- Institute continuous cardiac monitoring, as ordered.
- If prescribed, premedicate the patient with atropine to help prevent vasovagal bradycardia and hypotension.
- Help the patient into a supine position.

DURING THE PROCEDURE

- As ordered, assist in preparing the skin over the fifth to sixth intercostal space at the left sternal margin.
- Help connect an ECG lead to the pericardial needle with a clip. As the needle enters the pericardial sac, observe the ECG; report ST-segment elevation, which signals that the needle is in contact with epicardial tissue.

- The physician then aspirates pericardial fluid into a 50-ml syringe and places it in each of several containers. Label the containers with your patient's name and a note that they contain pericardial fluid, and send them to the laboratory promptly.
- If your patient has recurrent cardiac tamponade, the physician may leave a catheter in the pericardial space for several days to drain fluid.

AFTERCARE

- Monitor your patient's vital signs frequently according to your facility's protocol—for example, every 15 minutes for the first hour, every hour for the next 4 hours, and then every 4 hours. Report an elevated temperature, which could signal infection.
- If a catheter has been left in the pericardial space, provide appropriate care, using sterile technique. Cover the catheter with a sterile dressing and maintain a closed drainage system.
- Observe the ECG for myocardial ischemia and needle-induced arrhythmias.
- Be aware that cardiac tamponade may develop if the myocardium has been punctured and hemorrhages into the pericardial sac. Stay alert for signs and symptoms: hypotension, narrowing pulse pressure, and pulsus paradoxus.
- Also watch for pneumothorax, another possible complication. Report suggestive signs and symptoms: decreased or absent breath sounds, chest pain, and dyspnea.
- Stay alert for signs of hemorrhage—cool and clammy skin, tachycardia, and hypotension—which may occur if the liver has been lacerated.

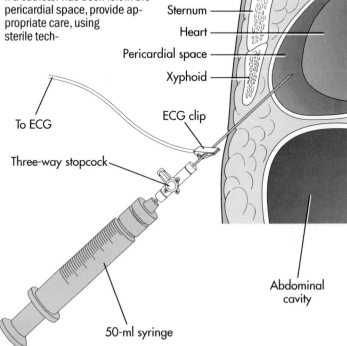

- Continue to assess his vital signs, heart sounds (including checking for a pericardial friction rub), peripheral pulses, skin temperature, and capillary refill. Also check for signs and symptoms of cardiac tamponade.
- Encourage your patient to cough, deep breathe, and use an incentive spirometer frequently. Before these treatments, administer pain medications, as prescribed and needed.
- Assist him to a comfortable position, such as sitting upright and leaning forward. To help him lean forward, place a pillow on his overbed table. Reposition him at least every 2 hours.
- Expect to give corticosteroids, as prescribed, if the patient doesn't respond to NSAIDs. Administer these drugs with food or milk to reduce adverse GI effects. Assess for other adverse effects, such as peptic ulcer disease, sodium retention, hyperglycemia, hypokalemia, and Cushing's syndrome.
- Monitor the patient's hourly fluid intake and output, and report a decrease in output.
- If the patient has constrictive pericarditis, prepare him for a pericardiectomy, as ordered. If prescribed, administer digoxin (Lanoxicaps) and diuretics and provide a low-sodium diet.
- Be aware that a patient with chronic suppurative effusions may require a pericardial window (a type of pericardiectomy) to open and drain the pericardium.

FOLLOW-UP CARE
- Continue to assess your patient's ECG for changes. His ST segments should return to baseline within 7 days of onset and T waves should normalize in 7 to 14 days.
- If your patient is receiving corticosteroids, taper doses as ordered when discontinuing therapy.
- Continue to enforce bed rest until your patient regains hemodynamic stability. For comfort, keep the head of his bed elevated.
- Encourage fluid intake if your patient has a fever.
- Monitor laboratory test results, including white blood cell count, hematocrit, erythrocyte sedimentation rate, and serum electrolyte and hemoglobin levels. Remember that declining hematocrit and hemoglobin level may indicate hemorrhage, whereas elevated blood urea nitrogen and serum creatinine levels may indicate a uremic cause of pericarditis. A positive tuberculin skin test suggests tuberculous pericarditis.
- Remember—pericarditis commonly recurs. Regularly assess your patient for suggestive signs and symptoms.

SPECIAL CONSIDERATIONS
- If your patient has a pericardial catheter for drainage, inspect it frequently to make sure it's patent. If you suspect an obstruction, call the physician immediately—fluid accumulation can lead to cardiac tamponade.

P

- Before discharge, teach your patient about signs and symptoms of pericarditis recurrence, and advise him to report them immediately.

PERITONITIS

An inflammation of the peritoneum—the serous membrane that lines the abdominal cavity—peritonitis is always serious, even if it seems minor at first. The peritoneum is composed of two layers—the parietal peritoneum, which covers the abdominal wall, and the visceral peritoneum, which covers the abdominal organs. A potential space between these layers typically contains less than 50 ml of serous fluid. Normally sterile, the peritoneal membranes and fluid can become infected from invasion of bacteria or chemicals from the nonsterile GI tract or through bacteria borne by blood and lymph. For instance, bacterial organisms may enter the peritoneal cavity through an opening in the intestinal wall. (See *What precipitates peritonitis?*)

Once the inflammation arises, blood vessels in the peritoneal cavity dilate, capillary membrane permeability increases, and a fibrinous, purulent exudate develops. Usually the infection spreads quickly throughout the peritoneal cavity. Sympathetic nervous stimulation decreases peristaltic activity, resulting in paralytic ileus. Hypovolemia and hemoconcentration ensue from heavy loss of fluid from the intravascular space into the peritoneal cavity. These conditions in turn may lead to shock, oliguria, and, possibly, acute tubular necrosis. Septicemia may arise if the infection enters the general circulation.

Resolution of peritonitis may take various forms. In some patients, the exudate disappears without residual effects. In others, walled-off abscesses remain, eventually either healing or serving as the seed of a new infection. In still other patients, adhesions form, binding abdominal tissues together and interfering with normal function.

Despite today's more effective treatments, peritonitis still carries a high mortality risk. To improve your patient's odds, make sure you know how to recognize and respond to this emergency effectively.

WHAT TO LOOK FOR
Clinical findings in peritonitis may include:
- severe abdominal pain that intensifies with movement
- abdominal guarding and rigidity
- nausea and vomiting
- sudden spike in body temperature
- tachycardia
- tachypnea
- dyspnea
- hypotension
- oliguria
- diaphoresis
- pallor.

Diagnostic tests

Diagnostic findings may include:

- leukocytosis
- decreased serum sodium, chloride, and potassium levels
- metabolic alkalosis
- free air in the peritoneal cavity, as shown on abdominal X-ray
- polymorphonuclear leukocytes and bacteria in abdominal fluid, revealed by paracentesis.

WHAT TO DO IMMEDIATELY

If your patient shows signs and symptoms of peritonitis, notify the physician. Then carry out these measures:

- Obtain the patient's baseline vital signs.
- Institute and maintain strict intake and output documentation.
- Assess his abdomen for distention, diminished or absent bowel sounds, tenderness, and rigidity.
- Evaluate the patient's pain status, noting his precise description of the pain's character, intensity, and location.
- ➡ **NurseALERT** Throughout his illness, report any changes in the patient's description of the nature, severity, or location of abdominal pain. A sudden change in the nature or severity of the pain may signal organ rupture or other serious complications. Also, keep in mind that pain may paradoxically decrease after rupture.
- Establish I.V. access, and administer I.V. fluids and antibiotics, as prescribed. Expect the physician to order broad-spectrum agents.
- Insert a nasogastric (NG) tube and attach it to low intermittent suction for gastric decompression.
- If your patient has significant peritoneal contamination, assist with continuous peritoneal lavage, using saline solution or an antibiotic solution, as ordered.
- Insert an indwelling urinary catheter, as ordered, to monitor the patient's hourly urine output.
- Assess his respiratory status carefully, noting the rate, depth, and character of respirations; also auscultate breath sounds. If his respiratory status deteriorates, prepare for endotracheal intubation and mechanical ventilation, if indicated.
- Assess the patient's oxygen saturation by way of arterial blood gas values or pulse oximetry. Administer supplemental oxygen, as indicated and prescribed.
- Obtain blood samples to measure complete blood count, hematocrit, and serum electrolyte and hemoglobin levels.
- If indicated, assist with insertion of a central venous or pulmonary artery catheter to monitor hemodynamic parameters.

WHAT PRECIPITATES PERITONITIS?

Peritonitis may result from bacterial invasion of the peritoneum by such organisms as *Escherichia coli*, *Staphylococcus aureus*, and alpha-hemolytic and beta-hemolytic streptococci. Causes of such invasion include:

- abdominal tumors
- acute salpingitis
- appendicitis
- continuous ambulatory peritoneal dialysis
- diverticulitis
- duodenal ulcers
- stab wounds
- strangulated intestinal obstruction
- ulcerative colitis.

CHEMICAL IRRITATION

In other cases, peritonitis stems from chemical irritation caused by GI secretions that enter the peritoneal cavity. Such irritation may occur with:

- acute hemorrhagic pancreatitis
- bladder or fallopian tube rupture
- leakage of an internal suture line after surgery involving the liver, pancreas, stomach, or intestine
- perforation of the stomach or duodenum (as from cancer or peptic ulcer disease).

P

- Begin continuous cardiac monitoring, as ordered, and evaluate the ECG for ischemic changes caused by hypovolemia.

WHAT TO DO NEXT
After taking initial steps, follow these guidelines:
- Monitor his vital signs every 2 to 4 hours or more often if indicated.
- Assess his hemodynamic status, and observe the ECG for changes as often as hourly.
- Place the patient in semi-Fowler's position to minimize discomfort and help localize the infection to the abdominal area.
- Continue to assess the patient's pain status for changes.
- Assess the patient's abdomen at least every 4 hours; auscultate bowel sounds, check for increasing rigidity, and measure abdominal girth.
- Monitor the patient's laboratory test results and report significant changes.
- Regularly assess his hydration status, including skin turgor.
- Evaluate fluid intake and output every 4 hours; make sure to include NG drainage as output.
- Maintain NG tube decompression and suction, irrigating the tube to keep it patent. Be sure to inspect drainage for color.
- ➡ **NurseALERT** Be aware that NG tube decompression may contribute to stress ulcers and GI hemorrhage, especially in a critically ill patient. Stay alert for bright red drainage or for dark drainage that resembles coffee grounds; test drainage for occult blood.
- Administer analgesics, as prescribed, and evaluate their effectiveness.
- Prepare the patient for surgery, if indicated and ordered. Surgery typically is indicated to remove an inflamed appendix, repair a leaking suture line, or resect a necrotic intestine. However, surgery to resolve abscesses usually is delayed until the patient is stable. To manage intestinal disease, a temporary ostomy may be the initial procedure of choice.

FOLLOW-UP CARE
- Continue to monitor the patient's vital signs, hemodynamic parameters, ECG, and fluid intake and output.
- Continue I.V. antibiotic therapy, as prescribed.
- Continue to maintain NG tube decompression and suction. Inspect the patient's nares for irritation. To prevent drying and cracking, apply a water-soluble lubricant to his lips and around the nares. Provide oral hygiene as needed to ease discomfort from the NG tube.
- Assess for the return of bowel sounds. When peristalsis returns, start the patient on clear fluids, as ordered, and progress his diet as tolerated and prescribed. Monitor his tolerance of food and carefully assess for bowel movements, noting stool amount and characteristics.
- Provide preoperative and postoperative care and teaching tailored to the specific procedure your patient undergoes. Anticipate the need for home care follow-up, especially if wound care must continue after discharge.

SPECIAL CONSIDERATIONS

- After peritonitis, some patients develop fibrous adhesions, which may lead to intestinal obstruction. Before discharge, instruct the patient to seek medical care if he experiences abdominal pain, a change in bowel habits, nausea, or vomiting.
- Teach the patient to check his temperature daily and to report a sudden fever with or without abdominal pain; this may indicate abscess development.

PNEUMONIA, ACUTE

In acute pneumonia, lung tissue becomes inflamed after invasion by bacteria, viruses, fungi, *Mycoplasma* organisms, or protozoans. Some patients face a higher risk of developing pneumonia than others. (See *Risk factors for pneumonia.*)

Usually, pneumonia results from infection with pneumococcal bacteria, especially *Streptococcus pneumoniae*. However, hospitalized patients may develop pneumonia from other bacteria, such as *Pseudomonas aeruginosa*. (See *An inside look at pneumonia,* page 288.)

In viral pneumonia, usually a milder illness, the patient develops interstitial inflammation and infiltrates in the walls of the alveoli rather than exudates or consolidation. In either case, pneumonia often resolves without crisis.

Pneumonia also can have potentially ominous complications, including pleurisy, pleural effusion, empyema, atelectasis, and lung abscess. If the infection spreads, the patient could develop septic arthritis, meningitis, endocarditis, or even septic shock. If atelectasis or tenacious secretions impair gas exchange in the alveoli, she could develop respiratory insufficiency and, possibly, respiratory arrest.

Because of these potential complications, you'll need to be ready to respond rapidly and accurately any time you care for a patient with pneumonia.

WHAT TO LOOK FOR

Clinical findings for a patient with pneumonia differ based on whether she has a bacterial or viral infection.

Bacterial pneumonia

Findings for a patient with bacterial pneumonia may include:
- a recent upper respiratory tract infection
- fever
- chills
- a cough with green, bloody, or rust-colored sputum
- pleuritic chest pain
- dyspnea
- tachypnea

P

RISK FACTORS FOR PNEUMONIA

Many factors can increase the risk of pneumonia, including:
- decreased level of consciousness
- reduced cough and gag reflexes
- old age
- malnutrition
- chronic illness, including lung disease, heart disease, diabetes, and cancer
- immunosuppression, as from steroids, chemotherapy, organ transplantation, and infection with the human immunodeficiency virus
- prolonged exposure to air pollution
- smoking and secondhand smoke exposure
- upper respiratory tract infection
- artificial airway, such as endotracheal intubation or tracheostomy, and mechanical ventilation
- prolonged immobility.

AN INSIDE LOOK AT PNEUMONIA

In bacterial pneumonia, the invading organisms typically enter the alveoli in infected droplets or saliva. In response to this bacterial invasion, the alveolar walls become inflamed, causing adjacent pulmonary capillaries to dilate and leak serum and red blood cells into the alveoli. In addition, polymorphonuclear leukocytes move into the alveoli to engulf and kill the bacteria on the alveolar walls, and macrophages migrate to the area to remove cellular and bacterial debris. As the infection worsens, the alveoli fill with more serum, red blood cells, polymorphonuclear leukocytes, and macrophages and the area becomes consolidated. Increasing consolidation can seriously interfere with alveolar gas exchange, causing the patient to develop hypoxemia.

**Cross section
of alveoli**

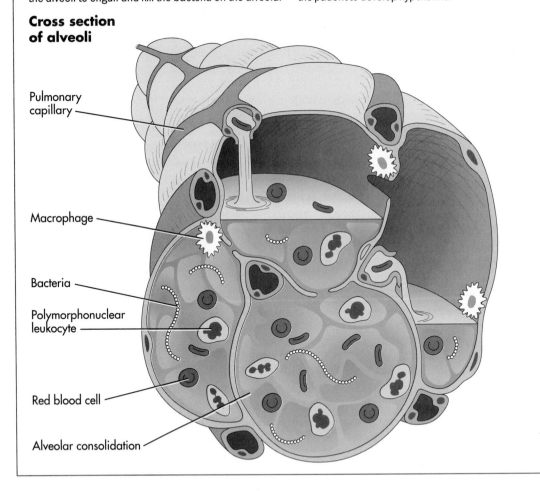

- tachycardia
- crackles
- decreased or bronchial (loud, high-pitched) breath sounds over the affected lung area
- dullness over the affected lung area when percussed

- pleural friction rub
- malaise
- weakness.

Viral pneumonia

Findings for a patient with viral pneumonia are milder and may include:
- fever
- cough
- headache
- anorexia
- myalgia
- sneezing and nasal congestion.

WHAT TO DO IMMEDIATELY

If your patient develops signs of acute pneumonia, notify the physician and follow these measures:

- Obtain her vital signs, watching especially for fever. Also note her level of consciousness and her skin color and temperature.
- Assess the patient's respiratory status frequently. Note the rate, rhythm, depth, and character of her respirations. Auscultate for diminished or adventitious breath sounds. Watch for use of accessory muscles, dyspnea, and paradoxical breathing, in which part of a lung deflates with inspiration and inflates with expiration.
- Assess oxygen saturation using pulse oximetry and arterial blood gas (ABG) values, as ordered. Give supplemental oxygen, as indicated.
- ➡ **NurseALERT** Watch for signs of increasing respiratory distress, including a respiratory rate above 30 breaths/minute, increasing dyspnea, and changes in level of consciousness. Anticipate endotracheal intubation and mechanical ventilation if your patient develops severe respiratory distress.
- Provide continuous ECG monitoring, as indicated. Stay especially alert for arrhythmias caused by hypoxemia.
- Collect a sputum sample for culture and sensitivity testing. To avoid delaying treatment while waiting for culture results, also send a sample for a Gram stain for a preliminary identification of the causative organism and begin antibiotic therapy, as prescribed. If your patient can't produce a sputum specimen, anticipate obtaining one by suction or bronchoscopy.
- Send blood samples to the laboratory for culture and sensitivity testing and a complete blood count, as ordered.
- Obtain a chest X-ray, as ordered.
- Start an I.V. line, if the patient doesn't already have one, to administer prescribed fluids and medications.
- When the sputum culture and sensitivity testing results are available, expect to administer anti-infective agents, as prescribed.

P

WHAT TO DO NEXT

After your patient has stabilized, take these steps:

- Monitor her vital signs every 2 to 4 hours or more often if indicated. If she develops hypotension, keep in mind that it may stem from septic shock. Question her about chills and watch for diaphoresis. Monitor her white blood cell count and report abnormal values.
- Continue to assess your patient's respiratory status, including her breath sounds, respiratory rate and rhythm, level of consciousness, skin color and temperature, and capillary refill. Assess her oxygen saturation levels and monitor serial ABG measurements, as indicated. Pay special attention to how difficult it is for her to breathe and whether she's using accessory muscles to do so.
- ➡ **NurseALERT** Stay alert for signs and symptoms of respiratory failure. Report dyspnea, restlessness, tachypnea, partial pressure of arterial oxygen under 60 mm Hg, partial pressure of arterial carbon dioxide over 50 mm Hg, and pH under 7.35. (See *Interpreting ABG values*, page 253.)
- Place your patient in semi-Fowler's position to maximize her lung expansion and ventilation.
- Check her gag and cough reflexes. If they're reduced or absent, keep in mind that she has an increased risk for aspiration.
- Perform chest physiotherapy and postural drainage to help your patient mobilize secretions. Also, teach her to cough, deep breathe, and use incentive spirometry at least every 2 hours. If she's in pain, you may need to show her how to splint her chest.
- Note the amount, color, and thickness of the patient's sputum.
- Continue the patient's antibiotic therapy, as ordered, and administer an antipyretic—such as acetaminophen—for fever. If she has a high fever, anticipate using a hypothermia blanket. Once her temperature falls to 102.2° F (39° C), turn off the blanket to avoid reducing her temperature too much. That could cause her to shiver, thus raising her metabolic and oxygen needs.
- Provide expectorants to liquefy the patient's secretions and help her cough them up. If she has trouble doing so, you may need to suction her.
- ➡ **NurseALERT** Never give a cough suppressant to a patient who has a productive cough. Remember: Coughing is a protective mechanism to help clear the airway.
- Watch your patient carefully for signs of septic shock, including fever, hypotension, tachycardia, decreased level of consciousness, and reduced urine output.

FOLLOW-UP CARE

- Continue to assess the patient's respiratory status. As ordered, obtain a chest X-ray to verify resolution of the infection.
- Anticipate switching to an oral antibiotic before discharge.
- Help your patient to plan her activities and rest periods to reduce her oxygen demands.

- Make sure she has plenty of tissues and a convenient place to discard them. After she coughs up sputum, help her clean her mouth.
- As appropriate, encourage the patient to drink 3 L of fluid daily to liquefy secretions. If she can't, you'll need to provide I.V. fluids.
- Provide mouth care before meals to help make them more palatable. If helpful, give smaller, more frequent meals. Consider consulting with a dietitian if your patient is malnourished.
- Assess for adverse antibiotic effects, such as nephrotoxicity and GI effects, including nausea, vomiting, and diarrhea. Also stay alert for hypersensitivity or allergic reactions.

SPECIAL CONSIDERATIONS
- To reduce the risk of transmitting the pathogen to other patients, wash your hands frequently. Urge the patient to cover her mouth and nose when she coughs or sneezes and to discard tissues properly.
- Make sure the patient understands the importance of finishing her antibiotic prescription.
- Discuss the importance of pneumococcal and influenza vaccines with all chronically ill and elderly patients.

PNEUMOTHORAX

When air accumulates in the potential space between the visceral and parietal pleura (called the pleural space), the adjacent lung can collapse in a condition called a pneumothorax. In an *open pneumothorax*, air enters the pleural space through an opening in the chest wall. In a *closed pneumothorax*, the patient has no chest wall opening; instead, air enters the pleural space when the surface of the lung, weakened by emphysema, cancer, pneumonia, or a congenital defect, suddenly ruptures. (See *Closed and open pneumothorax*, page 292.)

A closed pneumothorax also may result from an iatrogenic lung injury, such as barotrauma (secondary to mechanical ventilation with positive end-expiratory pressure); subclavian catheter insertion; or traumatic injury, such as a rib fracture. In pneumothorax, air collects in the pleural space, but other substances—including blood and lymphatic drainage—may accumulate in the pleural space as well. (See *Understanding hemothorax and chylothorax*, page 293.)

A tension pneumothorax is a potentially life-threatening condition in which air enters the pleural space with each inspiration but can't escape during expiration. Consequently, so much air collects in the pleural space that the lung on the affected side collapses. As air continues to collect, pressure becomes so great that the mediastinal contents are pushed toward the unaffected side, eventually compressing the once unaffected lung and twisting the heart and great vessels.

Many times, a small pneumothorax will resorb on its own. However, if enough lung collapses to significantly decrease ventilation, your patient

P

CLOSED AND OPEN PNEUMOTHORAX

The illustrations below show a closed pneumothorax and an open pneumothorax.

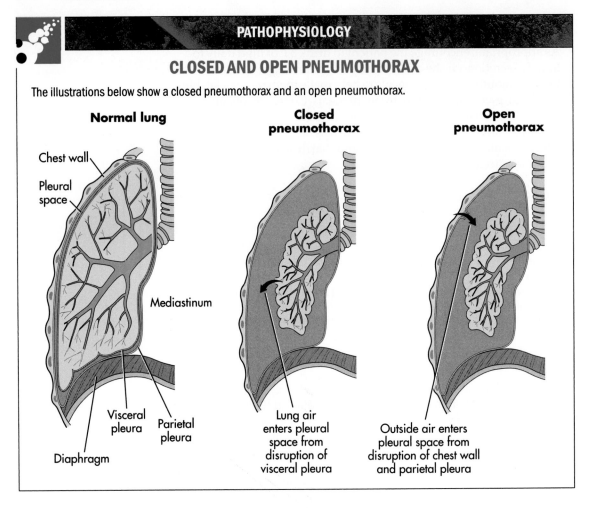

Normal lung

Chest wall

Pleural space

Mediastinum

Visceral pleura

Parietal pleura

Diaphragm

Closed pneumothorax

Lung air enters pleural space from disruption of visceral pleura

Open pneumothorax

Outside air enters pleural space from disruption of chest wall and parietal pleura

will quickly develop respiratory distress, possibly even respiratory arrest. Your timely assessment and prompt intervention can help to alleviate a pneumothorax quickly, or at least to prevent its progression to complete lung collapse and possible life-threatening tension pneumothorax.

WHAT TO LOOK FOR

If your patient develops a pneumothorax, clinical findings may include:
- dyspnea
- sudden, sharp pleuritic chest pain
- decreased or absent breath sounds over the area of lung collapse
- decreased chest-wall movement on the affected side
- shallow, rapid respirations
- cough or hemoptysis.

Tension pneumothorax

Clinical findings in tension pneumothorax may include:
- severe dyspnea

UNDERSTANDING HEMOTHORAX AND CHYLOTHORAX

Air is not the only substance that can collect in the pleural space. Hemothorax occurs when blood accumulates in the pleural space. When lymphatic drainage collects, the disorder is known as chylothorax.

HEMOTHORAX
Usually, hemothorax results from penetrating or blunt chest trauma. It also can develop as a complication of thoracic surgery, lung biopsy, pulmonary infarction, a dissecting thoracic aneurysm, anticoagulation therapy, and a neoplasm.

CHYLOTHORAX
Chyle is a milky fluid that contains lymph and fat globules produced by the GI tract. Normally, it passes from the GI tract into the thoracic lymphatic ducts for transport to the central circulation. In chylothorax, chyle leaks from the thoracic ducts into the pleural space. Chylothorax may arise after certain types of thoracic surgery, trauma, inflammation, or malignant infiltration that obstructs or injures the thoracic ducts.

ASSESSMENT CHARACTERISTICS
A small accumulation of fluid or chyle may produce no signs or symptoms and resorb without treatment. As the amount of accumulated fluid rises, so does the pressure exerted on nearby lung tissues, the heart, and great vessels. In addition to causing lung collapse, rising intrathoracic pressure causes blood to back up in the venous system, reducing venous return and, eventually, cardiac output.

If your patient has a large amount of fluid in the pleural space, you may observe these signs and symptoms:
- dullness on percussion over the area of fluid accumulation
- decreased or absent breath sounds in the area of fluid accumulation
- tachypnea
- mild to severe dyspnea
- anxiety
- restlessness
- chest pain
- hypotension
- stupor
- cyanosis
- shock
- milky drainage from the chest tube (in chylothorax)
- bloody drainage from the chest tube (in hemothorax)
- history of traumatic injury, thoracic surgery, or cancer.

- no breath sounds on the affected side
- restlessness
- distant heart sounds
- tachycardia
- hypotension
- distended neck veins
- tracheal shift toward the unaffected side
- cyanosis
- subcutaneous emphysema.

WHAT TO DO IMMEDIATELY
If you think that your patient has developed a pneumothorax, notify the physician and follow these measures:
- If your patient has an open pneumothorax, as may occur if a chest tube is inadvertently removed, cover the puncture site with an occlusive dressing, such as petroleum gauze or sterile gauze, and cover the dressing completely with adhesive tape.
- ➡ **NurseALERT** Know that patients with open pneumothorax can quickly develop tension pneumothorax. Tension pneumothorax develops if

P

air is sucked into the chest with inhalation but can't escape with exhalation.

- Place your patient in Fowler's position to maximize his ventilation.
- Assess his respiratory status and auscultate his lungs. Note a decrease in breath sounds. Assess oxygen saturation by way of pulse oximetry and arterial blood gas values. Give supplemental oxygen, as ordered.
- Obtain a chest X-ray, as ordered, to confirm the presence, location, and size of the pneumothorax.
- Have emergency equipment readily available.
- Obtain and set up chest tube equipment, and assist with chest tube insertion. Provide your patient with a simple, brief explanation of the procedure and what's expected of him. He'll need to know that it's important for him not to move during the insertion procedure.
- ➡ **NurseALERT** If a chest tube can't be inserted right away, obtain a large-bore needle and assist the physician with its insertion to release trapped air.

WHAT TO DO NEXT

After your patient has stabilized, take these actions:

- Obtain a chest X-ray, as ordered, to check chest tube placement.
- Connect the chest tube to the drainage system and apply suction, as ordered. Make sure all connections are securely fastened and taped to prevent accidental disconnection.
- Apply a sterile occlusive dressing over the insertion site.
- Monitor chest drainage hourly, and report a significant increase or decrease to the physician. Record the time and corresponding fluid level on the collection chamber.
- Check for bubbling in the water-seal chamber. If you see continuous bubbling, air is leaking into the drainage system. Check all connections to make sure they're tight; check the collection device for cracks. Keep in mind that intermittent bubbles are expected in the water-seal chamber when the patient has a closed pneumothorax. This results from air that continues to escape from the lung's damaged surface. When the site of the air leak heals, you shouldn't see any air bubbles in the water-seal chamber.
- Make sure the drainage tubing is free of kinks; kinked tubing can cause a tension pneumothorax because air accumulates in the intrapleural space and can't escape.
- ➡ **NurseALERT** Never clamp the chest tube of a patient with a closed pneumothorax and a persistent air leak because you could cause a tension pneumothorax.
- Assess your patient's respiratory status for improvement after chest tube insertion, including breath sounds, respiratory rate and effort, use of accessory muscles, skin color and temperature, and vital signs.
- Encourage your patient to deep breathe to help reinflate his lung. Teach him to splint the chest tube insertion site to reduce discomfort. Administer analgesics, as prescribed and needed.

FOLLOW-UP CARE

- Prepare your patient for chest tube removal once the air leaks from the lung's surface have stopped (indicated by the absence of bubbling in the water-seal chamber) and drainage has stopped. Several hours before removal, clamp the tube, as ordered, and watch carefully for signs of respiratory distress, which suggest recurring pneumothorax.
- After the tube is removed, keep a petroleum gauze dressing over the insertion site until it closes (usually within 24 to 48 hours). Then, monitor the puncture site daily as it heals, watching for signs of infection.
- Continue to assess the patient's respiratory status, and encourage him to cough, deep breathe, and use the incentive spirometer to maintain lung expansion.

SPECIAL CONSIDERATIONS

- If the pneumothorax doesn't resolve, the patient may require pleurodesis, a sclerosing procedure that creates adhesions between the pleural layers. This procedure involves instilling an irritating substance, such as tetracycline, into the pleural space. The substance causes inflammation of the pleural membranes, which then fuse together as they heal, thus sealing the air leak.
- ➡ **NurseALERT** Pleurodesis is painful, so be sure to give the patient pain medication before the procedure. If the procedure is ineffective, the patient may need to have a portion of the affected lung removed (a lobectomy).

PSYCHOSIS, ACUTE

Usually an exaggerated defensive response to an extreme psychological or physical stressor, acute psychosis is a mental disorder characterized by a loss of grasp on reality. Indeed, the psychotic person incorrectly perceives and responds to reality on the basis of hallucinations, delusions, and disordered thinking. Trying to talk the person out of that erroneously conceived reality is inevitably unsuccessful.

A psychotic episode can stem from such organic causes as drug intoxication or withdrawal, delirium, or even a seizure disorder. Psychiatric causes include schizophrenia, bipolar disorder, schizoaffective disorder, and personality disorders.

A diagnosis of acute psychosis is made when an episode lasts from a few hours to a month. It includes at least one of the following symptoms: hallucinations, delusions, loose associations, or catatonia. (See *Recognizing the symptoms of psychosis*, page 296.)

After an acute psychotic episode and in the absence of another psychiatric disorder, the patient typically returns to a full functional level with a good prognosis. In the interim, you must respond carefully and skillfully to protect the patient and those around her, including yourself and other staff members and patients.

RECOGNIZING THE SYMPTOMS OF PSYCHOSIS

Psychosis is characterized by the presence of at least one of the following symptoms.

HALLUCINATIONS
A hallucination is a sensory perception that doesn't stem from an external stimulus. For example, the patient may see objects that are not present in the room (a visual hallucination). She may hear a voice when no one is talking (an auditory hallucination). If the voice tells her to do something (kill herself or harm someone else, for example), she is having a command hallucination. Your patient may say that she smells something burning or that someone nearby has body odor (an olfactory hallucination). She may even feel something touching her, such as the sensation of bugs crawling on her (a tactile hallucination).

DELUSIONS
A delusion is a false, fixed belief not shared by others. For example, your patient may believe that she is more powerful than or superior to other people (a grandiose delusion). She may believe that she is in imminent danger of harm—from the FBI, for example—and she may have a clear idea of how that harm will occur (a persecutory delusion). Many psychotic patients experience symptoms of paranoia in which they have an irrational and overwhelming suspicion that people intend to exploit or harm them. At times, you may find that a psy-

chotic patient's paranoia stems from a small bit of reality but that it has escalated into the realm of the irrational. For example, a patient who had a negative experience with one health professional may now believe that all health professionals want to harm or even kill her. When her paranoia becomes systematic and specific, it's called a paranoid delusion. She may believe that her body has died (a somatic delusion). Or she may believe that forces outside herself are controlling her thoughts and actions (a delusion of control).

LOOSE ASSOCIATIONS
Also called loosening, this symptom is characterized by a disturbance in the association of ideas and concepts. If your patient has loose associations, her thinking seems haphazard and her conversation unclear. Consecutive sentences lacks a logical sequence or a natural progression of thought. They don't relate to previous sentences. In fact, in severe cases, the patient's speech may be incoherent.

CATATONIA
In this state of psychologically induced immobility, your patient is unresponsive and tends to remain in a fixed, stiffened position. She'll seldom move or talk, although her immobility may be interrupted by agitation or excitement.

WHAT TO LOOK FOR
Clinical findings for a patient with psychosis may include:
- agitation
- auditory hallucinations
- visual hallucinations
- tactile hallucinations
- olfactory hallucinations
- delusional thoughts
- paranoia
- disordered thinking
- loose associations
- catatonia.

WHAT TO DO IMMEDIATELY
If your patient develops acute psychosis, notify the physician and follow these measures:
- Ask your patient to describe what she's experiencing, including what she's hearing, seeing, smelling, and feeling.

- Reassure the patient that she is safe.
- If she asks for validation of her psychosis, tell her you believe that she is experiencing the symptoms she describes to you.
- Try to pinpoint which of her issues and ideas are not based on reality. Does she have a consistent concern, comment, or complaint that doesn't reflect her environment or condition?
- ➡ **Nurse ALERT** Remember that excessive worrying, repeated questions, and overblown fears do not necessarily constitute psychosis; on the contrary, they may be realistic responses to the stress of hospitalization. If the patient's concern or fear is grounded in reality and her thoughts and reasoning about the situation are logical and realistic, she is not psychotic.
- Some psychotic patients trust only certain people with their information. Consequently, you may need to rely on a trusted person to talk with the patient about her concerns and fears.
- Assess the level of fear and agitation experienced by the patient during her psychotic episode so that you can ensure the safety of the patient, staff, other patients, and visitors.
- If your patient's psychosis seems to be focused on a particular person, limit her contact with that person.
- Document the patient's psychotic episode in detail, including her behavior and mental status.

WHAT TO DO NEXT
Once your patient has been stabilized, take these actions:
- Gather information about her psychiatric history and any recent stressful or traumatic events. Consult the patient, her family, her chart, and other professionals as needed to obtain necessary data.
- Note previous psychiatric problems that could underlie the current psychosis, including schizophrenia, schizoaffective disorder, bipolar disorder, borderline personality disorder, schizoid personality disorder, and psychotic depression.
- Review the patient's medication history for anticonvulsants, recreational drugs, and antipsychotic medications. As needed and ordered, obtain blood samples for drug screening, which may provide clues to the cause of the psychotic event.
- Continue to offer reassurance about the patient's safety.
- Request a psychiatric consultation.
- If your patient recently experienced a traumatic event, gently initiate an open-ended conversation about it. Let the patient set the pace, and avoid offering her advice, opinions, or explanations.
- Assess the family's reaction to the patient's mental status. Reassure family members and explain as much as possible about the patient's condition. As needed, guide them in appropriate interactions with the psychotic patient.
- The patient may ask if everyone thinks that she's crazy. If so, tell her that what she's experiencing does not make her crazy. Also reassure her that you understand how stressful the situation is for her.

P

- Try to distract the patient by engaging her in conversation that has nothing to do with the psychotic episode.
- ➡ **NurseALERT** Be careful about trying to use a television or radio as distraction during psychosis; they may worsen the situation.

FOLLOW-UP CARE
- Continue to assess the patient's behavior and mental status.
- Offer nonjudgmental reassurance to establish a trusting relationship, which in turn will help in managing the psychosis.
- Implement the prescribed treatment plan based on psychiatric consultation.
- Administer antipsychotic medication, as prescribed. Keep in mind that the drug, dose, and frequency ordered will vary with the extent to which the psychosis affects the patient's behavior. Most patients require only short-term therapy if they have no other psychiatric problems.

SPECIAL CONSIDERATIONS
- Remember that you can't talk a psychotic patient out of her hallucinations or delusions, no matter how clearly you think you're presenting reality.
- Also remember that talking about the psychotic event will not worsen the patient's symptoms or imply that she's thinking correctly.
- When documenting your patient's mental status and behavior, be as precise and consistent as possible. Avoid generalized, judgmental terms to describe her behavior, such as *weird* or *crazy*.

PULMONARY EDEMA

This potentially life-threatening accumulation of extravascular fluid in the lungs develops from an imbalance between pulmonary capillary hydrostatic pressure and colloid oncotic pressure. Either pulmonary capillary pressure rises or colloid oncotic pressure falls.

Commonly, the imbalance stems from heart failure, myocardial ischemia (possibly with left-sided heart failure), mitral stenosis, chronic mitral regurgitation, severe aortic regurgitation or stenosis, acute mitral regurgitation from ruptured chordae tendineae, barbiturate or opioid poisoning, and overhydration. Here's what happens.

As pressures rise on the left side of the heart, as with left-sided heart failure, pressures in the pulmonary veins and capillaries also rise. Increased pressure in the pulmonary capillaries forces fluid to exit the vessels and accumulate in interstitial tissue around the lungs. For a time, the lymphatic system prevents an increase in interstitial volume by removing excess fluid. Eventually, fluid accumulates in the alveoli faster than the lymphatic system can drain it. Alveolar flooding and pulmonary edema result, impairing gas exchange and leading to hypoxemia.

If colloid oncotic pressure decreases, as in hypoalbuminemia caused by malnutrition, the capillaries can't hold fluid in the blood vessels and fluid flows easily into the lung tissue, causing pulmonary edema.

Pulmonary edema may be a chronic disorder, or it may develop suddenly and progress rapidly. Unless you recognize the problem quickly and respond appropriately, your patient may suffer severe respiratory insufficiency, which could lead to profound hypoxemia, respiratory failure, and death.

WHAT TO LOOK FOR
Because pulmonary edema causes severe respiratory distress, clinical findings may be dramatic, possibly including:
- agitation, restlessness, confusion
- anxiety
- feelings of suffocation and drowning
- severe dyspnea
- crackles, wheezes, and rhonchi (see *Assessing crackles*, page 300)
- sitting bolt upright, using accessory muscles to breathe
- nasal flaring
- respiratory rate above 30 breaths/minute
- diaphoresis
- cold, clammy skin
- pallor or cyanosis
- tachycardia
- third (S_3) heart sound
- neck vein distention
- decreased level of consciousness, progressing to stupor and coma
- blood-tinged, frothy sputum
- hypoxemia
- diminished breath sounds (advanced)
- thready pulse (advanced)
- hypotension (advanced).

WHAT TO DO IMMEDIATELY
If you think that your patient has pulmonary edema, notify the physician and follow these measures:
- Place your patient in high-Fowler's position to improve lung expansion and reduce venous return. If indicated, position his overbed table so that he can lean forward onto it. If possible, help the patient sit with his legs dangling over the side of the bed to promote venous pooling and reduce venous return.
- Assess carefully your patient's respiratory status, including nasal flaring and the use of accessory muscles. When listening to his breath sounds, note the level at which you hear crackles. If his pulmonary edema worsens, the crackles will move up bilaterally from the lung bases. You may even be able to hear gurgling without a stethoscope.
- Assess oxygen saturation by pulse oximetry or arterial blood gases (ABG) analysis, as ordered, and provide supplemental oxygen by

P

TIPS AND TECHNIQUES

ASSESSING CRACKLES

To assess for crackles, listen carefully to the patient's anterior and posterior chest, using the diaphragm of your stethoscope. If you hear short, discrete popping sounds during inspiration, they could be crackles. If you can still hear them after your patient coughs, they probably are crackles.

When documenting what you hear, specify whether the crackles are fine, medium, or coarse and whether they occur early or late in inspiration. Usually, fine crackles sound something like hair rubbing together next to your ear. They reflect the closure of small airways. Medium crackles have a low-pitched, moist sound. Coarse crackles make a low-pitched, bubbling sound something like blowing air through a straw under water. They typically reflect bronchitis or pneumonia. In general, crackles heard early in inspiration reflect obstructive pulmonary disease. Those heard late in inspiration reflect restrictive pulmonary disease.

WHERE YOU'LL HEAR CRACKLES
Usually, you'll first hear crackles at the base of the patient's lungs if he's sitting. That's because gravity draws fluids to dependent areas. As pulmonary edema worsens, crackles may gradually be heard higher in the lungs.

nasal cannula or face mask. (See *Understanding pulse oximetry,* page 219.)

- Begin I.V. therapy at a keep-vein-open rate to avoid fluid volume overload.
- Obtain a chest X-ray, as ordered. Typically, it will reveal cardiomegaly (when pulmonary edema results from chronic heart failure) and diffuse haziness in all lung fields.
- Give morphine I.V., as ordered, to reduce the patient's anxiety, respiratory rate, and venous return. Morphine dilates pulmonary and systemic blood vessels and reduces preload and afterload.
- ➡ **NurseALERT** Watch your patient's respiratory rate closely because morphine can cause respiratory depression. Keep naloxone (Narcan) readily available to reverse narcotic-induced respiratory depression.
- Begin continuous ECG monitoring, and assess for arrhythmias. Electrolyte imbalances (from diuretics) and hypoxia increase the likelihood of arrhythmias. Also monitor the patient for ischemic changes, such as ST-segment and T-wave changes.
- As ordered, give sublingual nitroglycerin if an I.V. line is not in place.
- Give I.V. vasodilators, such as nitroprusside sodium (Nitropress) or, possibly, nitroglycerin, to reduce preload and afterload. (See *Giving nitroprusside sodium safely,* page 195.)
- ➡ **NurseALERT** Monitor the patient's blood pressure and heart rate carefully because vasodilators can cause hypotension and reflex tachycardia. Use them cautiously in a patient who's already hypotensive or at risk for cardiogenic shock.

- As ordered, give diuretics (such as furosemide [Lasix] and bumetanide [Bumex]) to reduce intravascular volume, venous return, and preload.
- Give inotropic drugs to increase myocardial contractility, such as digoxin (Lanoxicaps), dobutamine (Dobutrex), milrinone (Primacor), and amrinone (Inocor).
- ➡ **NurseALERT** Unlike digoxin, dobutamine and amrinone can increase contractility without increasing oxygen consumption.
- If the patient develops bronchospasm, give I.V. aminophylline (Aminophylline), as prescribed, and assess for such adverse effects as tachyarrhythmias, nausea, vomiting, headache, and hypotension.
- If your patient's respiratory status deteriorates, anticipate transfer to a critical care setting, insertion of a pulmonary artery catheter, and endotracheal intubation and mechanical ventilation. Add positive end-expiratory pressure, as ordered, to maintain positive pressure in his airways. (See *What is PEEP?* page 302.)
- Use the intra-arterial line to directly and continuously monitor the patient's blood pressure and to obtain blood samples for ABG analysis.
- Keep in mind that the procedures your patient must undergo will be frightening to him and his family. Do your best to keep them calm (and reduce his respiratory rate) by offering reassurance and simple explanations of all procedures.

WHAT TO DO NEXT
- Titrate medications, as prescribed, to achieve the desired hemodynamic parameters, including blood pressure, cardiac output, heart rate, and pulmonary artery wedge pressure.
- Monitor the patient's response to therapy, including respiratory rate, use of accessory muscles, skin color, and level of consciousness. Auscultate his lungs for adventitious sounds, such as crackles and wheezes. Treatment should reduce his respiratory rate and ease his breathing.
- Assess his vital signs, heart sounds, peripheral pulses, capillary refill, urine output, and level of consciousness frequently.
- Monitor his ABG values and report abnormal results to the physician.
- Monitor the patient's fluid intake and output closely. Reduced cardiac output decreases blood flow to the kidneys, which can cause a decrease in urine production. You'll also want to monitor urine output to evaluate the patient's response to diuretic therapy.
- As ordered, limit the patient's fluid intake to less than 2 L/day.
- Urge him to rest so that he can reduce his work of breathing and oxygen demands. Keep in mind that it may be easier for him to breathe if he sits up and dangles his feet. Maintain a calm environment to minimize his anxiety.
- If medical therapy fails to help your patient, anticipate the use of intra-aortic balloon counterpulsation to reduce afterload.

P

WHAT IS P.E.E.P.?

Positive end-expiratory pressure (PEEP) is a mechanical ventilator setting that maintains a set level of positive pressure (5 cm H_2O, for example) in the patient's lungs during expiration—a time when airway pressure normally drops to zero. By maintaining pressure during expiration, PEEP increases functional residual capacity. If your patient with pulmonary edema has hypoxemia that doesn't improve with oxygen therapy, anticipate an order for PEEP.

BENEFITS OF PEEP

PEEP improves oxygenation in several ways. It prevents alveoli from collapsing, reinflates some alveoli that have already collapsed, and increases the size of alveoli. It also exerts an opposing force against fluid leaking into the alveoli from the capillaries. And finally, by reducing the patient's required fraction of inspired air,

PEEP can reduce the amount of oxygen that must be administered to your patient.

DRAWBACKS OF PEEP

PEEP also has some drawbacks. For example, by increasing intrathoracic pressure, PEEP compresses blood vessels in the chest, thus decreasing venous return (preload) and cardiac output and causing hypotension. (Some researchers think that reduced preload may benefit patients with impaired left ventricular function.) PEEP also impairs venous return from the cerebrovascular system, which may increase intracranial pressure. Finally, the patient may sustain barotrauma if overdistended alveoli rupture, allowing air to leak into subcutaneous tissue, pleural tissue, and the mediastinum and, possibly, resulting in pneumothorax.

FOLLOW-UP CARE

- Keep your patient on bed rest until he's hemodynamically stable. During that time, help him to change positions often. Also encourage him to cough, deep breathe, and use the incentive spirometer.
- Keep the patient in Fowler's position to ease the work of breathing.
- Weigh him daily; gradual weight increase may indicate that fluid is reaccumulating.
- Track the patient's laboratory results and report abnormalities. If he receives diuretics, watch for electrolyte imbalance. Elevated blood urea nitrogen and creatinine levels suggest reduced renal perfusion. Elevated lactate levels indicate anaerobic metabolism.
- If your patient receives diuretics, watch for signs and symptoms of hypokalemia, including muscle weakness, tetany, and arrhythmias. Maintain continuous cardiac monitoring to detect changes that suggest electrolyte imbalance.

SPECIAL CONSIDERATIONS

- Explain to your patient and his family how pulmonary edema develops and the need to immediately report increased shortness of breath, anxiety, frothy pink sputum, and feelings of drowning and suffocation.
- Teach your patient about the medications he'll need to take at home, including doses, frequency, and adverse effects.
- Teach the patient about a low-sodium diet, fluid restrictions, and the need for potassium supplements, as appropriate. Tell him to weigh himself daily at the same time of day, wearing the same type of clothing, and using the same scale. Advise him to report a weight gain of more than 3 lb (1.36 kg) in 1 week to his physician .

PULMONARY EMBOLISM

When undissolved substances—fat globules, tumor fragments, air, amniotic fluid, foreign matter, bacterial debris, or, most commonly, a thrombus—circulate in the bloodstream, they may eventually lodge in a small vessel in the patient's lung. If this occurs, the patient has what is called a pulmonary embolism. Because impaired perfusion reduces alveolar gas exchange, the patient may develop severe respiratory distress. The ischemic lung tissue may become necrotic, and pulmonary infarction may occur, especially if a large arterial branch is occluded. (See *What happens in a pulmonary embolism,* page 304.) Because a pulmonary embolism can increase pulmonary artery and right ventricular pressures, it also may lead to right-sided heart failure and reduced cardiac output.

Pulmonary emboli commonly arise from deep vein thrombosis. Such thrombi are most likely to develop in patients with abnormal or damaged blood vessel walls, hypercoagulability, and venous stasis—a set of factors commonly known as Virchow's triad. Additional risk factors include old age, obesity, recent surgery, immobility, traumatic injury, atrial fibrillation, and mitral stenosis. Women who are pregnant or taking oral contraceptives also face increased risk.

Keep in mind that the extent of the embolization and the patient's cardiac and respiratory status are strong determinants of her outcome. If she has underlying cardiac and respiratory problems, she may die within a few hours of suffering a pulmonary embolism. But if she had normal cardiac and respiratory function before the event, she may survive with prompt treatment unless more than one-half of her pulmonary vasculature is occluded. If your patient develops a pulmonary embolism, your rapid detection and response could save her life.

WHAT TO LOOK FOR
Clinical findings for a patient with pulmonary embolism may include:
- dyspnea, usually sudden and unexplained
- sudden, severe pleuritic chest pain
- anxiety, apprehension, and restlessness
- a sense of impending doom
- diaphoresis
- tachycardia
- tachypnea
- cough and hemoptysis
- crackles
- pleural friction rub
- fourth (S_4) heart sound
- confusion, altered level of consciousness
- hypoxemia
- cyanosis

P

WHAT HAPPENS IN A PULMONARY EMBOLISM

When an embolus lodges in the pulmonary circulation, it blocks or reduces blood flow to lung tissues distal to the obstruction and initiates a series of physiologic changes in the body. Platelets, which degrade at the time of the embolism, release histamine, serotonin, prostaglandins, and thromboxane, which cause the pulmonary arterioles and bronchi to constrict.

Because of the actions of these substances, pulmonary vascular resistance rises and perfusion is further compromised. Typically, ventilation is adequate but perfusion isn't, creating an imbalance that eventually leads to hypoxemia. In an attempt to compensate for this imbalance, the patient typically breathes faster, which blows off carbon dioxide.

The hemodynamic consequences of a pulmonary embolism can be severe. Decreased arterial blood flow through the lungs causes pulmonary pressures to rise, which may cause right ventricular hypertrophy and right-sided heart failure. Cardiac output eventually decreases from right-sided heart failure and decreased left ventricular preload. Systemic hypotension and shock follow. Occasionally, the embolus may lead to pulmonary infarction, with subsequent infection and abscess formation in the lung tissues.

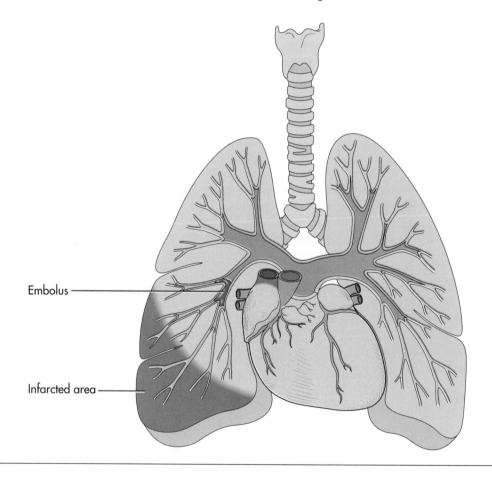

Embolus

Infarcted area

- syncope
- fever (low grade).

If the embolism stems from deep vein thrombosis, the patient may have additional clinical findings at the site of the thrombus, often in the calf, including:
- swelling
- warmth
- redness
- tenderness.

WHAT TO DO IMMEDIATELY

If you think that your patient has a pulmonary embolus, quickly evaluate her airway, breathing, and circulation. Then notify the physician and take these steps:
- Obtain the patient's vital signs and assess her cardiopulmonary status closely. Auscultate for a fourth (S_4) heart sound. Also note the rate, depth, and character of her respirations. Auscultate for crackles and a pleuritic rub.
- ➡ Nurse**ALERT** Signs common to pulmonary embolism are also common to other serious problems, such as myocardial infarction (MI) and pneumonia. Consider all your patient's signs and symptoms carefully, including other health conditions and risk factors, before concluding that pulmonary embolism has caused her distress.
- Assess the patient's level of consciousness and degree of anxiety.
- ➡ Nurse**ALERT** Pulmonary embolism commonly creates a strong feeling of impending doom that is out of proportion with other signs and symptoms.
- Assess oxygen saturation levels by way of pulse oximetry and arterial blood gas (ABG) analysis, as ordered. Give supplemental oxygen, as indicated, and elevate the head of the bed at least 45 degrees to maximize lung expansion and ease the work of breathing.
- Obtain a 12-lead ECG to rule out MI, and begin continuous ECG monitoring, as indicated. Watch for changes that suggest pulmonary embolism, such as tall, peaked P waves in leads II, III, and aVF; nonspecific ST-segment and T-wave changes; and arrhythmias.
- Establish I.V. access if a line isn't already in place. Also anticipate insertion of a pulmonary artery or central venous catheter to evaluate hemodynamic status.
- If the pulmonary embolus originates from a thrombus, obtain baseline coagulation studies. Expect to give a bolus of heparin to begin anticoagulation and then follow with a continuous infusion, as prescribed. Monitor later test results to evaluate the drug's effectiveness. Prepare the patient for possible thrombolytic therapy, as ordered.
- If the patient has evidence of shock, give vasopressors, as ordered.

P

CONFIRMING A PULMONARY EMBOLISM

If you suspect that your patient has a pulmonary embolism, you'll need to prepare her for one or more diagnostic tests, including ventilation-perfusion ($\dot{V}/\dot{Q}$)scan, pulmonary angiography, and, possibly, chest X-ray, arterial blood gas analysis, ECG, echocardiography, Doppler ultrasonography, venography, or impedance plethysmography. Keep in mind that a positive test result doesn't necessarily mean that your patient has a pulmonary embolism. Both clinical signs and symptoms and the confirmation of a source, such as deep vein thrombosis, support the reliability of a positive test result.

$\dot{V}/\dot{Q}$ SCAN
As part of the diagnostic workup for a possible pulmonary embolism, $\dot{V}/\dot{Q}$ scans may be performed. Neither test alone is conclusive in confirming or ruling out whether your patient has a pulmonary embolism. But when reviewed together, the test results can help the physician make the diagnosis.

Purpose and procedure
A perfusion scan is used to detect an obstruction in pulmonary blood flow. In this test, human serum albumin particles, bonded to the radioisotope technetium, are injected into the patient's peripheral vein. These radioactive particles flow through the right side of the heart and temporarily lodge in the narrower pulmonary capillaries. A nuclear scanner then detects the distribution of the radioactive particles within the pulmonary capillary bed. Areas with normal blood flow, or *hot spots,* show a high uptake of the radioactive substance and appear in a uniform pattern. Areas with reduced blood flow, or *cold spots,* show a low uptake of radioactivity and indicate poor perfusion. They also suggest the presence of an embolism.

To increase the reliability of the perfusion scan results, a ventilation scan is also usually performed. A ventilation scan evaluates abnormalities in ventilation throughout the lung tissue. In this procedure, the patient inhales a small amount of air that's mixed with a radioactive gas, such as xenon or krypton, for several minutes through a face mask affixed with a mouth piece. The lungs are then scanned to evaluate the distribution of the gas during three phases: the wash-in phase, when the gas builds up; the equilibrium stage, when the gas reaches a constant level; and the wash-out phase, when the gas is exhaled from the lungs. Normally, the gas is equally distributed throughout the lungs during the wash-in and wash-out phases.

Expected test results
The $\dot{V}/\dot{Q}$ scan results are evaluated together for a mismatching. Normal, healthy lung tissues are adequately perfused and ventilated. In pulmonary embolism, the embolism obstructs blood flow to the lung area supplied by the affected vessel. This shows up on the perfusion scan as a *cold spot,* an area with a low saturation of radioactive particles. In the patient with a pulmonary embolism, as in the healthy patient, the ventilation scan indicates an equal distribution of the inhaled radioactive gas. This mismatching—decreased or absent perfusion in normally ventilated areas of the lung—suggests a pulmonary embolism.

$\dot{V}/\dot{Q}$ scan results are graded as normal, low probability, indeterminate, or high probability. If the patient has normal results, indicating that both scans are normal, then she doesn't have a pulmonary embolism. If the results show high probability, there's about a 90% chance that she has a pulmonary embolism.

PULMONARY ANGIOGRAPHY
After completing the $\dot{V}/\dot{Q}$ scan, the physician may order pulmonary angiography to rule out or confirm the diagnosis of pulmonary embolism. The only diagnostic test that provides information about abnormalities in the anatomy of the pulmonary vasculature, pulmonary

WHAT TO DO NEXT
Once your patient has stabilized, take these steps:
- Prepare her for diagnostic tests to confirm the pulmonary embolism. (See *Confirming a pulmonary embolism.*)
- Continue to assess her cardiopulmonary status, oxygen saturation levels, and serial ABG values to detect changes in her condition.
- Monitor the patient for signs and symptoms of a developing pulmonary infarction, including severe pleuritic chest pain, pleural friction rub, hemoptysis, fever, and cyanosis.

(angiography is considered the gold standard for detecting pulmonary perfusion defects.

Purpose and procedure
Using fluoroscopy as a guide, the physician inserts a pulmonary artery catheter into a vein and threads it through the right side of the heart into the pulmonary artery. Once the catheter is in place, the physician obtains and evaluates important hemodynamic information, such as the pulmonary artery and wedge pressure readings as well as cardiac output. Then, after a radiopaque contrast agent is injected through the catheter, X-rays of the pulmonary vessels are taken in timed sequence to visualize the pulmonary vasculature.

Expected test results
If a pulmonary embolus is present, the affected pulmonary vessel will show either a filling defect or an abrupt cut-off at the point of embolism. Generally, a filling defect is found because complete obstruction of the pulmonary vessel is uncommon.

RELATED TESTS
Other tests frequently used in ruling out a suspected pulmonary embolus include chest X-ray, arterial blood gas analysis, 12-lead ECG, and echocardiography. In addition, studies to confirm deep vein thrombosis, the most common cause of a pulmonary embolus, may be ordered; they may include Doppler ultrasonography, venography, and impedance plethysmography.

Chest X-ray. An elevated hemidiaphragm, an enlargement of either of the chambers of the right side of the heart or pulmonary artery, linear basal atelectasis, and the presence of infiltrates or pleural effusions are chest X-ray abnormalities suggestive of pulmonary embolus.

Arterial blood gas values. A partial pressure of arterial oxygen of less than 80 mm Hg and a partial pressure of arterial carbon dioxide of less than 36 mm Hg on room air are arterial blood gas findings suggestive of pulmonary embolus. Keep in mind that normal results don't imply the absence of a pulmonary embolus. That's because the embolism may not be large enough to cause a significant alteration in gas exchange.

ECG. In the presence of a pulmonary embolus, a 12-lead ECG may reveal such changes as tall, peaked P waves in leads II, III, and aVF; nonspecific ST-segment and T-wave changes; and a right bundle-branch block or right axis deviation caused by right ventricular hypertrophy. Sinus tachycardia is also common, and atrial fibrillation or flutter may be seen.

Echocardiography. Findings in a two-dimensional echocardiogram that suggest a pulmonary embolus (especially when evaluated together with the 12-lead ECG) include right atrial or ventricular enlargement, tricuspid regurgitation, and, possibly, a thrombus in the right side of the heart or proximal pulmonary artery.

Doppler ultrasonography. Venous thrombosis can be detected through Doppler ultrasonography and confirms the diagnosis if venous blood flow velocity does not change with respirations, increases after compression has been applied, or is absent.

Venography. Using a contrast medium, venography uses X-rays to show filling or occluding defects and the subsequent development of collateral circulation in the area affected by deep vein thrombosis.

Impedance plethysmography. Electrodes attached to the patient's leg enable a plethysmograph to monitor changes in electrical impedance (resistance) in response to blood volume variations induced by inflating a pneumatic thigh cuff. In the patient with occlusive proximal deep vein thrombosis, electrical impedance changes will be minimized. However, remember that the results may be influenced by variables stemming from such conditions as heart failure and severe arterial insufficiency and from the effects of mechanical ventilation.

- Also watch for signs of pleural effusion, such as decreased chest movement and breath sounds and dullness over the affected lung.
- ➡ **NurseALERT** If the patient has jugular vein distention, peripheral edema, and Kussmaul's sign, she's probably developing right-sided heart failure. Check for increased central venous pressure, right atrial pressure, and right ventricular pressure to corroborate.
- Assess the patient for pain and provide analgesics, as prescribed.
- Monitor for development of emboli to other organs. (See *Signs of other emboli*, page 308.)

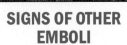

SIGNS OF OTHER EMBOLI

As your patient recovers from a pulmonary embolism, stay vigilant for signs of emboli to other organs, especially these:

- *Cerebral embolism*: decreased level of consciousness, confusion, aphasia, muscle paralysis, paresis, altered sensation (numbness, tingling, paresthesias), and seizures.
- *GI embolism*: abdominal pain, reduced or absent bowel sounds, and nausea and vomiting.
- *Renal embolism*: hematuria, rising blood urea nitrogen and creatinine, and reduced urinary output.

- If your patient's pulmonary embolus is caused by deep vein thrombus or other thrombi, monitor your patient's activated partial thromboplastin time (APTT) results and titrate the heparin infusion, as prescribed, to maintain the APTT at 1½ to 2½ times the control. Assess the patient for signs and symptoms of bleeding.
- ➡ **NurseALERT** Be on the lookout for complaints of abdominal pain and changes in level of consciousness; they may indicate internal bleeding.
- If your patient is scheduled for surgery, teach her and her family about the planned procedure—probably embolectomy, vena caval clipping, or insertion of a vena caval filter.

FOLLOW-UP CARE

- Keep the patient on bed rest in a comfortable position. Pace her activities to reduce oxygen demand. Assess oxygen saturation levels in response to activity, and slowly increase her activity level as tolerated.
- Reposition the patient at least every 2 hours and urge her to cough and deep-breathe.
- If she received anticoagulation or thrombolytic therapy, continue to assess her for evidence of bleeding. Look for bleeding gums or incisions, blood in her stool or urine, abdominal pain, a falling hemoglobinlevel or hematocrit, or a change in level of consciousness. Take measures to prevent injury, such as avoiding intramuscular injections and providing the patient with a soft toothbrush.
- ➡ **NurseALERT** Avoid aspirin and aspirin-containing products because they alter platelet function and may increase the patient's risk for bleeding.
- Anticipate beginning oral anticoagulant therapy while your patient is still receiving heparin; monitor her prothrombin time.
- If the patient has an arterial line in place, use it to obtain blood specimens. If you must perform a venipuncture, apply direct pressure to the site for 10 to 15 minutes and then apply a pressure dressing. When discontinuing an I.V. or arterial line, apply pressure for 20 to 30 minutes before applying the pressure dressing. Monitor all invasive procedure sites for bleeding or hematoma formation.

SPECIAL CONSIDERATIONS

- If your patient is at risk for deep vein thrombosis, provide preventive interventions, as ordered, including sequential pneumatic compression devices or antiembolism stockings, early ambulation, and anticoagulants (such as subcutaneous heparin). Also, urge her not to stand or sit for long periods and not to smoke. Tell her to perform leg and foot exercises while sitting.
- If the patient will go home on oral anticoagulant therapy, teach her about the regimen, about ways to prevent bleeding, and about the need for a stable intake of foods high in vitamin K. Remind her to obtain follow-up blood tests, as prescribed, to evaluate her drug therapy.
- Keep in mind that the physician may prescribe histamine-2-receptor antagonists to prevent GI bleeding and stool softeners to prevent rectal bleeding from straining.

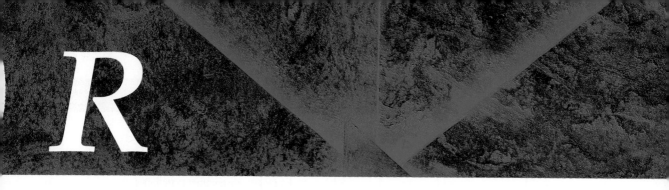

RENAL FAILURE, ACUTE

A sudden reduction in renal function, acute renal failure can develop over several hours or several days. Depending on the underlying cause, it's classified as prerenal, intrarenal, or postrenal. (See *Classifying acute renal failure*, page 310.)

Clinical effects of acute renal failure include:

- uremia from accumulation of waste products in the blood
- fluid overload
- electrolyte imbalances (especially hyperkalemia)
- metabolic acidosis from impaired acid-base regulation
- faulty blood pressure regulation
- changes in red blood cell production from lack of erythropoietin.

If detected and treated in time, acute renal failure can be reversed. If treatment comes too late, the patient may develop end-stage renal disease and die; even in acute-care settings, the condition has a mortality rate of 40% to 50%. Your expert assessment and rapid response can tip the scales in your patient's favor.

WHAT TO LOOK FOR

Clinical findings in acute renal failure may include:

- oliguria (urine output below 30 ml/hour over 2 to 4 hours or less than 400 ml in 24 hours)
- anuria
- azotemia (retention of nitrogenous substances in the blood)
- hypotension, especially orthostatic hypotension (an early sign)
- hypertension (a later finding)
- arrhythmias
- Kussmaul's respirations (an attempt to compensate for acidosis)
- apathy, drowsiness, and changes in mental status (from uremia)
- anorexia
- nausea and vomiting
- pruritus
- jaundice
- purpura, bleeding disorders, and thrombocytopenia
- neutropenia.

R

CLASSIFYING ACUTE RENAL FAILURE

Acute renal failure may be classified as prerenal, intrarenal (intrinsic or parenchymal), or postrenal.

PRERENAL FAILURE
Prerenal failure results from conditions that reduce blood flow to the kidneys, such as:
- hypovolemia (as from diuretics, hemorrhage, burns, and prolonged diarrhea or vomiting)
- decreased cardiac output (as from cardiomyopathy, myocardial infarction, arrhythmias, shock, and cardiac tamponade)
- decreased renal perfusion (as from vascular obstruction and interruption of renal blood flow during surgery).

INTRARENAL FAILURE
With intrarenal failure, the kidneys themselves are damaged. Precipitating conditions include:
- medullary damage, as from nephrotoxic drugs and other substances (including antibiotics nonsteroidal anti-inflammatory drugs, amphotericin, angiotensin-converting enzyme inhibitors, and radiographic contrast material)
- ischemic medullary injury (as from shock, gram-negative bacteremia, crush injuries, trauma, and transfusion reactions)
- cortical damage (as from systemic lupus erythematosus, glomerulonephritis, and Goodpasture's syndrome)
- uncorrected prerenal or postrenal failure.

POSTRENAL FAILURE
In postrenal failure, urine flow out of both kidneys is obstructed. It can be caused by:
- renal calculi
- prostatic hypertrophy
- prostate cancer
- abdominal and bladder tumors
- neurogenic problems, such as spinal cord disease.

WHAT TO DO IMMEDIATELY

If you that suspect your patient is developing acute renal failure, notify the physician. Then take these actions:
- Insert an indwelling urinary catheter if one is not already in place.
- Obtain the patient's pulse rate and blood pressure to establish a baseline. Be sure to check for orthostatic blood pressure changes.
- If your patient has oliguria and hypotension, expect to infuse 250 ml of normal saline solution over 15 to 30 minutes, as prescribed. During and after the infusion, assess the patient's response by measuring his blood pressure, heart rate, and urine output.
- Assist with insertion of a central venous or pulmonary artery catheter, as ordered, to evaluate the patient's hemodynamic status. Then obtain central venous pressure or cardiac output readings as often as the physician directs.
- Obtain blood samples to measure blood urea nitrogen (BUN) and serum creatinine and electrolyte levels. Monitor the patient's serum potassium level for potentially life-threatening hyperkalemia.
- Collect a urine specimen for urinalysis and electrolyte measurement.
- Institute continuous cardiac monitoring; check the patient's ECG often for arrhythmias.
- Keep meticulous intake and output records.
- If the patient has postrenal failure, prepare him for urologic interventions, as ordered.
- Administer inotropic drugs, as prescribed, if renal failure stems from decreased cardiac output.

- Withhold diuretics and nephrotoxic drugs, such as aminoglycosides, until the underlying problem is identified and the patient's renal function can be evaluated with blood and urine tests.

WHAT TO DO NEXT
Once your patient has stabilized, follow these guidelines:
- Assess his heart rate and rhythm, blood pressure, and hemodynamic parameters every 2 to 4 hours. Watch for hypotension, hypertension, and arrhythmias (related to electrolyte imbalances and acidosis).
- Monitor the patient's fluid intake and output hourly, and weigh him at least daily. Be sure to include diarrhea and, if appropriate, nasogastric drainage as output.
- Watch for changes in the patient's mental status; as needed, initiate safety measures.
- Auscultate his heart and breath sounds every 2 to 4 hours. Report evidence of fluid overload, such as the development of a third or fourth heart sound or crackles in the lung fields.
- Expect to administer diuretics, as prescribed, to correct oliguria. This is a primary goal of therapy because nonoliguric renal failure (output of at least 1,000 ml in 24 hours with rising BUN and serum creatinine levels) carries a lower mortality than oliguric failure.
- Expect to give lower doses or lengthen dosing intervals when administering drugs excreted primarily through the kidneys. To help detect drug toxicity, monitor the patient's serum creatinine level closely.
- If the patient doesn't respond to treatment, expect to prepare him for hemodialysis, peritoneal dialysis, or another type of renal replacement therapy. (See *Understanding renal replacement therapy*, page 312.)

FOLLOW-UP CARE
- Continue to monitor the patient's fluid intake and output, and weigh him daily to guide fluid management.
- Monitor laboratory results to help assess the effectiveness of treatment and track improvements in the patient's baseline renal function.
- Maintain adequate nutrition—given orally or parenterally as indicated—to promote healing.
- Maintain fluid restrictions to avoid fluid overload. To ease dry mouth, provide ice chips or hard candy.
- During the diuretic phase of intrarenal failure, anticipate replacing most of the patient's urine volume (3 to 10 L/day) with I.V. fluids, based on serum electrolyte levels, to help prevent prerenal failure.
- ➡ **Nurse ALERT** Be aware that a patient with renal failure is especially vulnerable to infection. Use strict aseptic technique, and check closely for signs and symptoms of infection (such as fever), especially during the diuretic phase of renal failure.

SPECIAL CONSIDERATIONS
- If your patient is scheduled for diagnostic studies that use contrast dyes, make sure he receives adequate hydration (such as 1 L of I.V.

R

UNDERSTANDING RENAL REPLACEMENT THERAPY

A patient with acute renal failure who doesn't respond to other treatments aimed at controlling uremic symptoms may require hemodialysis, peritoneal dialysis, or continuous renal replacement therapies.

HEMODIALYSIS
Hemodialysis is preferred in acute renal failure because it rapidly removes toxins, wastes, and excess electrolytes from the blood. The procedure, which uses an external pump and extracorporeal filter, shunts the patient's blood through a machine, filters it, and then returns it to his circulation. The treatment takes 3 to 4 hours. Because hemodialysis may cause rapid fluid shifts within the body, it's usually not tolerated well by hemodynamically unstable patients.

PERITONEAL DIALYSIS
Slower than hemodialysis, peritoneal dialysis uses the peritoneum as the semipermeable membrane that filters waste products from the body. Dialysate is infused into the peritoneal space, left there to dwell for a specified period, and then drained. This procedure, called an exchange or cycle, is repeated a number of times.

Because it doesn't require blood to be withdrawn from the body, filtered, and then returned to the body, peritoneal dialysis is better tolerated by hemodynamically unstable patients. However, peritoneal dialysis carries with it the risk of infection (peritonitis) and respiratory compromise. In addition, its slow filtration rate makes the procedure less than ideal in acute renal failure.

CONTINUOUS RENAL REPLACEMENT THERAPIES
Continuous arteriovenous hemofiltration with dialysis (CAVHD) and continuous venovenous hemofiltration (CVVH) are reserved for patients who are hemodynamically unstable because they involve slow, continuous removal of fluid.

In CAVHD, the patient's blood is slowly directed through an arterial catheter into an external hemofilter or dialyzer. A dialysate, infused into the hemofilter, flows in the opposite direction of the patient's blood. This infusion removes wastes and fluid. Then the blood is returned to the patient through a venous catheter. Replacement fluid is also infused through the venous catheter.

CVVH requires a double-lumen venous catheter, as opposed to an arterial and a venous catheter during the dialysis procedure.

fluid) before the procedure to help prevent intrarenal failure.

➡ **NurseALERT** Certain contrast agents are contraindicated for patients with renal insufficiency or failure.

RESPIRATORY ACIDOSIS

An acid-base imbalance characterized by retention of excessive carbon dioxide (CO_2), respiratory acidosis results from any condition that causes alveolar hypoventilation and thus interferes with pulmonary gas exchange. The excess CO_2 combines with water to form carbonic acid, thereby increasing acid levels in the blood. (See *Causes of respiratory acidosis*.)

Respiratory acidosis can be an acute or a chronic condition. Acute respiratory acidosis begins suddenly with high partial pressure of arterial carbon dioxide ($PaCO_2$) levels and a severe decrease in serum pH before the renal system can neutralize or compensate for the increasing acidity. In chronic (or compensated) acidosis, the renal system compensates for elevated CO_2 levels, retaining bicarbonate and returning pH toward normal.

Depending on the severity of its underlying cause, respiratory acidosis may lead to central nervous system depression, respiratory arrest, arrhythmias, and myocardial depression with subsequent cardiogenic

CAUSES OF RESPIRATORY ACIDOSIS

Conditions that lead to respiratory acidosis can be grouped into one of the following categories:
- *Airway obstruction.* Examples include aspiration, foreign-body obstruction, severe bronchospasm, obstructive sleep apnea, and pulmonary or laryngeal edema.
- *Respiratory center depression.* Examples include drug use (including narcotics, anesthesia, and sedatives), meningitis, and medullary tumors.
- *Neuromuscular respiratory disorders.* Examples include myasthenia gravis, Guillain-Barré syndrome, and spinal cord injury.
- *Pulmonary diseases.* Examples include pneumonia, atelectasis, asthma, bronchitis, emphysema, and smoke inhalation.
- *Thoracic cage disorders.* Examples include flail chest and pneumothorax.

shock and cardiac arrest. You'll need to recognize and respond promptly to this potentially life-threatening imbalance.

WHAT TO LOOK FOR

Early signs and symptoms of respiratory acidosis are related to central nervous system depression. Clinical findings may include:
- pH less than 7.35
- $PaCO_2$ greater than 45 mm Hg
- decreased respiratory rate and depth
- dyspnea
- tachypnea
- dull headache
- apprehension, restlessness (early sign)
- decreasing level of consciousness; drowsiness and lethargy progressing to coma
- arrhythmias
- muscle twitching
- warm, flushed skin
- dehydration
- cyanosis (late sign)
- papilledema (late sign).

WHAT TO DO IMMEDIATELY

If your patient develops respiratory acidosis, notify the physician and follow these measures:
- Obtain his vital signs and assess his level of consciousness and cardiopulmonary status. Make sure he has a patent airway. Assess his respiratory rate, depth, and character, and auscultate his breath sounds for changes characteristic of his underlying condition. Help him into high Fowler's position to facilitate gas exchange.
- Begin continuous cardiac monitoring, and watch the patient's ECG for ischemic changes and arrhythmias.

R

- Obtain arterial blood gas (ABG) measurements to establish a baseline and assess future changes. (See *Interpreting ABG values*, page 253.) Assess the patient's oxygen saturation continuously by way of pulse oximetry to detect hypoxemia.
- ➡ **NurseALERT** Because severe respiratory acidosis is secondary to respiratory failure, it's often accompanied by hypoxemia.
- Give supplemental oxygen, as indicated.
- ➡ **NurseALERT** Use extreme caution when giving supplemental oxygen to a patient with chronic respiratory acidosis. Remember that chronically elevated $PaCO_2$ levels suppress the brain's respiratory drive center. In a patient with chronic respiratory acidosis, hypoxemia becomes the primary respiratory stimulant. By elevating his $PaCO_2$ level above normal, you may eliminate the patient's respiratory drive.
- Repeatedly check for declining level of consciousness, a sign of worsening acidosis.
- Monitor for signs that the patient is tiring (he'll grow sleepy and his respirations will become weaker and slower, progressing to apnea.) Anticipate endotracheal intubation and mechanical ventilation if this occurs.
- If the patient has copious secretions, suction him as necessary.
- Give bronchodilators to dilate smooth muscles in his large airways.
- ➡ **NurseALERT** Avoid giving narcotics and sedatives because they increase respiratory depression.
- Establish I.V. access if a line isn't already in place. Give fluids to moisten the patient's secretions and ease their removal. Also give antibiotics, as prescribed.
- Obtain a chest X-ray and blood samples for testing, including complete blood count (CBC) and serum electrolyte levels.
- ➡ **NurseALERT** Monitor the patient's laboratory values closely, especially his serum potassium level. As his acidosis is reversed, the serum potassium level may decrease, and the patient may become hypokalemic.
- Give emotional support to decrease the patient's fear and anxiety.

WHAT TO DO NEXT
Once your patient has stabilized, take these steps:
- Continue to assess and document his ECG rhythm; vital signs; mental status; heart, breath, and bowel sounds; and urine output. Report any significant changes.
- Keep the patient in high Fowler's position to ease gas exchange.
- Maintain hydration with I.V. and oral fluids, as appropriate.
- If the patient has required mechanical ventilation, monitor his $PaCO_2$ levels closely and watch for alkalosis.
- ➡ **NurseALERT** When $PaCO_2$ levels are reduced too rapidly, the kidneys may be unable to eliminate bicarbonate quickly enough to prevent alkalosis. Monitor end-tidal CO_2 levels carefully.
- Continue to monitor serial ABG values for hypoxemia as well as improvement or worsening of acidosis.

- Obtain follow-up chest X-rays and blood tests, including CBC and serum electrolyte levels.
- Continue to monitor laboratory values, especially serum potassium level.
- Have the patient turn, cough, deep breathe, and use the incentive spirometer every 2 hours to promote optimal ventilation.
- To promote rest and decrease oxygen demands, keep the patient on bed rest, minimize activities and procedures, and help him with activities of daily living. Use his oxygen saturation levels to evaluate the effects of activity on his respiratory status.
- Continue to provide emotional support.

FOLLOW-UP CARE
- Continue to keep your patient on bed rest until his respiratory status is stable. Then gradually increase his activity level as tolerated, based on oxygen saturation levels.
- Elevate the head of the bed 45 degrees for comfort and to promote optimal lung expansion and aeration.
- Continue to have your patient turn, cough, deep breathe, and use incentive spirometry every 2 hours.
- Monitor the patient's hydration status, intake and output, and daily weight, if appropriate. Encourage the oral intake of fluids.
- Continue to assess and document continuous ECG rhythm; vital signs; level of consciousness; heart, breath, and bowel sounds; and intake and output.
- Continue to monitor daily chest X-rays, blood tests, and ABG values.
- Teach your patient techniques he can use to improve his respiratory function, such as pursed-lip breathing.

SPECIAL CONSIDERATIONS
- Keep in mind that patients with chronic respiratory acidosis have a chronically elevated $PaCO_2$ level. Use the patient's baseline values to determine when an acute episode has resolved. Typically, an elevation of 5 to 10 mm Hg in $PaCO_2$ signals an acute problem.

R

RESPIRATORY ALKALOSIS

When alveolar ventilation increases in the absence of a similar increase in carbon dioxide (CO_2) production, the affected patient may develop an acid-base imbalance called respiratory alkalosis. Hyperventilation causes CO_2 (an acid) to be eliminated (blown off) by the lungs. Partial pressure of arterial carbon dioxide ($PaCO_2$) decreases to less than 35 mm Hg (normal $PaCO_2$ is 35 to 45 mm Hg) and arterial pH increases above 7.45 (normal pH is 7.35 to 7.45).

Respiratory alkalosis may be an acute or a chronic condition. (See *Causes of respiratory alkalosis,* page 316.) Early signs and symptoms of

CAUSES OF RESPIRATORY ALKALOSIS

Respiratory alkalosis can result from various pulmonary or nonpulmonary conditions.

PULMONARY CAUSES

Pulmonary conditions that can lead to respiratory alkalosis include:
- pneumonia
- pulmonary embolus
- pulmonary edema
- fibrotic lung disease
- acute asthma
- conditions that cause hypoxia (such as heart failure)
- excessive mechanical ventilation.

NONPULMONARY CAUSES

Nonpulmonary causes that can lead to respiratory alkalosis include:
- fear, anxiety, panic, and other psychogenic disorders
- pain
- toxicity from drugs that stimulate respiration, such as salicylates and epinephrine
- fever
- gram-negative sepsis
- central nervous system disorders, such as meningitis, encephalitis, and head injury
- damage to the brain's respiratory center (as from trauma, stroke, and tumor)
- chronic hepatic insufficiency
- pregnancy (progesterone increases sensitivity of the brain's respiratory center to carbon dioxide).

acute respiratory alkalosis stem from decreased cerebral blood flow and hyperexcitability of the peripheral and central nervous systems. As a result, the patient may develop life-threatening arrhythmias, hypocalcemic tetany, and seizures. Your expert rapid response could be responsible for saving her life.

WHAT TO LOOK FOR

Because of a compensatory decrease in serum bicarbonate level, which normalizes pH, chronic respiratory alkalosis usually produces no symptoms. Clinical findings in acute alkalosis may include:
- pH over 7.45
- $PaCO_2$ under 35 mm Hg
- decreased serum bicarbonate levels (a compensatory response to chronic alkalosis)
- increased rate and depth of respirations ("blowing off" of CO_2)
- dizziness
- numbness or tingling in the fingers and toes
- muscle weakness and cramping
- tetany
- syncope
- arrhythmias
- palpitations
- diaphoresis
- dyspnea
- feelings of anxiety, fear, or panic
- tetany, seizures, and apnea (with severe alkalosis).

WHAT TO DO IMMEDIATELY

If your patient develops respiratory alkalosis, notify the physician and follow these measures:

- If the patient is hyperventilating, have her breathe slowly and steadily into a paper bag, if appropriate. Breathing her own expired CO_2 will raise her $PaCO_2$ level and slow her respirations.
- Position the patient to prevent injury and maximize lung expansion. Have her sit in a chair or lie in semi-Fowler's or high Fowler's position.
- Stay with the patient and offer support and guidance. Keep the patient and her environment as calm and quiet as possible.
- Assess the patient's vital signs, level of consciousness, and cardiopulmonary status. Auscultate her lungs for adventitious sounds.
- Obtain immediate arterial blood gas (ABG) measurements to establish a baseline and assess future changes. (See *Interpreting ABG values*, page 253.)
- Assess oxygen saturation levels continuously by way of pulse oximetry, and administer supplemental oxygen, as indicated.
- Use a nonrebreather mask or reservoir mask to increase the $PaCO_2$ level.
- Begin continuous cardiac monitoring, and assess for changes that suggest ischemia or hypoxemia.
- Repeatedly assess level of consciousness for changes that suggest worsening alkalosis. Institute seizure precautions, as indicated.
- Obtain a chest X-ray and blood samples for testing, including a complete blood count and serum electrolyte levels.
- Monitor for signs that the patient is tiring, including weaker respirations, increasing sleepiness, seizures, and, possibly, respiratory arrest. Anticipate endotracheal intubation and mechanical ventilation.
- Monitor the patient's laboratory results and report all abnormal values.
- ➡ **NurseALERT** Watch serum potassium levels closely because as alkalosis resolves, potassium levels may increase, causing hyperkalemia.
- If the patient has an anxiety-related disorder, give sedatives or tranquilizers, as prescribed.

WHAT TO DO NEXT

Once your patient has stabilized, take these steps:

- Provide emotional support to decrease anxiety, fear, and panic. Continue to keep the environment calm and quiet.
- Maintain the patient in high Fowler's position to facilitate gas exchange.
- Continue to assess oxygen saturation levels, and give supplemental oxygen by way of mask or nasal cannula. Assess and document the patient's vital signs; mental status; heart, breath, and bowel sounds; and urine output.
- Repeatedly monitor for progression of alkalosis by checking for dizziness, palpitations, tetany, and seizures.

R

- Follow the patient's serial ABG values, and monitor for hypoxemia and worsening acid-base disturbances.
- Continue to administer sedatives or tranquilizers, if prescribed.
- Institute safety precautions and maintain bed rest if the patient has weakness, dizziness, or syncope.

FOLLOW-UP CARE
- Continue to limit your patient to bed rest until her respiratory status is stable. Gradually increase her activity as tolerated, using oxygen saturation levels as a guide.
- Elevate the head of the bed to 45 degrees for comfort and to promote optimal lung expansion and aeration.
- Continue to assess and document vital signs; mental status; heart, breath, and bowel sounds; and urine output. Note any significant changes.
- Continue to provide emotional support.
- Monitor laboratory tests, including serial ABG values. Report all abnormal values.
- With the patient, try to identify factors that could have precipitated the episode. Teach the patient how to identify possible triggers and warning signs of hyperventilation. Teach her relaxation techniques to decrease anxiety, and help her identify positive coping behaviors.
- Help her learn to counteract hyperventilation with controlled breathing and CO_2 rebreathing. Have the patient simulate breathing into a paper bag to learn rebreathing.

SPECIAL CONSIDERATIONS
- Keep in mind that one of the most common causes of respiratory alkalosis is hyperventilation in response to anxiety, fear, or panic. Suspect respiratory alkalosis in anxious or agitated patients who complain of such seemingly vague symptoms as tingling, numbness, and dizziness in the absence of other physiologic disorders.

RESPIRATORY ARREST

A patient in respiratory arrest is not breathing, and his heart may or may not be beating. This condition can arise for a number of reasons. (See *Causes of respiratory arrest*.) No matter what the cause, respiratory arrest requires emergency intervention because it can rapidly progress to full cardiac arrest. Your prompt and targeted actions will help prevent permanent injury to your patient, including cardiac arrest and, possibly, death.

WHAT TO LOOK FOR
Your patient may have distinctive clinical findings both before and after respiratory arrest.

CAUSES OF RESPIRATORY ARREST

Although many disorders can lead to respiratory arrest, they represent just four major mechanisms.

OBSTRUCTED AIR MOVEMENT
When air can't move through the respiratory system, gas exchange can't take place and respiratory arrest may ensue. Causes of obstructed air movement include:
- airway obstruction
- acute exacerbation of chronic airway disease
- status asthmaticus.

DEPRESSED RESPIRATORY CENTER
When the brain's respiratory center becomes severely depressed, it stops sending impulses that control respiratory muscles, and pulmonary function ceases. Causes of depressed respiratory center include:
- suppression from narcotics or other drugs
- head injury involving the brain stem
- lesion involving the brain stem.

INADEQUATE BLOOD FLOW
When blood stops flowing to the brain, respirations cease within seconds. (In contrast, the heart can beat for several minutes after respirations cease.) Causes of inadequate blood flow in respiratory arrest include:
- shock
- cardiac arrest
- drowning or near drowning
- electrical shock
- suffocation.

IMPAIRED OR DAMAGED RESPIRATORY STRUCTURES OR MUSCULATURE
When pulmonary structures are damaged or the muscles of respiration can no longer function, the patient may stop breathing. Causes of impaired or damaged respiratory structures or muscles include:
- chest trauma
- inhalation of fire or smoke
- effects of myasthenia gravis, Guillain-Barré syndrome.

Before arrest
Clinical findings just before respiratory arrest may include:
- a feeling of impending doom
- restlessness, anxiety
- tachypnea
- dyspnea
- use of accessory muscles for breathing
- nasal flaring during inspiration (a sign of respiratory distress)
- uncoordinated or paradoxical breathing patterns
- audible wheezing
- stridor
- cessation of previously audible breath sounds
- altered level of consciousness, including irritability, agitation, disorientation, lethargy, stupor, or coma
- tachycardia
- diaphoresis
- hypertension (acute), deteriorating to hypotension
- cyanosis (distal extremities, lips, mucous membranes).

After arrest
Clinical findings after respiratory arrest may include:
- no respiratory effort
- no air movement from mouth or nose
- generalized cyanosis

R

- unresponsiveness
- lack of palpable carotid pulse
- lack of audible or palpable blood pressure
- arrhythmias, including ventricular tachycardia, ventricular fibrillation, asystole, or pulseless electrical activity.

WHAT TO DO IMMEDIATELY

If your patient is in respiratory arrest, activate your facility's emergency system, have a colleague notify the physician, and begin cardiopulmonary resuscitation (CPR) according to the American Heart Association guidelines:

- Open the patient's airway using the head-tilt, chin-lift maneuver. Quickly remove any foreign matter or vomitus visible in his mouth.
- Assess his breathing. Look for rising and falling of his chest and air movement from his mouth or nose.
- ➡ **NurseALERT** If you cannot detect breathing, begin rescue ventilations with a pocket face mask. Give two ventilations over 2 to 4 seconds, making sure you maintain the proper head tilt so that each breath can be exhaled. If you can't ventilate the patient, his airway may still be obstructed. Reposition his head and try to ventilate again. If you still can't ventilate him, administer an abdominal thrust (the Heimlich maneuver) followed by a finger sweep. Then ventilate again.
- Check for a carotid pulse on the side closer to you for 5 to 10 seconds. If you find it, begin giving breaths at a rate of 12 times/minute. If you don't find it, begin external chest compressions at a rate of 15 compressions for every two breaths if you're performing CPR alone or 5 compressions for every breath if someone is helping you with CPR.
- After four cycles of compressions and breaths (or after 1 minute if someone is helping you), stop and check to see if the patient's spontaneous respirations have returned and palpate for the presence of a carotid pulse. If present, stop CPR and monitor the patient closely. If not, continue CPR and check again every few minutes.

Additional steps

While you're performing CPR, have team members do the following:

- Place the patient on continuous cardiac monitoring to evaluate the rhythm and check for arrhythmias. Prepare for possible defibrillation.
- Establish I.V. access if a line isn't already in place. Keep in mind that you may need more than one access site. Give fluids and medications, as ordered.
- ➡ **NurseALERT** If the patient doesn't already have I.V. access, establish a peripheral line rather than a central line; although a peripheral line provides lower peak drug levels and increased circulation time, it allows you to continue CPR uninterrupted.
- Insert or assist with insertion of a nasogastric or orogastic tube to prevent aspiration of gastric contents and aid in gastric decompression.
- ➡ **NurseALERT** Without a nasogastric tube in place, artificial respirations can fill the stomach with air and distend the abdomen, hampering

continued respirations.
- Document the therapy given and the patient's responses to it.
- Prepare for possible endotracheal intubation and mechanical ventilation.
- After intubation, assess for bilateral breath sounds.
- Obtain a chest X-ray to verify endotracheal tube position. Also obtain arterial blood gas (ABG) values to evaluate pulmonary status.
- Prepare your patient for transfer to the intensive care unit.

WHAT TO DO NEXT
Once your patient has stabilized, take these steps:
- Continuously assess his cardiopulmonary status. Monitor vital signs and oxygen saturation by way of pulse oximetry and ABG values. Continue supplemental oxygen, as indicated. Maintain continuous cardiac monitoring, looking for ischemic and hypoxemic changes. Treat arrhythmias according to advanced cardiac life support guidelines.
- If spontaneous respirations and circulation do not occur after initial drug administration, prepare for insertion of a central venous line to evaluate hemodynamic parameters and administer medication.
- Give bronchodilators to dilate smooth muscles of the large airways. Suction as needed to remove secretions.
- Support the family, and prepare them to see the patient by describing changes in the patient's appearance, the endotracheal tube, the mechanical ventilator, and other invasive equipment. Provide emotional support to decrease their fear and anxiety.

FOLLOW-UP CARE
- Determine the underlying cause of the patient's respiratory arrest, and take corrective actions, as prescribed, to prevent a recurrence.
- Limit your patient to bed rest until his respiratory status is stable. Continue supplemental oxygen, as indicated. Use oxygen saturation levels to evaluate his activity tolerance.
- Elevate the head of the bed to 45 degrees or more for comfort and to promote optimal lung expansion and aeration.
- Assess your patient at least every 2 hours for bilateral breath sounds, respiratory rate and depth, response to mechanical ventilation, vital signs, pulse oximetry, and mental status. Monitor daily chest X-rays, blood tests, and ABG values for changes.
- Assess and document continuous ECG rhythm; heart, breath, and bowel sounds; and urine output.
- Provide frequent mouth care while the patient is intubated to keep his mucous membranes moist and prevent tissue breakdown. Suction as necessary. As his status improves, prepare for extubation.
- Encourage your patient to sit in a chair as soon as possible to promote alveolar expansion and prevent complications of bed rest.
- Provide emotional support to the patient and significant others to decrease their fear and anxiety.

R

SPECIAL CONSIDERATIONS

- Assess the psychological impact of respiratory arrest on the patient. Some patients vividly recall the resuscitation effort, and most fear a recurrence. Provide support and referrals, as appropriate.
- After resuscitation, watch for possible complications, such as aspiration pneumonia (from vomiting); oral, tracheal, or laryngeal edema (from improper airway placement or repeated attempts at placement); and cervical neck injury (from hyperextension to open the airway). Notify the physician and provide treatment, as prescribed.

RETINAL DETACHMENT

The light-sensitive lining in the back of the eye, the retina consists of 10 layers. In retinal detachment, a portion of the inner sensory layer separates from the outer retinal pigment epithelium. This leads to partial or complete loss of vision in the affected eye—possibly permanently.

Retinal detachment can take one of three main forms:

- *Rhegmatogenous detachment*, the most common form, is associated with a retinal hole or tear that allows vitreous fluid to seep beneath the sensory layer and separate it from the retinal pigment epithelium. Retinal holes or tears may result from traumatic eye injury. Two of every three rhegmatogenous detachments occur among near-sighted people between ages 50 and 60.
- *Tractional detachment* results from vitreous bands or membranes that pull the sensory retina away from the retinal pigment epithelium. Typical causes include proliferative diabetic retinopathy, sickle cell hemoglobinopathy, and retinopathy of prematurity. Tractional detachment also may occur when a foreign body penetrates and tracks through the eye.
- *Exudative detachment*, the rarest form, is marked by the accumulation of subretinal fluid. It develops secondary to an inflammation, such as posterior uveitis; leaking retinal vessels; or such disorders as eclampsia. Other causes include choroidal and retinal tumors.

No matter which type of retinal detachment your patient has, your prompt response could mean the difference between sight and possibly permanent blindness in the affected eye.

WHAT TO LOOK FOR

Clinical findings in retinal detachment may include:

- seeing showers or floating spots
- seeing flashing lights or lightning streaks, possibly even when the eye is closed
- seeing a veil, cloud, curtain, or cobweb over the field of vision
- visual field deficits
- immediate loss of vision when a blood vessel breaks, causing a vitreous hemorrhage.

WHAT TO DO IMMEDIATELY

If you suspect that your patient has a retinal detachment, notify the physician. Then carry out these interventions:

- Anticipate a referral to an ophthalmologist. Keep in mind that some ophthalmologists specialize in retinal problems.
- ➡ **NurseALERT** Don't try to manipulate the patient's eye to see what's causing the problem.
- If you have access to a Snellen visual acuity chart, obtain a baseline assessment of the patient's visual acuity. If you don't have a Snellen chart, shine a flashlight toward the patient's eye from the six cardinal positions of gaze. Have him tell you if the light disappears in any of the positions; if it does, keep in mind that the affected portion of his retina is inverted from the position where the light disappears.
- If the patient can't see in the lower nasal quadrant, have him lie down to stop subretinal fluid from flowing downward into the macular area. Such vision loss suggests that his macula (the retinal area responsible for central vision and sharp focus) is at risk. Remember that a detached macula may lead to permanent loss of acute vision.
- If the patient can't see in the upper nasal quadrant of the visual field, gravity will cause subretinal fluid to settle. Have him sit up to keep the fluid in a dependent position.

WHAT TO DO NEXT

Once retinal detachment is confirmed, take these steps:

- Prepare the patient for surgical correction by an ophthalmologist. (See *Repairing a detached retina,* page 324.)
- Before surgery, dilate the patient's pupil fully by instilling cycloplegic drops (typically, tropicamide 1% [Mydriacyl], cyclopentolate 1% [Cyclogyl], and phenylephrine 2.5% [Neo-Synephrine]), as prescribed.

FOLLOW-UP CARE

After surgery to correct retinal detachment, follow these guidelines:

- Instill prescribed eyedrops (a cycloplegic, a steroid-antibiotic combination) two to four times daily (or possibly more), as prescribed.
- Make sure the patient understands and follows the surgeon's instructions to lie in a particular position. If the surgeon placed gas or silicone oil in the eye to hold the retina in place, the patient may need to lie face-down or facing right or left, maintaining the position for 1 to 4 weeks.
- Apply cold compresses four times daily to ease ocular swelling and pain.
- ➡ **NurseALERT** Avoid commercial cold packs because they could leak into the eye.
- Assess the patient's pain carefully. For persistent pain unrelieved by pain medication, notify the physician in case the intraocular pressure is elevated. Give acetaminophen, 650 mg (two tablets every 4 hours), or acetaminophen with codeine #3 (one tablet every 4 to 6 hours), as prescribed.

R

REPAIRING A DETACHED RETINA

Techniques used to repair a detached retina include scleral buckling, vitrectomy, and cryopexy. No matter which procedure your patient undergoes, you'll need to prepare him for it both physically and psychologically. Above all, make sure he understands the importance of maintaining a specific position after surgery if the physician requests it.

SCLERAL BUCKLING

If the ophthalmologist suspects macular involvement, expect the patient to undergo an immediate surgical procedure called a scleral buckle. In this technique, the surgeon seals the tear with a cryoprobe to scar the retinal and choroidal layers together and then places a silicone patch over the area. Finally, he places a band around the outside of the eye and tightens it enough to buckle the sclera inward, as shown in the illustration. The inward buckle prevents vitreous traction on the retina.

VITRECTOMY

If the detachment resulted from a giant tear or from vitreous bands and membranes, the surgeon may perform a vitrectomy, removing the vitreous and replacing it with saline solution. Occasionally, gas or silicone oil may be used to tamponade the retina.

CRYOPEXY

In less severe cases, the surgeon may repair a retinal hole or tear by cryopexy. In this procedure, a coolant is circulated through a metal probe called a cryoprobe. The moist retinal tissue adheres to the cold metal of the probe and freezes; cells are destroyed, their membranes burst, and scar tissue forms over the hole in the retina, sealing it.

Scleral buckling

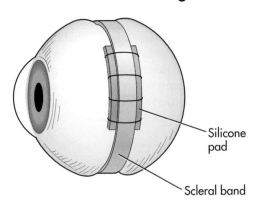

Silicone pad

Scleral band

- Prepare to implement treatments to correct the underlying cause of exudative detachment. For example, with posterior uveitis, expect to administer anti-inflammatory agents. If the detachment stemmed from a tumor, radioactive plaque therapy or even surgical eye removal may be indicated.

SPECIAL CONSIDERATIONS

- Warn the patient not to drive, bend over, or lift heavy objects immediately after surgery. Describe signs and symptoms of increased intraocular pressure, such as pain and visual changes, and instruct the patient to notify the physician immediately if they occur.
- Encourage the patient to comply with follow-up medical visits.
- If gas was applied to the eye, advise the patient not to fly in an airplane until the gas is absorbed because gas molecules expand at high altitudes.
- Instruct the patient to protect the affected eye by wearing a shield at night and eyeglasses during the day to avoid bumping the eye while it's healing.

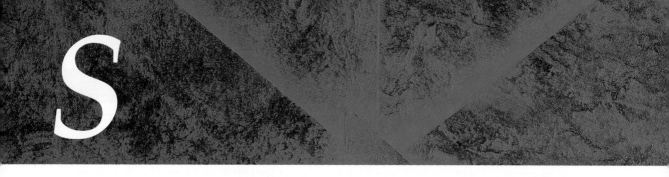

S_3 AND S_4 HEART SOUNDS

As you know, cardiac function is reflected in a series of sounds you can hear by auscultating your patient's chest. If the heart is functioning normally, you'll hear two major sounds, called S_1 and S_2. If it's not functioning normally, you may hear more than two heart sounds. In fact, you might hear up to two extra heart sounds, called S_3 and S_4. (See *Assessing extra heart sounds*, page 326.)

S_3

Produced by the vibration of valves and supporting structures, S_3 results from a large volume of blood flowing quickly into the ventricles during diastole. This sound is normal in children, young adults, and women in the third trimester of pregnancy; in these cases, it's called a physiologic third heart sound. If you hear an S_3 heart sound in other adult patients, it's called a ventricular gallop. Usually, it signals such disorders as mitral or tricuspid insufficiency, hyperthyroidism, volume overload, hypertension, and anemia. It also may signal early decompensation in heart failure, ventricular septal defect, and papillary muscle rupture.

S_4

Also called an atrial gallop, S_4 occurs when the atria contract to force blood into a noncompliant, stiff ventricle. It may be a normal finding in pregnant women, athletes, and older adults. In most other adults, an S_4 heart sound signals underlying pathology, such as aortic or pulmonic stenosis, hypertension, myocardial infarction (MI), pulmonary hypertension, coronary artery disease, and cardiomyopathy.

WHAT TO LOOK FOR

Clinical findings for a patient with S_3 or S_4 heart sounds vary widely, depending on what's causing the sounds.

Heart failure

If the patient has heart failure, clinical findings may include:
- crackles
- orthopnea

S

ASSESSING EXTRA HEART SOUNDS

Auscultating heart sounds is a crucial aspect of a complete cardiovascular assessment. Not only must you be able to identify normal heart sounds (S_1 and S_2), but you also must be able to detect extra sounds (S_3 and S_4) that may provide early warning of potentially serious heart problems.

S_3 and S_4 are commonly called gallops because they sound something like a galloping horse. When S_3 and S_4 occur too close together to be heard as separate sounds, they're called a summation gallop.

Use these guidelines to help assess S_3 and S_4 heart sounds accurately.

- Have the patient lie on his back, and use the diaphragm of your stethoscope to locate the high-pitched S_1 and S_2 heart sounds. Listen in all the locations (see illustration below at left). Then palpate the carotid artery while you listen in the tricuspid and mitral areas, where you'll hear S_1 and S_2 most clearly. Because the carotid pulsation occurs almost simultaneously with S_1, palpating the carotid pulse is a good way to distinguish S_1 from other heart sounds.

- Listen to S_1 and S_2 until you can recognize their sounds, and then switch to the bell of your stethoscope. Press lightly against the skin to hear the low-pitched S_3 and S_4 sounds (see illustration below at right).

- Generally, if the sound is coming from the *left* ventricle, you'll hear S_3 loudest over the heart's apex, at the fourth or fifth intercostal space, left midclavicular line. If the sound results from a rush of blood into the *right* ventricle, you'll hear S_3 best at the lower left sternal border during inspiration, with the patient lying on his left side. S_3 occurs early in diastole, just after S_2. The sequence S_1-S_2-S_3 sounds like *lub-dubb-dee* and has a cadence like the word *ken-tuc-key*.

- Typically, if your patient's S_4 is produced by the *left* atrium, you'll hear it best over the apex during expiration, with your patient lying on his left side. While not as common, an S_4 that originates in the *right* atrium is heard best at the lower left sternal border during inspiration, with your patient lying on his back. S_4 occurs late in diastole, just before S_1. The sequence S_4-S_1-S_2 sounds like *te-lub-dubb* and has a cadence like the word *ten-ne-see*.

Heart sound locations

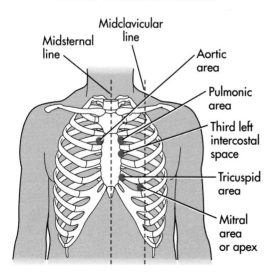

Visualizing heart sounds

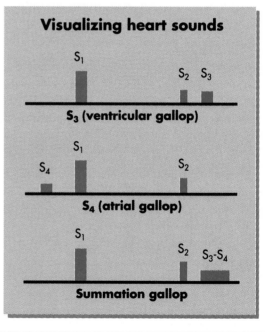

- dyspnea
- peripheral edema
- S$_3$ heart sound
- S$_4$ heart sound.

MI

If the patient has an acute MI, clinical findings may include:
- severe chest pain
- ST-segment and T-wave changes on the ECG
- anxiety
- diaphoresis
- S$_3$ heart sound (with left-sided heart failure)
- S$_4$ heart sound.

Papillary muscle rupture

If the patient has a papillary muscle rupture (a potential complication of an inferior-wall MI), clinical findings may include:
- abrupt onset of a loud holosystolic murmur
- signs of left-sided heart failure, such as crackles and dyspnea
- S$_3$ heart sound
- S$_4$ heart sound.

Hyperthyroidism

If the patient has hyperthyroidism, clinical findings may include:
- tachycardia
- bounding pulses
- tremors
- tachypnea
- S$_3$ heart sound.

Aortic stenosis

If the patient has aortic stenosis, clinical findings may include:
- crescendo-decrescendo systolic murmur
- signs of heart failure, such as dyspnea, orthopnea, and crackles in lung bases
- exertional syncope
- angina
- prominent S$_4$ heart sound.

WHAT TO DO IMMEDIATELY

If you hear new S$_3$ or S$_4$ heart sounds, notify the physician and follow these measures:
- Describe the extra heart sound as fully as you can, including whether it's louder with the bell or the diaphragm of your stethoscope, where you heard it best, the patient position in which you heard it best, and whether it was louder on inspiration or expiration.

S

- Perform a complete cardiovascular assessment, including vital signs, peripheral pulses, capillary refill, skin color and temperature, jugular vein distention, urine output, and level of consciousness. Listen for murmurs of aortic, mitral, and tricuspid regurgitation. Auscultate the patient's lungs for adventitious sounds that accompany heart failure, such as crackles.
- Question your patient about such symptoms as shortness of breath, fatigue, chest pain, weight gain, and activity intolerance.
- Obtain laboratory studies and a 12-lead ECG, as ordered.
- ➡ **NurseALERT** If you see ST-segment and T-wave changes on the ECG, the S$_3$ or S$_4$ sounds you heard probably stem from an MI. If you detect atrial fibrillation and supraventricular tachycardia, the S$_3$ sounds you heard may result from hyperthyroidism.

WHAT TO DO NEXT

Once the patient's abnormal heart sounds have been confirmed, carry out these actions:
- Monitor laboratory results to help detect the underlying cause of the extra heart sound. For example, elevated triiodothyronine (T$_3$) or thyroxine levels, increased T$_3$ resin uptake, and reduced thyroid-stimulating hormone levels may point to hyperthyroidism. Reduced serum hemoglobin level and hematocrit may suggest anemia as the cause of your patient's S$_3$ heart sound.
- Prepare to treat the underlying cause of the S$_3$ or S$_4$ sounds, if possible. For example, treat heart failure with inotropic agents, vasodilators, diuretics, and supplemental oxygen, as ordered. Papillary muscle dysfunction may require afterload reduction with nitroprusside sodium (Nitropress) or intra-aortic balloon counterpulsation therapy.
- After treating the underlying cause, continue to monitor your patient's heart sounds. With successful treatment, they may disappear.
- Perform ongoing assessments of your patient's cardiovascular status to track the effect of treatment on his heart sounds and general condition.

FOLLOW-UP CARE

- Continue to listen for S$_3$ and S$_4$ heart sounds and to assess for signs and symptoms of cardiac decompensation. Notify the physician if they recur.
- Explain the cause of the extra heart sounds to your patient. Make sure he understands the importance of treating the underlying cause—for example, taking antithyroid drugs for hyperthyroidism.
- Discuss with your patient the medications he'll be taking at home, including their names, indications, doses, frequency, and adverse effects.
- Tell the patient what to report to his physician, including shortness of breath, chest pain, and activity intolerance (which may suggest heart failure).

SPECIAL CONSIDERATIONS

- If you hear an S_3 or S_4 heart sound, look at the whole clinical picture before concluding that the extra sound has a pathologic cause. Questioning your young adult patient may reveal that he's an athlete, in which case his S_4 is probably normal.
- If your patient has atrial fibrillation, you won't be able to hear an S_4 sound because his atria quiver instead of contracting.

SEIZURES

Reflecting sudden, excessive electrical discharge of neurons in the brain, seizures may trigger involuntary muscle contractions, alterations in consciousness, and sensory abnormalities. Seizure disorder, sometimes called *epilepsy*, refers to a condition marked by susceptibility to recurrent seizures.

About half the time, seizures have no known cause. With seizures of new onset, the most common precipitating conditions are brain tumors, arteriovenous malformation, traumatic head injury, central nervous system infection (such as encephalitis), and metabolic disturbances (such as electrolyte or acid-base imbalances).

Seizures may be generalized or partial. In a generalized seizure, the abnormal electrical discharge spreads through the entire brain. Types of generalized seizures include absence, myoclonic, tonic, clonic, generalized tonic-clonic, and atonic seizures.

In a partial seizure, the abnormal electrical discharge remains localized to one brain region. Sometimes a partial seizure spreads to other parts of the brain, becoming generalized. Types of partial seizures include simple and complex seizures.

Most seizures stop on their own within a few seconds or minutes. Until they do, airway obstruction and traumatic injury can threaten the patient's life. *Status epilepticus*, prolonged seizure activity, may impede cardiac function as well as imperil breathing.

Regardless of the type of seizure a patient experiences, your prompt and targeted actions can help him avoid residual effects. Your nursing care also must focus on preventing seizures—and the injuries that can ensue—whenever possible.

S

WHAT TO LOOK FOR

Although some clinical findings are common to seizures in general, many findings vary with the type of seizure the patient experiences. What's more, you may need to question witnesses about signs and symptoms that arose before the patient sought treatment. (See *Questioning a seizure witness*, page 330.)

QUESTIONING A SEIZURE WITNESS

If you didn't witness a seizure yourself, obtain a description of the patient's behavior just before, during, and after it from someone who did witness it—for instance, a family member, friend, or bystander. Ask questions such as the following:

- Did the patient complain of any unusual feelings or sensations just before the seizure occurred?
- What was he doing immediately before the seizure began?
- Which parts of his body were affected by seizure activity first?
- How long did the seizure last?
- Did the patient fall?
- Did he lose consciousness?
- Did he make odd or repetitive muscle movements? If so, describe the movements.

- Which parts of his body were affected by the unusual movements?
- Did he drool from or froth at the mouth?
- Did he make noises?
- Did he stop breathing?
- Did he lose bladder or bowel control?
- After the seizure ended, did he fall asleep? Was he groggy or confused? Did he complain of a headache? Did he have any residual weakness or paralysis? If so, what part of his body was involved and how long did it last?

By obtaining this information, you'll be better able to identify the type of seizure involved, help determine the underlying cause, and guide treatment.

Generalized tonic-clonic seizure (formerly called grand mal seizure)

If the patient experiences a generalized tonic-clonic seizure, clinical findings may include:

- report of an aura (an unusual sensory experience) just before seizure onset
- sustained, generalized muscle contraction with stiffening of the body, arm flexion, leg extension, and, possibly, arching of the back; breathing ceases, and cyanosis may occur (tonic phase)
- violent, repetitive jerking of muscles, which may begin in one part of the body but progresses to involve the entire body (clonic phase)
- loss of consciousness
- bladder and bowel incontinence
- postseizure lethargy, confusion, headache, muscle soreness, speech difficulty, transient paralysis, and paresthesias (postictal phase).

Absence seizure (formerly petit mal seizure)

If the patient experiences an absence seizure, clinical findings may include:

- brief (10 seconds or less) loss of awareness of and response to surroundings without loss of consciousness
- staring spells (person stares blankly into space, momentarily stopping all activity)
- eyelid flickering and jerking hand movements
- typically affects children
- recurrence possible many times a day.

Tonic seizure

If the patient experiences a tonic seizure, clinical findings may include:
- sudden increase in muscle tone in face and trunk, resulting in stiffening of face, neck, and jaw
- sustained generalized muscle contraction, with stiffening of extremities as well as face and neck, resulting in dystonic posturing (writhing and twisting of the body)
- sustained deviation of the eyes and head to one side
- brief (several seconds to minutes) loss of consciousness.

Clonic seizure

If the patient experiences a clonic seizure, clinical findings may include:
- repetitive, jerking contraction and relaxation of muscles that affect the arms, legs, or trunk
- brief (several seconds to minutes) loss of consciousness.

Myoclonic seizure

If the patient experiences a myoclonic seizure, clinical findings may include:
- brief, sudden muscle contractions that affect the arms, legs, or trunk that may be unilateral or bilateral
- very brief loss of consciousness (so short may not be noted).

Atonic seizure

If the patient experiences an atonic seizure, clinical findings may include:
- sudden loss of muscle tone
- brief alteration in level of consciousness
- brief duration (seizure lasts only a few seconds).

Simple partial seizure

If the patient experiences a simple partial seizure, clinical findings may include:
- *With motor partial seizures*: repetitive, jerking movements that involve one part of the body, such as an arm, a leg, or one side of the face
- *With sensory partial seizures:* abnormal sensory perception, such as an unusual tactile sensation (tingling, burning, paresthesias), smell (of burning, rotten eggs), or sound
- *With autonomic partial seizures:* flushing, pallor, tachycardia, elevated blood pressure, diaphoresis, nausea, vomiting, dilated pupils, and sudden incontinence
- *With psychic partial seizures*: sensory changes, such as hallucinations, anger, and feelings of déjà vu.

Complex partial seizure

If the patient experiences a complex partial seizure, clinical findings may include:

S

- automatisms (involuntary, repetitive, purposeless movements, such as lip smacking and hand wringing)
- facial grimaces or chewing movements
- altered level of consciousness or thought process
- speech disturbance (slurred speech, dysphasia) or nonverbal vocalizations (grunting, crying, shouting)
- postseizure amnesia
- loss of awareness of surroundings without loss of consciousness.

WHAT TO DO IMMEDIATELY

During a seizure, focus your interventions on maintaining a patent airway and preventing injury to the patient and others. Take the following measures:

- Move furniture and other objects away from the patient so he won't hurt herself.
- If possible, slip a blanket or towel under his head to prevent head trauma.
- If he's in bed, raise the side rails and remove the pillow.
- ➡ Nurse**ALERT** Don't try to restrain the patient—you're likely to injure him and, possibly, yourself in the process.
- Turn the patient to one side (if possible) so his tongue won't obstruct his airway.
- ➡ Nurse**ALERT** Don't try to insert an artificial airway during the seizure. Chances are you won't be able to pry his jaw open, and you may injure the patient or yourself by trying.
- Loosen tight clothing to aid respirations.
- Monitor and evaluate the adequacy of the patient's respirations throughout the seizure. Be prepared to assist with endotracheal intubation after the seizure if he experiences persistent respiratory distress.
- ➡ Nurse**ALERT** Know that during the tonic phase of a generalized tonic-clonic seizure, the patient's respirations temporarily cease and he may become cyanotic. Breathing should resume spontaneously when the tonic phase ends.
- To halt status epilepticus, expect to administer prescribed anticonvulsant medications. (See *Responding to status epilepticus.*)

WHAT TO DO NEXT

Once the seizure ends, follow these guidelines:

- Ensure a patent airway; if needed, suction oral secretions and insert an oral airway.
- Check the patient's pulse and respiratory rates and blood pressure. Evaluate his level of consciousness.
- If necessary, help him back to bed. To protect him from aspirating secretions, raise the head of the bed about 30 degrees.
- Assess him for obvious injuries, such as bruises and lacerations. Be sure to check his lips, mouth, cheeks, and tongue.

TREATMENT OF CHOICE

RESPONDING TO STATUS EPILEPTICUS

Most common in people with poorly controlled seizure disorders, status epilepticus is either a seizure that lasts at least 15 minutes or a continuous series of seizures with no return to consciousness in between. This patient needs immediate intervention to avoid anoxia, arrhythmias, brain damage, and death. Expect to take the following actions.

- Insert an I.V. line if one isn't already in place. Keep in mind that two I.V. lines are preferred, with one of the two running an infusion of normal saline solution.
- When the cause of a generalized seizure is not immediately apparent (such as in an adult with no history of seizures and no obvious injury or illness), the physician may first order I.V. administration of 20 to 50 ml of dextrose 50% in water.
- Next, anticipate giving diazepam (Valium), 5 to 20 mg I.V. at a rate of 2 mg/minute, as prescribed.
- The physician may also prescribe a loading dose of phenytoin (Dilantin), 10 to 15 mg/kg I.V., up to a total of 1,000 to 1,500 mg. Administer phenytoin at a rate not exceeding 50 mg/minute. Too-rapid administration can cause bradycardia.
- Remember that phenytoin is incompatible with glucose I.V. solutions. A heavy white precipitate will form on contact. Use only normal saline solution.
- As an alternative to phenytoin, the physician may prescribe fosphenytoin (Cerebyx), a new prodrug formulation of phenytoin. Fosphenytoin has several advantages over phenytoin, including compatibility with most I.V. solutions (including glucose solutions) and a less alkaline pH (which decreases the risk of phlebitis), and it can be administered intramuscularly if I.V. access can't be established.
- If phenytoin or fosphenytoin fails to halt the seizure, expect to give phenobarbital (Luminal), 3 to 20 mg/kg I.V., to a total dose of 700 mg.
- During drug therapy, monitor the patient closely for respiratory depression and other adverse effects.

- Help reorient the patient. Keep in mind that many patients seem confused or disoriented for a short time immediately after a seizure.
- Maintain a calm environment to minimize stimulation.
- If not already in place, institute seizure precautions according to your facility's policy.

FOLLOW-UP CARE

- Check the patient's level of consciousness frequently.
- Stay alert for signs and symptoms of impending seizure recurrence, such as a report of an aura.
- Administer anticonvulsants, as prescribed; monitor serum drug levels to evaluate therapeutic effectiveness and prevent toxicity.
- Review the patient's history for clues to the cause of the seizure, such as fluid and electrolyte imbalances, drug toxicity, hypoxemia, infection, and hemorrhage.
- Prepare your patient for diagnostic tests, such as magnetic resonance imaging and electroencephalography, as ordered.
- Reassure the patient that he'll be monitored closely for further seizures and protected from injury.

SPECIAL CONSIDERATIONS

- Make sure the patient has I.V. access so that anticonvulsant drugs can be administered if another seizure occurs.
- Keep oxygen and suction equipment within easy access, and tape an oral airway to the patient's bedside for use after a seizure, if one should occur.

S

- To prevent injury if a seizure should occur, don't use a glass thermometer when checking a patient's temperature.
- Keep the side rails up and padded, and keep the bed in the lowest position to avoid injury in case of another seizure.
- Make sure you keep the bed, wheelchair, or stretcher brakes in the locked position.
- Place the patient's call button within easy reach.
- Instruct the patient to call for help immediately and to sit down if he experiences an aura.
- Instruct the patient with a seizure disorder to obtain a medical alert bracelet or other identification and to keep it with him at all times.

SEPTIC SHOCK

When a microorganism invades the body and enters the bloodstream, it triggers a systemic inflammatory response and the patient develops a condition called sepsis. If the infection continues unabated, sepsis may progress to a life-threatening condition known as septic shock. Here's what happens.

A number of microorganisms can cause sepsis, the most common being gram-negative bacteria. (See *Causes of sepsis*.) Endotoxins, which are released from the invading organism as it is broken down, and chemical mediators, which are released by the body's immune system in response to infection and inflammation, cause massive vasodilation, selective vasoconstriction, increased capillary permeability, and decreased vascular resistance. Consequently, the patient experiences massive fluid shifts and profound hypovolemia and hypotension.

The chemical mediators also increase the adherence of granulocytes to blood vessels, stimulate the movement of white blood cells (WBCs) to sites of tissue injury and infecton, produce oxygen-free radicals to kill bacteria, and cause fever. Certain mediators also cause myocardial depression, decrease perfusion of some organs, and contribute to the patient's hemodynamic instability.

Septic shock is a common cause of mortality in the intensive care unit. In fact, despite medical advances, the mortality rate for patients with sepsis and septic shock has increased in recent years, possibly due in part to the increasing number of chronically ill and immunocompromised patients living for longer periods.

If you suspect that your patient has developed septic shock, you'll need to take quick action to save her life.

WHAT TO LOOK FOR

Clinical findings for a patient in septic shock may include:
- tachycardia (more than 90 beats/minute)
- increased or decreased temperature (greater than 100.4° F [38° C] or less than 96.8° F [36° C])

CAUSES OF SEPSIS

Causes of sepsis include the following:
- gram-negative bacteria, including *Escherichia coli*, *Klebsiella*, *Pseudomonas aeruginosa*, *Enterobacter*, *Serratia*, and *Proteus*
- gram-positive bacteria, including both alpha and beta hemolytic streptococci , and *Pneumococcus*
- viruses
- fungi
- yeast
- protozoa
- mycobacteria
- rickettsia.

- tachypnea (more than 20 breaths/minute)
- initially, respiratory alkalosis ($PaCO_2$ less than 35 mm Hg; pH above 7.45)
- leukocytosis or leukopenia (WBCs greater than 12,000/mm^3 or less than 4,000/mm^3)
- hypotension (systolic blood pressure less than 90 mm Hg or 40 mm Hg below baseline)
- changes in level of consciousness, including confusion (early sign) and stupor or coma (late sign)
- decreased urine output
- renal failure, evidenced by rising blood urea nitrogen (BUN) and serum creatinine levels
- bounding pulses
- high cardiac output (above 8 L/minute)
- low systemic vascular resistance (less than 800 dynes/sec/cm^{-5})
- decreased left ventricular ejection fraction (less than 50%)
- delayed capillary refill
- diaphoresis, flushed appearance, warm skin
- metabolic acidosis (pH below 7.35) with a base deficit of less than 22 mEq/L
- elevated serum lactate levels
- hyperglycemia
- prolonged prothrombin time (PT), activated partial thromboplastin time (APTT), and bleeding times.

WHAT TO DO IMMEDIATELY

If you suspect that your patient is developing septic shock, notify the physician and follow these measures:

- Assess her level of consciousness, vital signs, and cardiopulmonary status to establish a baseline, and then repeat every 15 minutes to detect changes. Anticipate insertion of an arterial line to monitor blood pressure directly.
- Establish I.V. access with one or two large-bore lines, if the patient doesn't already have them in place. Administer crystalloids (such as lactated Ringer's injection or normal saline solution) and colloids (such as albumin) as required to restore fluid volume. Anticipate blood transfusions to increase serum hemoglobin level and hematocrit and improve tissue perfusion.
- Begin to keep a meticulous record of the patient's intake and output. Insert an indwelling urinary catheter, as ordered, and monitor urine output hourly.
- Assess the patient's oxygen saturation levels by way of continuous pulse oximetry, and evaluate serial arterial blood gas (ABG) results to detect hypoxemia and acidosis (which affect myocardial contractility and may precipitate arrhythmias). Give supplemental oxygen, as indicated.
- ➡ Nurse**ALERT** Be aware that decreasing oxygen saturation may indicate a worsening of tissue perfusion and the onset of pulmonary dysfunc-

S

tion. Be prepared for endotracheal intubation and mechanical ventilation if the patient's respiratory status deteriorates.
- Obtain serial chest X-rays, as ordered, and use them to monitor the patient's pulmonary status.
- Assist with insertion of a pulmonary artery or central venous catheter to evaluate the patient's hemodynamic status. Assess her hemodynamic parameters—including mean arterial pressure (MAP)—at least every hour.

➡️ **Nurse ALERT** Know that an MAP that's under 60 mm Hg adversely affects cerebral and renal perfusion.

- Begin continuous cardiac monitoring and watch for ischemic changes and arrhythmias.
- Insert or assist with insertion of a nasogastric tube, if indicated; connect it to low intermittent suction for gastric decompression and to prevent aspiration.
- Obtain samples of blood, urine, and sputum for culture and antibiotic sensitivity testing. Obtain a complete blood count, as ordered, including a differential WBC count.
- Check the patient's serum hemoglobin level and hematocrit for evidence of her red blood cells' ability to carry oxygen. Assess BUN and serum creatinine and electrolyte levels to evaluate renal function.
- Give I.V. antibiotics or antifungal medications, as ordered.
- Anticipate giving inotropic drugs, such as dobutamine (Dobutrex) or dopamine (Intropin). Assess fluid therapy and hemodynamic parameters closely. Use I.V. infusion pumps, as indicated, to ensure accuracy of medication dosages and fluid volumes administered.

WHAT TO DO NEXT

Once the patient has stabilized, take these actions:
- Continue to monitor her vital signs, level of consciousness, cardiopulmonary status, and hemodynamic status at least hourly. Look for trends. Auscultate the patient's lungs for adventitious breath sounds, which may indicate pulmonary congestion. Also watch to see if she uses accessory muscles to breathe.
- Give vasoactive or inotropic medications, as needed, to maintain blood pressure. Monitor I.V. fluid replacement therapy, and give blood or blood products, as needed.
- Evaluate her ECG for ischemic changes and arrhythmias. Treat as ordered and necessary.
- Monitor her WBC count, ABG values, hematocrit, and serum electrolyte and hemoglobin levels. Also check for elevated levels of serum creatinine and liver enzymes, elevated BUN levels, and prolonged PT and APTT, which may indicate renal and hepatic dysfuntion.
- If the patient needed endotracheal intubation and mechanical ventilation, continue meticulous respiratory care. Prepare the patient for possible neuromuscular blockage to reduce oxygen consumption and improve ventilation.

- Regulate the patient's environment to maintain her body temperature between 97.7° and 100.4° F (36.5° and 38° C). Add extra linens or blankets if she has hypothermia; remove linens or apply tepid sponge baths or a hypothermia blanket if she has hyperthermia.
- Continue measures aimed at minimizing oxygen demands, such as decreasing anxiety, fever, shivering, and pain.
- Provide emotional support and clear, simple explanations to the patient and her family.

FOLLOW-UP CARE
- Provide adequate nutrition; anticipate the need for enteral or parenteral nutrition, as necessary.
- Maintain optimal pulmonary function. For example, position the patient to maximize lung expansion. If she isn't intubated, encourage coughing, deep breathing, and incentive spirometry at least every 2 hours. If she is intubated, suction her as necessary.
- Continue to give antibiotics, antifungals, and antipyretics for fever, as ordered.
- Assess any complications or residual organ dysfunction. For example, watch for multiple organ dysfunction syndrome, which may include acute respiratory distress syndrome, disseminated intravascular coagulation, and hepatic, GI, or renal problems. Administer treatments, as ordered.

SPECIAL CONSIDERATIONS
- Keep in mind that some patients in septic shock require surgery as part of their treatment to rid the body of potential sources of infection. Procedures commonly performed include closure of a bowel perforation, wound debridement, and drainage of abscesses. Remember that the patient's compromised condition increases the risk of surgical complications; monitor her closely after the procedure.
- A patient with septic shock is highly vulnerable to developing new infections. To prevent additional infections, wash your hands thoroughly and frequently, and use strict aseptic technique when giving wound care or handling invasive equipment, such as I.V. lines, endotracheal tubes, urinary catheters, and intestinal tubes.

S

SICKLE CELL CRISIS

An inherited autosomal hemolytic disease that primarily affects people of African descent, sickle cell anemia is characterized by an abnormal form of hemoglobin called hemoglobin S. Because of amino acid changes that render hemoglobin S different from the normal hemoglobin A, the affected person's red blood cells (RBCs) change from a round to a sickled shape in the presence of hypoxia. (See *Looking at a sickled cell*, page 338.)

PATHOPHYSIOLOGY

LOOKING AT A SICKLED CELL

The red blood cells of a person with sickle cell anemia contain an abnormal type of hemoglobin called hemoglobin S instead of the normal hemoglobin A.

This abnormality stems from a change in amino acids: In hemoglobin S, the amino acid valine is substituted for glutamic acid in the chain of the hemoglobin molecule.

In response to low oxygen tension, hemoglobin S molecules crystalize and acquire an inflexible, rodlike shape. This in turn changes the shape of the red blood cell into an elongated sickle, as shown in this illustration.

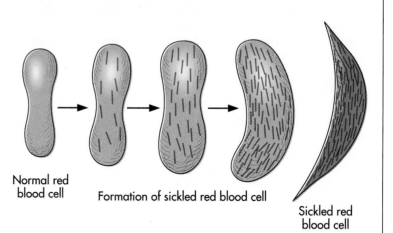

Normal red blood cell

Formation of sickled red blood cell

Sickled red blood cell

Because of the distorted shape and inflexibility of sickled RBCs, the patient is susceptible to a number of problems. Chief among them is the potential for erythrostasis and obstruction of the microvasculature, leading to thrombosis, ischemia, and infarction. In addition, because the life span of sickled RBCs is markedly reduced, the patient is chronically anemic.

Although sickle cell anemia is a chronic disease, you'll know it best in its crisis form because an exacerbation of sickle cell disease that causes severe pain is what brings the patient in for medical care. The average adult with sickle cell anemia has about four crises yearly. They may take several forms:

- vaso-occlusive (thrombotic) crisis, which is the most common type of crisis after age 5
- aplastic crisis (most common type in children)
- hemolytic crisis, which is rare and usually associated with drugs or infection
- acute sequestration crisis, which primarily affects children between ages 8 months and 2 years.

Typically, sickle cell crisis causes considerable pain in addition to potentially ominous clinical changes. Your rapid, expert response to this crisis can improve your patient's outcome in addition to increasing his comfort.

WHAT TO LOOK FOR

Clinical findings in sickle cell anemia vary, depending on whether the disease is in its chronic form and the specific type of crisis involved.

Chronic disease

If a patient has chronic sickle cell anemia, clinical findings may include:

- increased susceptibility to infection
- chronic hemolytic anemia (hemoglobin of 7 to 10 g/dl)
- reticulocyte count of 5% to 15%
- decreased pulmonary function
- history of flow murmurs, heart failure, cardiomegaly, and cor pulmonale
- icterus
- presence of bilirubin gallstones
- hepatomegaly
- splenomegaly (in children)
- presence of bony abnormalities
- hand and foot syndrome (dactylitis, which is painful swelling of hands and feet seen in young children).

Vaso-occlusive crisis

If your patient is in vaso-occlusive crisis, clinical findings may include:

- severe pain in the joints, bones, and muscles (usually worse in the humerus, tibia, femur, and lower back)
- severe abdominal pain of acute onset, diffuse and poorly localized
- pleuritic chest pain
- fever
- leukocytosis
- dyspnea
- headache
- dizziness
- cranial nerve palsies
- vestibular dysfunction
- hearing loss
- coliclike flank pain
- gross or microscopic hematuria
- priapism.

Aplastic crisis

If your patient is in aplastic crisis (an acute reduction in hemoglobin), clinical findings may include:

- pallor
- weakness and lethargy
- dyspnea
- fatigue
- worsening of heart failure
- shock.

Hemolytic crisis

If your patient is in hemolytic crisis, clinical findings may include:

- unexplained fever above 100.4° F (38° C)

S

- symptoms of pneumonia, meningitis, osteomyelitis, or urinary tract infection
- hepatic congestion and hepatomegaly.

Acute sequestration crisis

If your patient is in acute sequestration crisis, clinical findings may include:
- lethargy
- pallor
- cardiovascular collapse.

WHAT TO DO IMMEDIATELY

If you think that your patient is in sickle cell crisis, notify the physician and follow these measures:
- Take his vital signs, especially temperature and pulse rate, to check for evidence of infection and pain.
- Establish I.V. access if the patient doesn't already have a line in place. Begin giving fluids, as prescribed. Use the smallest-gauge I.V. catheter possible, and avoid multiple punctures to minimize the risk of infection. (Some patients need only oral fluids, depending on the level of pain and degree of dehydration.)
- ➡ **NurseALERT** Remember that patients in sickle cell crisis need 6 to 8 L of fluids daily.
- Assess the patient's level of pain, and administer analgesics as quickly as possible, as ordered. Keep in mind that the use of narcotic analgesics may be needed for effective pain relief.
- Assess respiratory status, and monitor the patient's oxygen saturation level by way of pulse oximetry. Obtain arterial blood gas values to monitor oxygenation levels and evaluate acid-base balance. Give supplemental oxygen, if indicated, and elevate the head of the patient's bed to increase lung expansion.
- Anticipate continuous cardiac monitoring, especially if the patient has a history of cardiopulmonary complications.
- Administer antipyretics for fever, as prescribed.
- Obtain laboratory tests, including complete blood count, reticulocyte count, electrolyte panel, liver function tests, erythrocyte sedimentation rate, and urinalysis. Also obtain a chest X-ray, as ordered, to check for possible pneumonia.

WHAT TO NEXT

After the initial crisis has passed and your patient is stabilized, follow these steps, based on the patient's presenting signs and symptoms:
- If the patient had hip pain, prepare him for aspiration and culture of joint fluid, if indicated.
- If he had localized bone tenderness, obtain X-rays, a bone scan, or magnetic resonance imaging, as ordered.
- If he had abdominal pain, prepare him for abdominal ultrasonography or computed tomography (CT).

- If he exhibited neurologic changes, prepare him for CT of the head or a lumbar puncture.
- Continue to administer fluid therapy, as prescribed. Assess the insertion site for signs of infiltration, such as redness and swelling.
- Evaluate the patient's response to analgesics, and switch to a stronger one if needed and ordered.
- Apply warm compresses or pads to painful areas.
- ➡ Nurse**ALERT** Be aware that if the compresses or pads are too hot or too heavy, you could worsen the patient's pain or even burn him. Never apply ice because vasoconstriction would worsen the occlusion and ischemia.
- Assess the patient's fluid balance. Monitor his intake, output, and daily weight for changes.
- Keep the patient on bed rest, and plan frequent rest periods to help prevent fatigue.
- Obtain blood, sputum, and urine samples for culture and sensitivity tests, as needed, for suspected infection. Administer antibiotics for infection, as ordered.
- If the patient has pulmonary compromise, prepare him for a ventilation-perfusion scan, if ordered.

FOLLOW-UP CARE
- Gradually increase the patient's activity level, as tolerated. Pace his activities and procedures, and continue his frequent rest periods.
- Urge him to consume adequate fluids. Continue to monitor his hydration and fluid balance.
- Monitor his vital signs, and stay alert for signs of infection.
- If he still has an I.V. line in place, continue to assess the site for signs of infiltration. Discontinue the I.V. as soon as the patient can take enough fluids orally.

SPECIAL CONSIDERATIONS
- Teach the patient about factors that could contribute to the development of a sickle cell crisis, including dehydration, exposure to extreme temperatures or high altitudes, and bacterial or viral infection. Urge him to seek medical care for increased pain, fever, or any change in symptoms.
- Educate the patient about his illness, and provide him with information about support groups. Offer support and encouragement to the patient and his family.
- Suggest genetic counseling for those patients who would like to have children.
- If your patient is a child, make sure he's been vaccinated against *Streptococcus pneumoniae, Haemophilus influenzae,* and hepatitis B. This is important because infections can precipitate a crisis, and patients with sickle cell anemia are more susceptible to infection. In the past, septicemia was a common cause of death among people with sickle cell disease, particularly children.

S

SPINAL CORD INJURY

Injury to the spinal cord can cause permanent, sometimes profound physical disability. Depending on the type and extent of damage, the patient may be left with partial or complete loss of motor, sensory, and autonomic function in all structures below the level of the injury. (See *Types of spinal cord injury.*)

Each year, more than 10,000 Americans sustain spinal cord injuries; most are men between ages 16 and 30. Most spinal cord injuries result from motor vehicle accidents; recreational accidents (such as diving and football) rank second. Care for patients affected by spinal cord injuries costs more than $10 billion yearly in the United States alone.

A patient with a spinal cord injury requires your immediate, expert response. What's more, he needs comprehensive care as his condition evolves. Keep in mind that a spinal cord injury causes edema and hemorrhage that in turn create hypoxia and necrosis at the site—a process that takes about 48 hours. Plus, the spinal cord may continue to swell for up to 1 week after the injury. You'll need to be ready to respond right away and then continue to give expert care until the extent of your patient's injury becomes clear.

WHAT TO LOOK FOR
Depending on the patient's injury, clinical findings may include:
- flaccid paralysis of skeletal muscles below the level of the injury
- loss of spinal reflexes at the level of the injury (during spinal shock, all reflexes are lost below the level of injury)
- loss of pain, temperature, and touch sensations below the level of the injury
- increased (hyperactive) spinal reflexes below the level of injury (after spinal shock subsides)
- loss of somatic and visceral sensations below the level of the injury
- inability to perspire below the level of the injury
- bowel and bladder dysfunction
- other signs of spinal shock, including hypotension, bradycardia, and hypothermia.

WHAT TO DO IMMEDIATELY
If you suspect that your patient has a spinal cord injury, notify the physician and take these steps:
- Immobilize the patient.
- ➡ **NurseALERT** If you need to move the patient, do your best to keep his vertebral column aligned. Don't flex, extend, or rotate his neck.
- Assess respirations.
- ➡ **NurseALERT** Be aware that if the patient's injury involves his cervical spine, diaphragm, and intercostal muscles, he'll have trouble breathing on his own. Prepare for endotracheal intubation and mechanical ventilation.

TYPES OF SPINAL CORD INJURY

The spinal cord can sustain direct or indirect injury as a result of hyperextension, hyperflexion, or compression.

In *hyperextension*, the neck bends sharply back, creating an arc that stretches the spinal cord against bony structures, causing contusions and ischemia. This injury most often arises at C4 and C5. In *hyperflexion*, a similar injury results when the neck bends sharply forward.

In *compression*, vertical pressure on the vertebral column narrows the spinal canal and bruises the spinal cord. It also may crush the vertebral bodies, possibly causing them to burst.

COMPLETE AND INCOMPLETE INJURIES

Spinal cord injuries also can be classified as complete or incomplete. As the name implies, a complete injury causes a complete loss of neurologic function below the level of the injury. An incomplete injury causes a varying amount of motor and sensory loss.

There are three common types of incomplete cord injuries. A *central cord injury* involves the center part of the cord and causes weakness that's more pronounced in the arms than in the legs. It typically results from hyperextension.

Anterior cord syndrome results from occlusion of the anterior spinal artery and causes complete paralysis and loss of pain and temperature sensation below the injury.

Brown-Séquard syndrome, also known as hemisection of the cord, is most common in stabbing and gunshot wounds. Because one side of the cord is damaged, the patient sustains loss of motor function on the same side as the injury, plus loss of pain, temperature, and touch sensation on the opposite side.

➡ **NurseALERT** If the patient has a cervical injury, don't hyperextend his neck for oral intubation. Use the chin-lift or jaw-thrust maneuver instead. If the patient has a complete spinal cord injury at C4 or above, loss of innervation to his diaphragm will render him permanently dependent on a ventilator.

- If the patient doesn't need immediate endotracheal intubation, obtain a baseline tidal volume, negative inspiratory force, and minute volume. These values will help you detect whether the patient is tiring from the work of breathing.
- Obtain vital signs; be especially alert for bradycardia and hypotension. Anticipate the need for continuous cardiac monitoring to check for arrhythmias secondary to hypoxemia.
- Assess the patient's oxygen saturation by way of pulse oximetry and arterial blood gas values. Give supplemental oxygen, as indicated.
- Perform a baseline neurologic assessment, including motor and sensory function, to document the level of the injury.
- Obtain spinal X-rays, both anteroposterior and lateral views, as ordered, to document bony displacement.
- Carefully assess for injury to other organs. Keep in mind that cardiac, intrathoracic, and abdominal injuries are commonly associated with spinal cord injury.
- Establish I.V. access, and prepare to start high-dose methylprednisolone (Solu-Medrol) treatment. (See *High-dose steroid therapy*, page 344.)

WHAT TO DO NEXT

Once the patient has stabilized, follow these measures:
- Continue to keep the patient's vertebral column aligned. If he's in

S

TREATMENT OF CHOICE

HIGH-DOSE STEROID THERAPY

A cornerstone of emergency care for spinal cord injuries, high-dose steroid therapy improves neurologic recovery when given shortly after the injury occurs. If it's ordered for your patient, take these steps:

- Take precautions by giving histamine-2-receptor antagonists, checking the patient's gastric contents and stools for blood, and monitoring blood glucose levels.
- Obtain a baseline weight.
- Calculate a methylprednisolone (Solu-Medrol) loading dose of 30 mg/kg and infuse it over 1 hour.

- Switch to an infusion of normal saline solution to keep the line open. Then, after waiting 45 minutes, begin a steroid infusion at a rate of 5.4 mg/kg/hour over 23 hours.

CONTRAINDICATIONS

Contraindications to high-dose steroid therapy include:

- an injury more than 8 hours old
- an injury below L2
- an injury to the cauda equina.

traction, make sure that the correct weights hang free and that the patient is properly aligned with the traction pulley.

- If the patient is a candidate for surgical stabilization, prepare him for the procedure as appropriate.
- Check the patient at least hourly for adequate oxygenation, stable blood pressure, and appropriate heart rate.
- If indicated, insert a nasogastric tube to decompress his stomach and prevent vomiting and aspiration.
- Insert an indwelling urinary catheter, and monitor the patient's urine output hourly. Remember that spinal shock renders the bladder temporarily atonic.
- Administer stool softeners, laxatives, and enemas, as prescribed, to avoid obstruction. Assess for abdominal distention and the presence of bowel sounds.
- Perform passive range of motion with the patient's limbs; then return them to functional positions.
- Provide frequent skin care, and turn the patient every 2 hours to prevent skin breakdown.
- Watch for the return of reflex function, which signals the end of spinal shock.
- Assess for signs of autonomic dysreflexia, and take appropriate actions immediately if it occurs. (See *Recognizing autonomic dysreflexia*.)
- To help prevent deep vein thrombosis (DVT), apply intermittent pneumatic compression boots or antiembolism stockings, as ordered.

FOLLOW-UP CARE

- Continue to assess the patient's neurologic and cardiopulmonary status for changes.
- Assess for signs of DVT.
- Continue to turn and reposition the patient every 2 hours.
- Monitor him carefully for signs of pulmonary embolism.

RECOGNIZING AUTONOMIC DYSREFLEXIA

After the acute phase of a spinal injury passes, patients with injuries above T6 are susceptible to a serious hypertensive event caused by simultaneous sympathetic and parasympathetic activity. Called autonomic dysreflexia, the condition may lead to cerebrovascular accident, seizures, myocardial infarction, and even death. It results most often from a distended bladder or bowel, a pressure ulcer, or an ingrown toenail. Here's what happens.

When a condition, such as from a distended bladder, produces a sensory stimulus, the neuropathways attempt to transmit that stimulus to the brain, but it's blocked at the level of spinal cord damage. This then triggers the sympathetic nervous system, which causes vasoconstriction below the level of the lesion. As a result, blood volume is shifted to the upper part of the body. This may produce severe hypertension and a pounding headache. Above the level of the lesion, the patient's skin is hot, flushed, and diaphoretic. Below the level of the lesion, his skin is pale, cool, and dry.

TREATING AUTONOMIC DYSREFLEXIA

Treatment of this emergency condition aims to immediately identify the noxious stimulus and remove it, thus lowering the patient's blood pressure. Start by raising the head of the patient's bed to help lower his blood pressure, and then look for possible causes. For example, if he has an indwelling urinary catheter, check it for kinks or occlusion. If you find an occlusion, replace the catheter. Also check for fecal impaction and, if present, try to clear it. Instill dibucaine (Nupercainal) ointment, as prescribed, to anesthetize the area.

Usually, one of these conservative measures will resolve the problem. If it doesn't, prepare to administer an I.V. vasodilator, such as hydralazine (Apresoline) or nitroprusside (Nitropress), as prescribed.

- Begin active physical and occupational therapy as soon as the patient is stable.
- If his spine has been surgically stabilized, provide wound care as indicated.
- If the patient is in halo traction, maintain the traction by making sure the frame remains tight. Never lift the patient by the traction device. Care for the skin under the vest, and make sure it isn't being pinched. Keep the wrench for the vest readily available at the patient's bedside in case of an emergency (for example, in case the vest must be removed to perform cardiopulmonary resuscitation).
- Especially if the patient has a cervical injury and is able, urge him to cough, deep breathe, and use the incentive spirometer to maintain lung function.
- Perform chest physiotherapy. If the patient has trouble coughing, anticipate the need to help him cough by using the quad cough maneuver. To perform this maneuver, have the patient inhale as deeply as possible, and tell him to hold it for 2 to 3 seconds. As the patient exhales and attempts to cough, apply upward pressure against his diaphragm.
- A patient with a high-level spinal cord injury won't be able to use a typical bedside call system; provide an appropriate alternate method.
- Provide time for the patient to express his feelings, and offer him emotional support.
- Provide a high-fluid, high-carbohydrate, high-protein diet to promote healing and enhance bowel elimination.
- Assess for spasticity, and administer medications, as prescribed.

- Teach the patient and his family about rehabilitation services and their importance; begin referrals for rehabilitation early.
- Help the patient and his family to identify and use all appropriate support services available in their area.
- Teach the patient and his family about risk factors for complications and strategies to avoid them.
- Also teach the importance of adequate nutrition, efficient bowel and bladder function, skin care, and infection prevention.

SPECIAL CONSIDERATIONS
- Be aware that because the life expectancy of a person with spinal cord injury is only 5 years less than that of an average person, quality-of-life issues take on crucial importance and underlie the need for extensive rehabilitation.
- Keep in mind that quadriplegic patients injured at C4 or above probably will need permanent ventilatory assistance. Instruct the patient and family in respiratory care measures.

SUBARACHNOID HEMORRHAGE

When blood enters the subarachnoid space around the brain, it quickly mixes with cerebrospinal fluid, circulates around the brain and spinal cord, and begins to create signs and symptoms of a growing problem. Usually, those signs and symptoms reflect meningeal irritation caused by the inflowing blood. If the hemorrhage is massive, signs and symptoms (including loss of consciousness) may reflect increased intracranial pressure as well. (See *Looking at a subarachnoid hemorrhage.*)

Most often, a subarachnoid hemorrhage results from a ruptured cerebral aneurysm—a condition that carries a guarded prognosis. Other causes include trauma, arteriovenous malformation, hypertension, and, rarely, infection.

Especially among patients whose hemorrhage stems from a ruptured aneurysm, vasospasm is a relatively common complication: It develops in about 40% of patients with subarachnoid hemorrhage and is the most common cause of death. Severe vasospasm can lead to cerebral infarction. Other complications include rebleeding and hydrocephalus.

Clearly, subarachnoid hemorrhage is a condition that allows no time for missteps or misdirected care. You'll need to be ready to respond swiftly and appropriately to help save your patient's life.

WHAT TO LOOK FOR
If your patient has a subarachnoid hemorrhage, your clinical findings may include:
- sudden explosive headache, often unresponsive to analgesics
- sudden transient decrease in level of consciousness
- nausea and vomiting
- stiff neck (nuchal rigidity)

PATHOPHYSIOLOGY

LOOKING AT A SUBARACHNOID HEMORRHAGE

In a subarachnoid hemorrhage, blood invades the sub-arachnoid space around the brain and mixes with cere-brospinal fluid. The blood coats nerve roots, irritating nerve tissues and causing inflammation. The patient may complain of neck stiffness, photophobia, and blurred vision.

In addition, the blood impairs cerebrospinal fluid re-absorption and impairs its circulation within the ventri-cles. As a result, intracranial pressure dramatically in-creases for about 10 minutes after the hemorrhage and then returns to baseline. During this time, the patient may experience nausea, vomiting, visual disturbances, motor deficits, and loss of consciousness.

If the hemorrhage continues to enlarge, the brain tis-sue becomes compressed and herniates through the foramen magnum, and the patient may die.

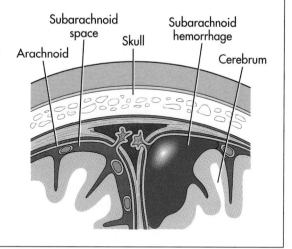

- positive Kernig's or Brudzinski's sign for meningeal irritation
- photophobia
- focal motor or sensory deficit that correlates with the extent and location of the hemorrhage
- seizures.

WHAT TO DO IMMEDIATELY

If you suspect that your patient is experiencing a subarachnoid hemor-rhage, notify the physician and follow these measures:

- Perform a complete neurologic assessment to establish a baseline. Check the patient's level of consciousness, the reaction of her pupils to light, and her bilateral motor strength. Also assess for signs of meningeal irritation.
- Use a standard grading scale to document the hemorrhage's severity and track changes in the patient's condition. (See *Grading a subarach-noid hemorrhage*, page 348.)
- Darken the room to ease the patient's photophobia and headache.
- If her level of consciousness is markedly decreased (stupor or coma), she may require endotracheal intubation and mechanical ventilation.
- Assess the patient's oxygen saturation level using pulse oximetry and arterial blood gas analysis. Give supplemental oxygen, as ordered.
- Prepare her for a computed tomographic (CT) scan, as indicated.
- If she has no signs of increased intracranial pressure, prepare to assist the physician with lumbar puncture to confirm blood in the sub-arachnoid space.
- ➡ **NurseALERT** Remember that a lumbar puncture must not be per-formed if the patient has increased intracranial pressure. During a

S

GRADING A SUBARACHNOID HEMORRHAGE

Use this grading scale to help document the severity of your patient's subarachnoid hemorrhage. Increase the apparent grade by one level if your patient is over age 70 or has significant systemic disease.

Grade I
A minimal bleed. The patient is alert with no focal neurologic deficit. She has a slight headache and minimal nuchal rigidity.

Grade II
A mild bleed. The patient is alert with a mild to severe headache. She has nuchal rigidity and may have a third nerve palsy.

Grade III
A moderate bleed. The patient is drowsy and may be confused. She has a more severe headache, nuchal rigidity, and a focal deficit.

Grade IV
A severe bleed. The patient is stuporous and has nuchal rigidity and hemiparesis.

Grade V
A severe bleed that's commonly fatal. The patient is in a deep coma and shows decerebrate posturing.

lumbar puncture, removal of cerebrospinal fluid from the spinal area may cause pressurized intracranial contents to shift, resulting in fatal brain stem herniation.
- Check the patient's blood pressure, pulse rate, and heart rhythm every 15 to 30 minutes.

WHAT TO DO NEXT
Once subarachnoid hemorrhage has been confirmed, take these actions:
- As prescribed, administer medication, such as calcium channel blockers, to minimize the severity of vasospasm.
- Anticipate giving crystalloids and colloids to maintain the patient's hemodynamic status, increase cerebral perfusion pressure, and improve cerebral microcirculation. If the patient's neurologic status doesn't improve, prepare to give vasopressors to improve it through controlled hypertension.
➡ **NurseALERT** Monitor serum electrolyte levels carefully during hypertensive and hypervolemic therapy. Sodium and potassium imbalances are common and alter the neurologic assessment.
- Prepare the patient for cerebral angiography to determine the cause of her hemorrhage and guide her treatment plan.
- Continue to monitor her vital signs, neurologic status, and cardiopulmonary status.
➡ **NurseALERT** Continue to perform frequent neurologic assessments, paying particular attention to possible signs of vasospasm, such as decreasing level of consciousness.
- Keep the patient on bed rest with the head of her bed elevated 30 to 45 degrees.
- Keep the environment quiet, the lights low, and the level of environmental stimuli minimized to reduce the risk of rebleeding.

- Monitor intake and output carefully. Anticipate insertion of an indwelling urinary catheter to assess hourly urine output.
- Assess the patient's ability to swallow before starting her prescribed diet.
- Provide the patient and her family with an explanation of her condition and the treatments she'll need. Provide support and encouragement.
- Institute seizure precautions in keeping with your facility's policy.
- Use analgesics as necessary to control headache. Codeine is the analgesic of choice because it has minimal effects on the level of consciousness.
- Control restlessness and agitation with mild sedation, as prescribed.
- Administer anticonvulsants, as prescribed, to prevent seizures.
- If the angiogram shows an aneurysm, prepare the patient for craniotomy to repair it, as ordered. If the angiogram doesn't show an aneurysm, the patient may still require bed rest for 7 days or more before repeat angiography can confirm a nonlocalized bleeding source.
- If the patient undergoes a craniotomy, provide appropriate postoperative care. For example, monitor her neurologic status at least every hour for the first 24 hours. Track her level of consciousness, looking for signs of increased intracranial pressure. Inspect the incision for drainage and swelling. Examine any drainage carefully for signs of bleeding, and maintain the patient's hypervolemic and hypertensive therapy to reduce the continued risk of vasospasm.

FOLLOW-UP CARE

- Because treatment for subarachnoid hemorrhage may involve prolonged bed rest, the patient has an increased risk for deep vein thrombosis and pulmonary embolism. Apply antiembolism stockings or intermittent pneumatic compression devices to decrease that risk.
- Give stool softeners to prevent constipation and straining.
- Provide frequent, meticulous skin care to prevent breakdown.
- Once the source of the hemorrhage has been treated, gradually begin to increase the patient's activity level.
- Assess carefully for neurologic deficits that require rehabilitation, and set up consultations as soon as possible.
- Prepare the patient and her family for follow-up care with a rehabilitation specialist.
- Encourage the patient to participate in her care and her activities of daily living as much as possible.
- Continue to perform neurologic assessments.
- ➡ **NurseALERT** Watch for subtle changes over time; they could signal the development of hydrocephalus, a common complication of subarachnoid hemorrhage.
- Prepare the patient for a follow-up CT scan, as necessary.
- Provide emotional support and a positive environment during the patient's recovery.

S

SPECIAL CONSIDERATIONS

- If the patient needed surgery for a cerebral aneurysm, teach her and her family about needed follow-up care, including incisional care, as ordered. If aneurysm clips were used, caution her about the need to obtain medical alert identification and to carry it with her. Explain that magnetic resonance imaging is contraindicated because the clips may migrate under the effects of the magnetic field.

SUBDURAL HEMATOMA

A subdural hematoma is a collection of blood under the dura mater, the tough outer covering of the brain. Blood can flow into the subdural space when bridging veins tear, small arterial branches rupture, or contusions or lacerations ooze or bleed. (See *Looking at a subdural hematoma*.)

Usually, a subdural hematoma results from traumatic head injury, and signs and symptoms commonly reflect the speed at which the blood collects. Many subdural hematomas develop slowly over days to weeks before producing symptoms. Sometimes the time between injury (which may be as minor as a bump on the head) and the appearance of symptoms may be so long that the patient and his family members can't recall the injury. That's why some experts advise you to suspect subdural hematoma in any patient with an unexplained gradual decrease in level of consciousness. (See *Classifying subdural hematoma*.)

Diagnosis of a subdural hematoma typically relies on computed tomographic (CT) scanning, and treatment varies with the severity of the problem. If the patient has a small hematoma, for example, treatment may simply involve observation and serial CT scans to verify the hematoma's gradual resorption. If the patient experiences a marked increase in intracranial pressure (ICP), treatment involves immediate surgery. Burr holes can relieve pressure by quickly evacuating an acute hematoma. In a subacute or chronic subdural hematoma, the patient usually needs a craniotomy to evacuate the hematoma and remove the membranes around it.

The prognosis for a patient with subdural hematoma depends largely on how rapidly diagnosis and intervention take place, on the extent of underlying brain damage, and on his neurologic status before surgery. Even when it develops slowly, a subdural hematoma can threaten your patient's life. By responding appropriately, you can help him get the care he needs to minimize the dangers of this potentially ominous condition.

WHAT TO LOOK FOR

Clinical findings in a patient with subdural hematoma may include:
- gradual decrease in level of consciousness
- papilledema (in chronic subdural hematoma)
- headache
- seizures
- ipsilateral dilated pupil with a sluggish to fixed light response (late)

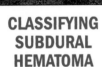

CLASSIFYING SUBDURAL HEMATOMA

The signs and symptoms of subdural hematoma relate largely to the rate at which the blood collects. That rate is reflected in the classifications of subdural hematoma listed here.
- An *acute subdural hematoma* produces signs and symptoms within 48 hours after an injury.
- A *subacute subdural hematoma* produces signs and symptoms between 48 hours and 2 weeks after the injury.
- A *chronic subdural hematoma* takes more than 2 weeks to produce symptoms.

LOOKING AT A SUBDURAL HEMATOMA

In a subdural hematoma, blood invades the subdural space between the dura mater and the arachnoid layer of the meningeal covering of the brain. Usually, the blood comes from torn bridging veins or ruptured small arterial branches.

If the source of the bleeding is the venous system, blood accumulation is slow and gradual. Consequently, signs and symptoms may not develop for several days or even weeks.

If the subdural hematoma develops as a result of an arterial hemorrhage, signs and symptoms develop faster—usually within 48 hours.

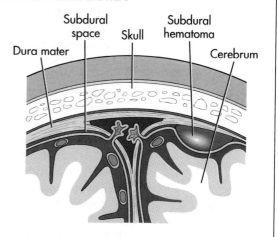

- hemiparesis, hemiplegia (late)
- changes in respiratory patterns.

WHAT TO DO IMMEDIATELY

If you suspect that your patient's declining neurologic status might be caused by an expanding subdural hematoma, notify the physician and follow these measures:

- Make sure the patient has a patent airway. If he loses consciousness, prepare for endotracheal intubation and mechanical ventilation.
- Assess his oxygen saturation by way of pulse oximetry and arterial blood gas analysis. Give supplemental oxygen, as indicated.
- Obtain a CT scan, as ordered.
- Monitor the patient's vital signs and neurologic status carefully.
- ➡ Nurse**ALERT** Pay particular attention to signs of increased ICP and impending cerebral herniation, including rising systolic blood pressure, widening pulse pressure, and bradycardia (Cushing's triad) as well as posturing and a unilateral fixed and dilated pupil.
- Prepare the patient for surgical intervention.

WHAT TO DO NEXT

When the patient returns from surgery, follow these measures:

- Continue to monitor his vital signs and neurologic status, initially every 15 to 30 minutes and then every hour.
- Keep the head of the patient's bed elevated between 15 and 30 degrees, depending on his blood pressure.
- ➡ Nurse**ALERT** Elevating the head of the bed promotes venous drainage but may also decrease cerebral blood flow by dropping blood pres-

S

sure. Determine the optimal elevation according to your patient's response.

- Provide pulmonary care and suction the patient as needed. Change his position frequently, and make sure he maintains adequate oxygenation.
- Maintain accurate intake and output records. Anticipate the need for an indwelling urinary catheter if the patient doesn't already have one in place. Your goal is to promote adequate systemic blood pressure by maintaining the patient's fluid volume status.
- Inspect the surgical dressing and drain (if present) for excessive drainage.
- If prescribed, give osmotic diuretics to help reduce ICP; monitor serum osmolarity and electrolytes during osmotic therapy.
- Institute seizure precautions according to your facility's policy, and watch carefully for signs of seizures.
- Use cool compresses to decrease facial swelling after surgery.
- If needed, give a mild analgesic, as prescribed, after surgery. Codeine is the analgesic of choice for patients who've had a craniotomy.
- ➡ **NurseALERT** Severe pain or headache after a craniotomy to evacuate a subdural hematoma is unusual. Notify the surgeon immediately if the patient has severe pain; it could indicate intracranial bleeding.
- Provide support to the patient and his family; explain procedures and treatments he'll undergo.

FOLLOW-UP CARE
- Continue to monitor the patient's respiratory function, including respiratory rate and volume.
- Continue to assess his neurologic status, watching for subtle changes in level of consciousness.
- Assess for signs of infection related to the surgery. Maintain normal temperature. Use hypothermia blankets and administer acetaminophen, as prescribed.
- ➡ **NurseALERT** Keep the patient from shivering to avoid increasing his ICP.
- If indicated, obtain referrals to appropriate acute or subacute rehabilitation facilities as quickly as possible so that rehabilitation can start early. Assist the family in decision making by encouraging them to visit the facilities and observe the therapies.

SPECIAL CONSIDERATIONS
- If the patient did not have surgery to remove the hematoma, monitor his neurologic status carefully until it stabilizes.
- ➡ **NurseALERT** An altered level of consciousness offers the most sensitive indicator of increasing ICP. If your patient becomes irritable, restless, or disoriented, suspect an expanding hematoma. If his pupils change size or their light reactions change, he could be experiencing dangerous, potentially fatal elevations of ICP. Altered vital signs are a late indicator of increased ICP.

- Keep in mind that chronic subdural hematoma is common in elderly patients and can result from a seemingly mild injury. That's because age-related cerebral atrophy increases traction on the bridging vessels, making them more likely to tear. The atrophy also provides more space in the intracranial vault, so the hematoma can become quite large before it causes signs and symptoms. Suspect chronic subdural hematoma in patients on anticoagulation therapy or patients with a history of chronic alcohol abuse if they become confused or show a gradual, unexplained decrease in level of consciousness.

SUICIDAL IDEATION

A patient with suicidal ideation—thoughts of killing himself—must be evaluated immediately. A suicide attempt is especially likely if suicidal ideation is accompanied by an intent to commit suicide and an organized plan for carrying out the act.

Because nurses commonly have more contact with patients than other members of the health-care team do, you may be responsible for observation of a suicidal patient and for intervening as necessary. You may even be directly responsible for keeping him safe. Your interventions focus on convincing the patient that suicide isn't a practical option and on keeping him alive until he decides he wants to live.

To ensure early intervention, you must be able to identify a patient who's contemplating suicide and to recognize a suicide threat in all its forms. Besides evaluating him for suicidal ideation, you'll need to assess the patient for specific risk factors that increase the likelihood that he'll attempt suicide. (See *Recognizing risk factors for suicide,* page 354.)

Keep in mind that most people who attempt suicide give clues to their suicidal thoughts beforehand. That's why you must always take a suicide threat—whether verbal or implied—seriously. Be especially wary if your patient has a history of multiple suicide attempts; with each attempt, the chance for success increases.

WHAT TO LOOK FOR
Suspect suicidal ideation in a patient who:
- expresses thoughts of suicide
- gives away personal objects
- takes steps to put his affairs in order, such as making a will
- behaves impulsively
- withdraws from others
- shows little or no future orientation (says he has nothing to look forward to, for example)
- expresses feelings of hopelessness, helplessness, worthlessness, loneliness, or isolation
- reports hearing voices that tell him to harm himself (command hallucinations)

S

RECOGNIZING RISK FACTORS FOR SUICIDE

The following factors increase a patient's risk for suicidal ideation or a suicide attempt.

Personal history
- Recent or current crisis
- Previous suicide attempt
- Substance abuse
- Limited support systems

Age
- Adolescence
- Old age

Marital status
- Widower

Occupation
- Air traffic controller
- Dentist
- Physician
- Police officer
- Unemployed

Racial background
- Caucasian
- Native American

Economic status
- Extremely poor
- Extremely wealthy

Medical history
- Chronic pain
- Chronic illness
- Terminal illness

Psychiatric history
- Antisocial personality disorder
- Borderline personality disorder
- Major depression
- Schizophrenia

Family history
- Suicide of a family member

- refuses to make a safety contract (an agreement not to harm himself) with the health-care team
- has attempted suicide in the past
- shows an increased energy level after starting to respond to antidepressant drug therapy because he'll have the necessary energy to carry out his plan
- makes such statements as "I wish I were dead," "Everyone would be better off if I were dead," "Life isn't worth living," and "Things will be better soon."

WHAT TO DO IMMEDIATELY

If you suspect that your patient has suicidal ideation, notify the physician. Then take these measures:
- Take safety precautions. For instance, remove harmful objects, such as scissors, sharp objects, string, medications, ties from gowns, and electrical cords, from the patient's environment. Search the patient and the room as necessary.
- Make sure someone stays with the patient at all times.
- Try to establish a rapport with the patient. Address him by name, and sit down and talk with him to show that you're willing to listen.
- Ask if he's going to harm himself or is thinking about suicide, wishes he were dead, or has a suicide plan. Find out if he's ever made a previ-

ous suicide attempt. Also ask if he'd tell a staff member if he felt the urge to harm himself. Don't be afraid to ask direct questions like these; doing so won't make him more likely to attempt suicide.

- If the patient tells you that suicide is his only option, negotiate with him for more time so you can get him the help he needs.
- Recognize your patient's feelings of desperation, anger, or frustration. Help him identify a reason to live (such as a loved one) and recognize alternatives to suicide. Reassure him that he's safe.
- Assess his willingness to make a written or verbal contract for safety—one that says he'll keep himself safe and that if he feels he can't keep himself safe, he'll seek help from a staff member.
- ➡ **NurseALERT** Arrange for one-on-one observation if the patient refuses to contract for safety.
- Check on your patient every 15, 30, or 60 minutes, as indicated—even if he has a safety contract or someone (such as a family member) is staying with him. Document your safety checks on a flow sheet or in your nursing notes. Be sure to include your patient's specific location and behavior.
- Arrange for a psychiatric consultation as soon as possible to evaluate the patient.
- Make sure your patient isn't stockpiling medication.
- Check visitors to make sure they don't bring the patient potentially dangerous objects.
- Administer antianxiety drugs if he's highly anxious, sleep-inducing drugs if he has insomnia, and antipsychotic drugs if he's having command hallucinations, as prescribed.

WHAT TO DO NEXT
After taking initial steps to safeguard your patient, follow these guidelines:
- Assess him frequently for threats to his safety. If he's impulsive, arrange for more intensive observation or have someone continue to stay with him so he's not alone.
- ➡ **NurseALERT** Be aware that even a minor setback may increase a suicidal patient's desire to die. So be sure to watch him closely if he receives news of a poor prognosis or an unsuccessful medical procedure or if he's in increasing pain that doesn't respond to analgesics.
- Use a team approach to deal with the patient's suicidal ideation. Ask the psychiatrist for help in establishing a plan of care.
- If another staff member has established a good rapport with the patient, ask that person to speak with the patient. Recognize that when this staff member goes off duty, the patient's suicide risk may rise.
- Instruct all staff members responsible for observing the patient one-on-one never to leave him alone. Keep him under direct observation even when he uses the bathroom, and arrange for someone to take your place when you must leave. Document the patient's statements and behavior. Make sure all health-care team members use a consistent policy when dealing with the patient.

S

FOLLOW-UP CARE

- Continue patient supervision, and record your observations.
- Encourage your patient to express his feelings. Empathize when he talks of his frustration, hopelessness, loneliness, or desperation.
- Avoid the urge to tell him "everything will be fine" because it may not. However, reassure him that you'll do what you can to help.
- Assist him in identifying coping methods that have worked for him in the past.
- Teach him about depression and its treatment. Administer antidepressants, if prescribed.
- ➡ **NurseALERT** Be aware that a patient's suicide risk may increase dramatically at the start of antidepressant therapy because the medication may give him the energy he needs to act on his suicidal urges. Therefore, monitor him especially closely when initiating antidepressant therapy. Keep in mind that the effect of some antidepressants may be noticed within 1 to 2 weeks. However, the effect of other antidepressants may not be noticed for up to 6 weeks.
- Review the patient's contract for safety with him, and reconfirm it once every 8 hours or as often as necessary. You can do this by simply asking him if he's able to keep himself safe.
- Evaluate the patient's need for continued one-on-one observation. If indicated, you may reduce observation to once every 15 minutes.
- Recognize that the suicidal patient may project his hostility onto you and other staff members. Don't take this personally; remember that his behavior reflects low self-esteem, frustration, or pain.
- Avoid unnecessary struggles with the patient. As his safety and condition allow, grant him privileges and let him make his own choices.
- Make necessary referrals to make sure the patient receives support and evaluation after discharge.

SPECIAL CONSIDERATIONS

- Have family members participate in one-on-one patient observation if your facility allows it. Teach all observers about relevant policies and regulations.
- Assess your own feelings about suicide. Self-preservation is a fundamental biological drive, and the preservation of life is a basic tenet of most religious, ethical, and philosophical systems. If your patient's suicidal thoughts or behavior evoke uncomfortable feelings, make a special effort to remain objective when dealing with him. Remember that your main goal is to keep him safe. Ask others for support in dealing with any negative feelings you may have toward the patient.
- If your patient has a chronic illness, be aware that underlying depression may be the primary reason for suicidal ideation. Anticipate administering treatments for depression.
- Be aware that although females make more suicide attempts, males are more successful in their attempts. Also, know that the rate of successful suicides is highest among elderly people.

SUPRAVENTRICULAR TACHYCARDIA

In supraventricular tachycardia, abnormal impulses from atria, junctional tissue, or the atrioventricular (AV) node reach the ventricles and raise the heart rate above 100 beats/minute. Types of supraventricular tachycardia include sinus tachycardia, atrial tachycardia, atrial flutter, atrial fibrillation, and junctional tachycardia. Depending on the type of arrhythmia, the ventricular response may be either regular or irregular. Usually, the QRS complex is of normal width—less than 0.12 second. The P waves may be visible or buried in the T wave of the preceding beat. If they're visible, they may be uniform in shape or variable, as in multifocal atrial tachycardia.

The most common cause of supraventricular tachycardia is AV nodal reentry, in which abnormal impulses stimulate repolarized AV nodal cells to cause repetitive depolarization of those cells. Less commonly, reentry can occur in atrial tissue. In some cases, the cause is abnormal automaticity—repetitive firing from an ectopic site.

Supraventricular tachycardia is either paroxysmal or nonparoxysmal. Paroxysmal supraventricular tachycardia starts and stops abruptly and usually lasts for short periods. When the arrhythmia doesn't start and stop abruptly, it's called nonparoxysmal supraventricular tachycardia.

Paroxysmal atrial tachycardia (PAT) and nonparoxysmal supraventricular tachycardia can arise—even in healthy hearts—from overexertion, emotional stress, position changes, smoking, thyroid medications, and alcohol ingestion. These arrhythmias also may result from coronary artery disease, digitalis toxicity, myocardial infarction (MI), pulmonary disease, rheumatic heart disease, and Wolff-Parkinson-White (WPW) syndrome. Because of their rapid rates, PAT and nonparoxysmal supraventricular tachycardia can reduce cardiac output and increase myocardial oxygen demand. Consequently, they can lead to heart failure and MI.

WHAT TO LOOK FOR
Clinical findings in supraventricular tachycardia include:
- ECG findings characteristic of atrial tachycardia
- palpitations
- hypotension
- syncope
- nervousness and anxiety
- chest pain
- light-headedness
- rapid peripheral pulse with a regular or an irregular rhythm
- reduced cardiac output.

S

TREATMENT OF CHOICE

ADMINISTERING ADENOSINE

Because adenosine (Adenocard) slows conduction and interrupts reentry pathways through the atrioventricular (AV) node, this drug is the treatment of choice for supraventricular tachycardia. Adenosine has a rapid onset and a short half-life (about 10 seconds). What's more, it causes few adverse effects. Here's what you need to know to administer this antiarrhythmic agent safely and effectively.

- Before initiating adenosine therapy, begin continuous ECG monitoring. If your patient has second- or third-degree heart block or sick sinus syndrome, *don't* give adenosine. Instead, consult with the physician.
- As prescribed, give 6 mg of adenosine by I.V. push over 1 to 2 seconds through a port near the insertion site of the I.V. line. Follow with a normal saline flush to make sure your patient gets the full dose.
- Remember that diazepam (Valium), dipyridamole (Persantine), and phenobarbital (Luminal) may enhance the effects of adenosine. If your patient is receiving one of these drugs, you'll need to reduce her adenosine dose.
- Expect to increase the adenosine dose if the patient is receiving a drug that antagonizes adenosine, such

as theophylline or another methylxanthine.
- If the sinus rhythm doesn't resolve in 2 minutes, give 12 mg of adenosine. Repeat this 12-mg dose, if needed.
- Assess the patient's ECG for heart rate and rhythm, PR interval, QRS complex, and QT interval.

MONITORING YOUR PATIENT DURING THERAPY
- Closely monitor the patient's ECG for arrhythmias induced by adenosine, including premature ventricular or atrial contractions, sinus bradycardia or tachycardia, AV block, atrial fibrillation or flutter, and ventricular tachycardia.
- Maintain continuous blood pressure monitoring.
- Frequently assess the patient's vital signs, level of consciousness, respiratory rate and depth, breath sounds, and skin color.
- If your patient has asthma, take extra care when monitoring her respiratory status because adenosine can cause bronchoconstriction.
- Stay alert for adverse effects of adenosine: chest pain, hypotension, dyspnea, nausea, facial flushing, headache, sweating, dizziness, arm tingling, metallic taste, groin pressure, and throat tightness.

WHAT TO DO IMMEDIATELY

If your patient develops supraventricular tachycardia, notify the physician. Then take the following steps:

- Assess the patient's vital signs, level of consciousness, breath sounds, and skin color.
- Begin continuous ECG monitoring. Assess the patient's heart rate and rhythm, P waves, PR intervals, and QRS complexes.
- Insert and maintain an I.V. line.
- Administer supplemental oxygen, as indicated and prescribed.
- Keep emergency equipment and medications nearby.
- Obtain a 12-lead ECG.
- If indicated, instruct the patient to perform vagal maneuvers, such as coughing or Valsalva's maneuver, to slow the heart rate. If the patient has no carotid bruits and no history of stroke, the physician may perform carotid sinus massage to stimulate parasympathetic fibers that slow conduction through the AV node.
- If supraventricular tachycardia doesn't resolve, give I.V. adenosine (Adenocard), as prescribed. (See *Administering adenosine.*) Also administer verapamil (Isoptin), diltiazem (Cardizem), digoxin (Lanoxi-

caps), and beta blockers (such as propranolol [Inderal]), as prescribed. For multifocal atrial tachycardia give verapamil, metoprolol
(Lopressor), or amiodarone (Cordarone), as prescribed.

➡ **NurseALERT** Be aware that supraventricular tachycardia sometimes
produces a wide QRS complex resembling that of ventricular tachycardia. If there's any chance your patient could have ventricular
tachycardia rather than supraventricular tachycardia, don't give verapamil; it could be fatal. Also, if your patient has WPW syndrome, remember that digoxin and calcium channel blockers can severely
compromise her hemodynamic status.

• If digoxin or theophylline is the cause of the supraventricular tachycardia, discontinue the drug, as ordered, and monitor the drug levels.

WHAT TO DO NEXT
If the tachycardia converts to a sinus rhythm, perform the following interventions:
• Continue to monitor your patient's ECG in case the arrhythmia returns or another one develops.
• Maintain a patent I.V. line.
• Assess the patient's vital signs, heart rate and rhythm, respiratory rate,
heart and breath sounds, and skin color.
• If supraventricular tachycardia persists despite treatment, prepare
the patient for overdrive pacing or electrical cardioversion, as ordered. (See *Caring for your patient during synchronized cardioversion*,
page 39.)

FOLLOW-UP CARE
• Continue to monitor the patient's heart rate and rhythm.
• Observe for adverse effects of antiarrhythmic medications.
• Continue to carry out interventions to treat the patient's underlying
disorder, as ordered.
• Monitor serum electrolyte levels and digitalis, theophylline, and an-
tiarrhythmic drug levels, as appropriate. Report abnormal values to
the physician.

SPECIAL CONSIDERATIONS
• After administering adenosine, watch for ECG changes; another arrhythmia or even asystole may develop. However, keep in mind that
adenosine has a short half-life, so any arrhythmia it causes is likely to
stop within seconds.
• Teach your patient ways to reduce the risk of recurring supraventricular tachycardia. For example, suggest that she cut back on coffee,
stop smoking, and reduce stress.

S

SYNCOPE

Also known as fainting, syncope is a sudden and temporary loss of consciousness that typically occurs within 10 seconds after a decrease in cerebral blood flow. Syncope can be benign, or it can signal a potentially dangerous underlying condition. In either case, if your patient has a history of syncope or experiences it while in your care, you'll need to respond rapidly to ensure his safety and help determine the cause of the problem. (See *Types of syncope*.)

WHAT TO LOOK FOR
Clinical findings with syncope vary, depending on its underlying cause, but may include:
- sudden, brief loss of consciousness
- bradycardia (heart rate less than 60 beats/minute)
- tachycardia (heart rate greater than 180 beats/minute)
- irregular heartbeat
- palpitations
- chest pain
- dizziness
- disorientation
- blurred vision.

Vasovagal syncope
Before an episode of vasovagal syncope, your patient may report symptoms that include:
- weakness
- nausea
- light-headedness
- pallor
- diaphoresis.

Transient ischemic attack
If your patient's syncope resulted from a transient ischemic attack (TIA), he may have transient focal neurologic deficits. Clinical findings may include:
- blurred vision or visual field deficits
- difficulty speaking
- dysphagia
- motor and sensory deficits.

Aortic stenosis
Syncope is one of the classic triad of symptoms associated with aortic stenosis. The others are:
- chest pain

TYPES OF SYNCOPE

Syncope arises from either cardiovascular or noncardiovascular sources. Cardiovascular sources stem from inadequate filling on the heart's right side (called a reflex source) or decreased output from the heart's left side (called a cardiac source).

Examples of reflex sources of syncope include:
- carotid sinus syncope
- coughing
- defecation
- dehydration
- drug effects
- micturition
- orthostatic hypotension
- sneezing
- swallowing
- vasovagal reactions.

Examples of cardiac sources of syncope include:
- aortic dissection
- aortic stenosis
- arrhythmias
- hypertrophic cardiomyopathy
- myocardial infarction
- pulmonary embolism.

Examples of noncardiovascular sources of syncope include:
- anemia
- hyperventilation
- hypoglycemia
- hypoxia
- medications, such as diuretics and vasodilators
- metabolic disorders
- transient ischemic attack
- subclavian steal syndrome.

- dyspnea.

Aortic dissection or subclavian steal syndrome
If syncope results from aortic dissection or subclavian steal syndrome (in which blood flow is diverted from the basilar artery to the subclavian artery), clinical findings may include:
- a difference in pulse strength between the patient's arms
- a difference in systolic blood pressure of more than 20 mm Hg between arms.

WHAT TO DO IMMEDIATELY
If your patient is experiencing syncope, notify the physician and follow these measures:
- Have the patient lie flat if he feels light-headed or dizzy or has fainted.
- If the patient has lost consciousness, make sure he has a patent airway, that he's breathing, and that he has a pulse.
- Check his vital signs, staying alert for abnormally low or high pulse rates, an irregular pulse, and hypotension.
- Give supplemental oxygen at a low flow rate, if ordered.
- Obtain an ECG to detect arrhythmias (such as bradycardias and tachycardias), to find ischemic ST-segment and T-wave changes, and to measure the QT interval. Start continuous cardiac monitoring, if indicated.

S

UNDERSTANDING E.P.S.

If your patient's syncope stems from an arrhythmia, he may need electrophysiology studies (EPS) to examine his heart's electrical activity, find defects in its conduction system, identify the mechanism and site of the arrhythmia, and assess the effectiveness of his antiarrhythmic medications.

In this invasive procedure, catheters typically are inserted into the femoral vein and advanced to the right side of the heart under fluoroscopy. The catheters record and map electrical activity at various sites in the heart while electrode catheters pace the heart in an attempt to induce arrhythmias.

If an arrhythmia arises, the physician may give various antiarrhythmic medications to determine which one best suppresses it. If ventricular tachycardia or ventricular fibrillation is induced, the patient may need cardioversion or defibrillation to convert back to a sinus rhythm. Other potential complications include a perforated myocardium, hemorrhage, phlebitis at the insertion site, and catheter-induced emboli.

Before EPS, explain the test to your patient and tell him that he'll need to fast for up to 8 hours. Afterward, he'll remain on bed rest with cardiac monitoring for 6 to 8 hours. Tell him to expect the test to take up to 4 hours, during which he'll need to lie still. If he feels any palpitations, light-headedness, or dizziness during the test, tell him to report it to the physician.

- Obtain a blood glucose measurement if your patient has diabetes. If he's hypoglycemic, administer treatment, as ordered.
- Establish I.V. access if a line isn't already in place, especially if the patient could be volume-depleted or shows signs and symptoms of dehydration.

WHAT TO DO NEXT
After your patient has gained consciousness and the initial crisis has subsided, follow these steps:
- Continue to monitor his vital signs. Report any difference in pulse strength or a difference of more than 20 mm Hg in systolic blood pressure between your patient's arms. Obtain blood pressure readings while the patient is sitting, lying, and standing. Note any changes.
- ➡ **NurseALERT** Be aware that carotid bruits may suggest that your patient's syncope results from a TIA, especially if he also has focal neurologic signs. Auscultate carefully for bruits.
- Review your patient's medications—especially diuretics and antihypertensives—with the physician and pharmacist to determine whether they could have caused his syncope. Discontinue medications, as ordered.
- To help determine the cause of syncope, ask your patient to describe the symptoms he had and the activity he was engaged in just before fainting. For example, fainting while having a bowel movement suggests reflex syncope, whereas fainting after arm exercises may be the result of subclavian steal syndrome. If family members were present, ask them what they observed.
- Continue to monitor blood glucose levels if your patient has diabetes.

- Obtain blood for testing—including hematocrit and serum electrolyte, hemoglobin, and cardiac enzyme levels—as ordered. Monitor the results.
- Administer I.V. fluids, as prescribed, to reverse volume depletion.
- Continue to monitor the patient's ECG for changes, including arrhythmias. Give antiarrhythmic medications, as ordered.
- Prepare the patient for possible electrophysiology studies (EPS) or the tilt-table test to determine the cause of an arrhythmia. (See *Understanding EPS*.)
- Anticipate insertion of a pacemaker if your patient's syncope results from carotid sinus sensitivity or certain arrhythmias.
- Take safety precautions to minimize the patient's risk of falling.

FOLLOW-UP CARE
- Do your best to protect your patient from injury. For example, if he's still having frequent syncopal episodes, explain the importance of calling for help before getting out of bed. Make sure his call button is within reach and that he knows how to use it.
- If the patient has orthostatic hypotension, have him rise to a sitting position and dangle his legs before standing up. Warn him not to stand up quickly, especially if he wakes at night to void. Also caution him against standing still for extended periods.
- Teach your patient how to put on antiembolism stockings, if ordered.
- Also teach him not to hold his breath and bear down but rather to exhale through his mouth when straining, as during defecation.

SPECIAL CONSIDERATIONS
- To take orthostatic vital signs properly, have your patient lie down for at least 5 minutes. Take his pulse and blood pressure in this position. Then ask your patient to stand. After he's been upright for 2 to 5 minutes, take his pulse and blood pressure again. Make sure you document the position in which you took each set of measurements.
- If your patient will have a continuous-loop ECG ambulatory recorder, you'll need to know and be able to explain the subtle differences between it and the Holter monitor. Like a Holter monitor, the continuous-loop ECG recorder continuously records the patient's ECG. But unlike the Holter monitor, it doesn't create a permanent recording of the patient's ECG. Rather, the tape loops back and is recorded over unless the patient activates the recording device. The patient activates the recording device if he experiences symptoms or immediately after regaining consciousness, if syncope has occurred. The recorder then preserves several minutes of the ECG leading up to activation.
- ➡ **NurseALERT** Tell your patient to lie down if he feels as though he might faint. If he can't lie down, he should sit down and put his head between his knees until the feeling passes.

S

- If your patient is scheduled for EPS, encourage him and his family to talk about their feelings and concerns. The events leading to EPS—such as syncope or sudden cardiac death—may have been frightening enough. Inducing them again, albeit under controlled and monitored conditions, can be equally frightening. What's more, the patient may need cardioversion or defibrillation to convert arrhythmias induced during EPS back to a sinus rhythm. Near-death experiences have been reported by some patients. Anticipate the need for premedication to promote your patient's relaxation and reduce his anxiety.

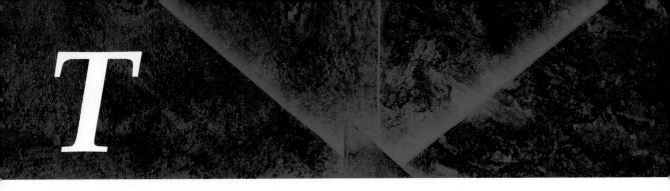

THYROID STORM

In a patient with hyperthyroidism, a stressful event can sometimes cause excessive amounts of thyroid hormones to suddenly be released into the bloodstream, sparking a life-threatening episode of severe hypermetabolism called thyroid storm. This condition results in excessive adrenergic activity, primarily in the cardiovascular, GI, and central nervous systems. Untreated, thyroid storm can quickly lead to exhaustion, coma, and death.

Factors that precipitate thyroid storm include infection, traumatic injury, surgery, and acute illness, such as acute myocardial infarction and pulmonary embolism. Patients who develop thyroid storm may not be aware of their chronic thyroid overactivity and thus have had no treatment for it. Others may develop thyroid storm after abruptly stopping their antithyroid medication or—less commonly today—after manipulation of the thyroid gland during surgery.

If you think that your patient is experiencing thyroid storm, you'll need to take quick action to prevent life-threatening complications. (See *Recognizing complications of thyroid storm*, page 366.)

WHAT TO LOOK FOR
Clinical findings for a patient experiencing thyroid storm may include:
- extreme nervousness
- agitation that progresses quickly to mania or psychotic behavior, followed by stupor and coma
- excessive sweating
- fever that can rapidly rise to 106° F (41.11° C)
- severe diarrhea
- nausea and vomiting
- tachypnea
- acute dyspnea
- severe tachycardia that may quickly rise to 300 beats/minute
- cardiac arrhythmias, most commonly atrial fibrillation.

WHAT TO DO IMMEDIATELY
If your patient develops thyroid storm, notify the physician and follow these measures:
- Quickly assess the patient's baseline cardiopulmonary status. Then start continuous ECG monitoring.

T

DANGER SIGNS AND SYMPTOMS

RECOGNIZING COMPLICATIONS OF THYROID STORM

Development of certain complications in a patient with thyroid storm can warn that her condition is deteriorating. If you detect the signs and symptoms listed in this table, notify the physician right away.

Signs and Symptoms	Complication
• Altered level of consciousness • Cool, clammy skin • Decreased urine output • Heart rate above 120 beats/minute • Systolic blood pressure below 90 mm Hg	Shock
• Pao_2 below 50 mm Hg • $Paco_2$ above 50 mm Hg • Paradoxical breathing • Respiratory rate above 30 breaths/minute • Restlessness	Respiratory failure
• Crackles • Dyspnea • Frothy sputum • Hypotension • Increased jugular vein pressure • S_3 heart sound • Tachycardia • Tachypnea	Heart failure and pulmonary edema

- Position the patient to facilitate respiration.
- Give oxygen by nasal cannula or mask. If her respiratory condition deteriorates, prepare for endotracheal intubation and mechanical ventilation.
- Quickly insert an I.V. line, and start fluid resuscitation measures with a dextrose solution to meet the patient's increased metabolic demands and to replace fluid lost through sweating, vomiting, and diarrhea. Expect to give at least 3 L during the first 24 hours, unless contraindicated.
- Administer propranolol (Inderal) I.V., as prescribed, to block peripheral beta-adrenergic activity.
- ➡ **NurseALERT** If you can't give the patient a beta-adrenergic blocker, expect to give reserpine (Serpalan, which depletes catecholamine stores) or guanethidine (Ismelin, which inhibits catecholamine release).
- Inhibit thyroid hormone synthesis by administering methimazole (Tapazole), as prescribed. Insert a nasogastric (NG) tube and use it to administer the drug, if necessary.
- Give acetaminophen to treat fever.

➡ **NurseALERT** Never give aspirin-containing products to a patient with thyroid storm because aspirin displaces thyroxine (T_4) from thyroid-binding globulin, which increases levels of free T_4 and exacerbates the patient's hypermetabolism.

- Take steps to keep the patient safe. Also keep the patient's environment as calm and quiet as possible to minimize agitation.
- Be prepared to administer additional emergency interventions in response to the patient's underlying condition.

WHAT TO DO NEXT

Once the patient has started treatment for thyroid storm, your continued care should include the following:

- Monitor her vital signs hourly, and continually observe her for respiratory distress, tachyarrhythmias, and signs of decreased cardiac output, such as hypotension and an altered level of consciousness. Be prepared to treat cardiopulmonary complications as they arise.
- Maintain fluid replacement therapy to prevent hypovolemia.
- Continue to give antithyroid hormone therapy (by mouth or NG tube) every 4 to 8 hours, as prescribed.
- Expect to start iodide therapy 1 hour after giving antithyroid hormone to inhibit further release of thyroid hormone. Either give 2 g/day of sodium iodide I.V. or 10 drops of potassium iodide saturated solution (SSKI) by mouth every 8 hours. When giving iodide orally, mix it with milk or fruit juice to make it more palatable. Have the patient drink it through a straw to avoid staining her teeth.
- Give acetaminophen every 3 to 4 hours, as needed. If you need to reduce her temperature quickly, use a hypothermia blanket or ice packs and fans. Be careful not to chill the patient or make her shiver because doing so will increase her metabolic rate.
- Continue to give propranolol every 3 to 4 hours I.V., as needed, until the patient's symptoms are under control. Then switch to oral therapy, as ordered (usually 20 to 40 mg every 6 hours).

FOLLOW-UP CARE

- Try to determine what precipitated the thyroid storm, and take steps to prevent a recurrence.
- When nausea and vomiting have subsided, remove the patient's NG tube and give her six high-calorie meals a day.
- Taper and discontinue the beta-adrenergic therapy, as ordered.
- Stress the importance of continuing antithyroid and iodide therapy in keeping with the physician's order until the patient's hyperthyroidism is controlled.
- Prepare the patient for radioactive iodine therapy or surgery, as prescribed.
- Assess the patient's and family's knowledge of hyperthyroidism and teach them about the condition, as indicated.
- Emphasize the importance of close follow-up care.

T

SPECIAL CONSIDERATIONS

- After thyroid storm, the patient's hyperthyroidism may need more aggressive management than it did before to keep the condition under control and prevent a recurrence.
- Because therapy for hyperthyroidism may induce hypothyroidism, you'll need to teach the patient about the signs and symptoms of hypothyroidism. Tell her to report them to her physician if they develop.

TRACHEOESOPHAGEAL FISTULA

An abnormal communication between the esophagus and trachea, a tracheoesophageal fistula (TEF) usually is a congenital anomaly seen in neonates. However, an adult may acquire TEF as a complication of esophageal cancer, esophageal perforation, long-term tracheal intubation, blunt chest trauma, corrosive esophageal burns, virulent infection (in an immunocompromised patient), and pressure necrosis caused by a cuffed endotracheal or tracheostomy tube (with long-term mechanical ventilation). (See *Looking at tracheoesophageal fistula*.)

If your patient is at risk for TEF, you'll need to stay alert for typical signs and symptoms—and then act swiftly to avoid respiratory compromise. Remember—in acute or severe cases, TEF may lead to respiratory arrest.

WHAT TO LOOK FOR

Clinical findings in a patient with TEF may include:

- cough associated with eating
- greenish material aspirated from a tracheostomy tube
- food-tainted sputum
- chronic, unproductive cough
- dyspnea
- hemoptysis
- stridor
- hoarseness
- weight loss
- weakness
- chest pain
- hypoxemia
- cyanosis.

WHAT TO DO IMMEDIATELY

If you think that your patient has developed TEF, notify the physician. Then take these steps:

- Position the patient to maximize respirations, typically in semi-Fowler's to high Fowler's position.
- Withhold oral intake.

LOOKING AT TRACHEOESOPHAGEAL FISTULA

In this cross section of the upper airway, you can see a tracheoesophageal fistula, an abnormal tubelike opening between the trachea and esophagus.

A tracheoesophageal fistula commonly develops in acute-care patients from long-term intubation with both a cuffed tracheal tube and a hard, plastic, large-bore nasogastric tube.

The cuffed tracheal tube, which rests in the trachea, exerts pressure against the anterior esophageal wall. With continuous pressure from the tubes, the posterior tracheal wall and the anterior esophageal wall weaken and become necrotic, causing the fistula to form.

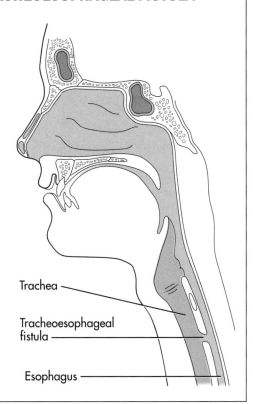

Trachea

Tracheoesophageal fistula

Esophagus

➡ **NurseALERT** If your patient has been receiving enteral feedings, stop them. Even though the tip of the feeding tube is positioned in the stomach or duodenum (below the esophagus), formula may reflux into the esophagus and pass through the TEF into the trachea.

- Suction secretions as necessary to maintain a patent airway and prevent aspiration. Gather emergency supplies, including a tracheostomy tube, in case they're needed to maintain the patient's airway.
- Assess the patient's vital signs and auscultate his lungs.
- Prepare the patient for ordered diagnostic studies, including X-rays, computed tomography, and radiologic contrast studies. (See *Confirming tracheoesophageal fistula,* page 370.)

WHAT TO DO NEXT

After your patient is stable, implement the following interventions:
- Continue to suction his mouth, pharynx, and trachea, as needed.
- Provide tracheostomy care, as indicated.

CONFIRMING TRACHEOESOPHAGEAL FISTULA

If you suspect that your patient has tracheoesophageal fistula (TEF), you may need to prepare him for one or more of the following diagnostic studies.

CHEST X-RAY

A chest X-ray may be used in combination with other studies to confirm TEF or reveal TEF complications. Both frontal and lateral views are obtained for better visualization of the trachea, esophagus, and lungs.

Expected results

A chest X-ray may confirm the presence of an opening or air-filled blind pouch in the proximal esophagus. It also may show TEF-related pneumonia or pneumonitis (for example, from aspiration of food from the esophagus into the trachea and lungs).

CONTRAST STUDIES

Radiologic or fluoroscopic studies using a contrast medium may help distinguish esophageal atresia (a pathologic closure of the esophagus, such as from a tumor) from TEF. Contrast medium, introduced into the esophagus through a catheter passed through the pa-

tient's nose, is tracked as it passes through the GI tract. Films are taken during its progression.

Expected results

The contrast medium helps define TEF. It also helps differentiate aspiration of liquids secondary to TEF from aspiration resulting from fluids that collect above an esophageal stricture or obstruction or that pool in a blind pouch in the esophagus.

ENDOSCOPY

Endoscopy usually is done in combination with other tests to confirm TEF. As the physician passes an endoscope through the patient's mouth and into the esophagus, a small fiber-optic camera on the endoscope's tip allows visualization of the area being explored. Video images are viewed as the endoscope is passed into the stomach, if necessary.

Expected results

Endoscopy may reveal the presence of TEF, a blind pouch, or esophageal stricture or obstruction.

- Continue to monitor the patient's vital signs and respiratory status, including breath sounds.
- Evaluate the patient for aspiration pneumonia by assessing his lungs for adventitious breath sounds and observing the amount and quality of his sputum.
- Continue to withhold oral intake, as ordered.
- Obtain blood samples for arterial blood gas analysis and routine preoperative tests, including complete blood count, prothrombin time, activated partial thromboplastin time, and blood type and crossmatch.
- As ordered, prepare your patient for surgery to correct TEF. Surgical options include fistula interruption and closure, creation of an artificial esophagus using a portion of intestine, and muscle-flap obliteration of the fistula. If your patient can't tolerate these approaches, a stent may be placed in his esophagus endoscopically to prevent aspiration or a gastrostomy or jejunostomy tube may be inserted to provide nutrition.

FOLLOW-UP CARE

- After fistula repair or stent placement, monitor the patient for signs and symptoms of leakage around the fistula site or stent.
- Administer I.V. solutions, as prescribed. Also give prescribed antibiotics and analgesics.

- Maintain strict fluid intake and output records.
- Withhold oral intake until the physician indicates otherwise. Then, gradually introduce fluids, and observe the patient for coughing and choking during feedings.
- Monitor for complications of TEF or corrective surgery, including stricture of the anastomosis or esophagus, pneumothorax, and fistula recurrence.
- If the patient has chest tubes, make sure to maintain the integrity of the closed drainage system and observe the color and amount of drainage.

SPECIAL CONSIDERATIONS
- To prevent the development of TEF, maintain endotracheal or tracheostomy tube cuff pressure at 18 to 22 mm Hg. Check the pressure at least every 8 hours.
- Keep in mind that about 5% of patients with esophageal cancer develop TEF. When caring for a patient with esophageal cancer, instruct him and his family about TEF signs and symptoms.

TRACHEOSTOMY OCCLUSION

If your patient's tracheostomy tube becomes occluded, she may suffer complete airway obstruction and respiratory arrest unless her condition is corrected promptly. Typically, tracheostomy occlusion results from thick mucus secretions, which may accumulate quickly in a patient with a tracheostomy because she lacks the humidity normally supplied by the upper airway. (See *Tracheostomy occlusion*, page 372.)

Your top priority in this emergency is to maintain a patent airway. But you'll also need to tailor your response to your patient's particular situation—mainly, whether her tracheostomy is new or long-standing and whether she's on a mechanical ventilator or breathing on her own.

WHAT TO LOOK FOR
Clinical findings in a patient with an occluded tracheostomy may include:
- distressed, panicked appearance
- acute dyspnea
- whistling noise through the tracheostomy with each breath
- decreased or absent breath sounds
- little or no airflow through the tracheostomy
- ineffective coughing
- pale, cyanotic skin
- diaphoresis
- use of accessory breathing muscles
- altered level of consciousness
- elevated blood pressure

T

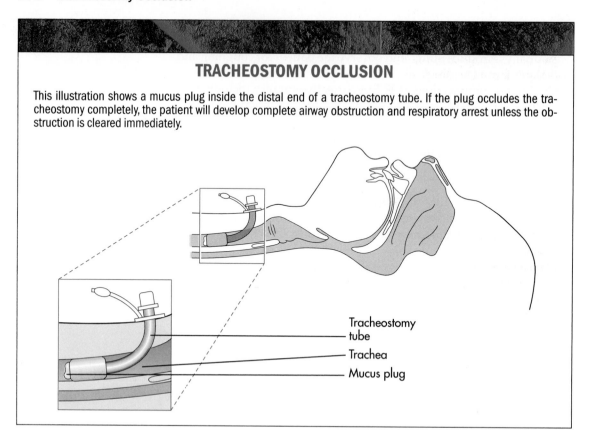

TRACHEOSTOMY OCCLUSION

This illustration shows a mucus plug inside the distal end of a tracheostomy tube. If the plug occludes the tracheostomy completely, the patient will develop complete airway obstruction and respiratory arrest unless the obstruction is cleared immediately.

Tracheostomy tube

Trachea

Mucus plug

- increased pulse rate
- oxygen saturation below 90%.

WHAT TO DO IMMEDIATELY

If you suspect that your patient has an occluded tracheostomy, notify the physician. Then carry out these measures:

- Place the patient in semi-Fowler's position, as tolerated, to keep her airway open and promote removal of mucus or other occluding material.
- Gently remove the inner cannula of the tracheostomy tube, if present, and inspect it. Discard the occluded cannula, if it's disposable, and insert a new one. If it's not disposable, clean it with hydrogen peroxide and normal saline solution according to your facility's policy, and then reinsert it.

If the inner cannula is absent or isn't occluded

- If your patient's tracheostomy tube doesn't have an inner cannula or if the inner cannula isn't occluded, suspect an occlusion farther down the tube or the patient's respiratory tract. To help dislodge the material causing the blockage, ask the patient to cough as forcefully as possible.

- If coughing fails to remove the obstruction, suction the tracheostomy tube.
- ➡ **NurseALERT** Never suction for more than 10 seconds at a time. Longer suctioning times may cause alveolar oxygen pressure to drop, possibly inducing hypoxemia. Between suctioning attempts, hyperoxygenate the patient by giving three breaths of 100% oxygen, if indicated, to minimize hypoxia.
- If these interventions fail to clear the blockage, notify the physician.
- ➡ **NurseALERT** Don't make further attempts to ventilate through an occluded tracheostomy tube because you could force air into tissue surrounding the stoma, causing subcutaneous emphysema, edema, and tracheal compression.

Inserting a new tube

- If your patient has a mature or healed tracheostomy, replace the tracheostomy tube if permitted by your facility. Because her tracheostomy tract is well established, replacement should be fairly easy. (See *Replacing a tracheostomy tube*, page 374.)
- If your patient has a new tracheostomy (less than 7 days old) and the tracheostomy tube must be removed because it's occluded, insert a hemostat or tracheal dilator to keep the airway open until the physician arrives.
- ➡ **NurseALERT** Don't try to replace a new tracheostomy tube yourself. Normally, a tracheostomy tract takes about 5 to 7 days to form; inserting a new tube before the tract heals may create a false passage or may cause tracheal compression or airway obstruction. Instead, prepare to assist the physician in replacing the tracheostomy tube. If retention sutures are present on either side of the stoma, you or the physician may grasp and pull them to spread open the stoma before inserting the new tube. Or the physician may open the stoma using tracheal dilators.

Establishing endotracheal intubation

- If a new tracheostomy tube can't be inserted and the patient progresses to respiratory arrest, assist with endotracheal intubation, as ordered. Keep in mind, though, that intubation is attempted only if the patient has no significant laryngeal trauma and no obstruction above the level of the tracheostomy site.
- Until endotracheal intubation is completed, ventilate the patient through the mouth and nose using a manual resuscitation device. As you do, watch for air escaping through the stoma; if it does, cover the stoma with a sterile occlusive dressing.
- After the endotracheal tube has been placed, expect the physician to reinsert the tracheostomy tube. Be sure to have a trach tray and replacement tube readily available.

T

TIPS AND TECHNIQUES

REPLACING A TRACHEOSTOMY TUBE

If you can't clear your patient's occluded tracheostomy tube, you may need to replace the tube—but only if the tracheostomy has healed and your facility allows you to do so. Using standard precautions, follow the steps below:

- Gather the necessary equipment. Then wash your hands.
- Elevate the patient's shoulders with a pillow and gently hyperextend her neck.
- Put on clean gloves.
- Cut the tracheostomy ties and deflate the tracheostomy cuff.
- Gently remove the tracheostomy tube. If the tube's sutured to the patient's skin, cut the sutures before trying to remove it.
- Using cotton-tipped applicators, clean the stoma—first with hydrogen peroxide and then with normal saline solution or according to your facility's policy.

- Remove your gloves and put on a new pair of sterile gloves.
- Insert the obturator into the new tracheostomy tube and apply a water-soluble lubricant to the tip of the tube.
- Ask the patient to take a deep breath. Then insert the tube into the stoma at a 45-degree angle to her neck.
- Once the tube is in the proper position, immediately remove the obturator so air can flow through the tube.
- Next, inflate the cuff (if present), check for bilateral breath sounds, and insert and secure the inner cannula.
- Secure the tube with ties and place a dressing under the tube. Make sure the dressing isn't too snug; you should be able to fit a finger comfortably between the patient's neck and the ties.
- Provide supplemental oxygen through a tracheostomy mask, if prescribed.

WHAT TO DO NEXT

Once your patient is stabilized and has a patent airway, take the following actions:

- Monitor her blood pressure, heart rate, and respiratory rate every 4 to 8 hours, as indicated. Watch for a rise or fall in blood pressure and an increase in her heart and respiratory rates—possible signs of tracheostomy reocclusion or improper tube placement.
- Stay alert for other signs of tracheostomy reocclusion, such as dyspnea and accessory muscle use.
- Monitor the patient's breath sounds every 4 to 8 hours; be sure to listen for decreased or adventitious breath sounds.
- Observe the patient for neurologic changes, such as anxiety, confusion, agitation, and mental sluggishness; they may indicate hypoxia or hypercapnia.
- Monitor arterial blood gas and pulse oximetry values, as indicated. Watch for decreased partial pressure of arterial oxygen, increased partial pressure of arterial carbon dioxide, and decreased blood pH.
- Keep the head of the patient's bed elevated, unless contraindicated.

FOLLOW-UP CARE

- Change the patient's position frequently to prevent pooling of respiratory secretions.
- Provide adequate humidification and hydration to loosen and aid removal of respiratory secretions.

- Monitor the patient's fluid intake and output. As prescribed, administer I.V. fluids to maintain hydration.
- Suction the tracheostomy tube as often as necessary to clear secretions and keep the airway open. Immediately after surgery, you may need to suction as often as every 5 minutes; after about 72 hours, expect to suction every 3 to 4 hours.
- Perform tracheostomy care as often as needed. If the inner cannula is disposable, be sure to change it according to your facility's policy.
- Regularly hyperinflate the patient's lungs to provide an artificial sigh that promotes lung expansion, enhances coughing, and helps remove tracheobronchial secretions.
- If ordered, perform chest physiotherapy to help remove secretions.

SPECIAL CONSIDERATIONS
- Keep a replacement tracheostomy tube of the same size as the patient's tube (or smaller) at the bedside at all times.
- If the patient has retention sutures, tape them to her skin for easy access in an emergency. Label them "left" and "right" to indicate which sides of the stoma they're attached to.

TRANSFUSION REACTIONS

Transfusion of blood or blood products can save a patient's life. It also can cause a range of adverse reactions that may threaten the patient's life. Reactions that arise during or within a few hours after the transfusion are called acute reactions. Those that arise days, weeks, or even years after the transfusion are called delayed reactions. In both cases, a reaction can result in either an immunologic response, such as a hemolytic reaction, or a nonimmunologic response, such as hypothermia caused by the infusion of cold blood. (See *Recognizing transfusion reactions*, page 376.)

Transfusion reactions can arise for a number of reasons, including:
- ABO incompatibility
- inaccurate crossmatching
- allergy (antigen-antibody response) to donor plasma proteins
- severe allergy (anaphylaxis, an immunoglobulin A–mediated response)
- the wrong blood or blood product
- infusing blood too rapidly, which can cause circulatory overload
- rough handling or chemical contamination, which can hemolyze red blood cells
- giving drugs or hypertonic solutions in the same line as the blood, which lyses red blood cells.

T

RECOGNIZING TRANSFUSION REACTIONS

If your patient has a transfusion reaction, the clinical effects reflect the type of reaction. Use this table to help familiarize yourself with different types of transfusion reactions and their effects.

Reaction	Clinical effects
Allergic (mild)	• Itching • Flushing • Rash • Urticaria • No fever
Anaphylactic	• Anxiety • Dyspnea • Wheezing • Urticaria • Difficulty swallowing • Hypotension • Tachycardia • Chest pain • Cyanosis • Cardiac arrest
Hemolytic	• Fever • Chills • Low back pain • Hypotension • Tachycardia • Tachypnea • Hemoglobinuria • Acute renal failure • Shock • Cardiac arrest
Febrile (pyrogenic)	• Anxiety • Flushing • Headache • Muscle pain • Sudden chills and fever
Serum sickness	• Fever • Joint pain • Rash • Splenomegaly • Swollen lymph nodes

Adverse reactions can arise even in autologous transfusions, in which the patient receives his own blood. They stem from such problems as coagulopathies, microemboli, hemolysis, and sepsis.

Not all transfusion reactions are life-threatening. If your patient develops one, however, you'll need to be ready to respond quickly and accurately.

WHAT TO LOOK FOR
Clinical findings vary with the type and severity of the transfusion reaction involved. An acute reaction may include the following:

With a mild transfusion reaction
- itching
- urticaria
- flushing
- rash.

With a severe transfusion reaction
- anxiety, feelings of impending doom
- chills
- temperature increased by more than 33.8° F (1° C)
- flushing
- muscle aches
- flank pain
- low back pain
- decreased urine output
- dark or red urine (hemoglobinuria)
- tachycardia
- dyspnea
- bronchoconstriction with wheezing
- stridor
- hypotension
- jaundice
- petechiae
- failure of blood to clot (oozing or frank bleeding)
- substernal chest pain.

WHAT TO DO IMMEDIATELY
If you think that your patient is having a transfusion reaction, notify the physician and follow these measures:
- ➡ **Nurse ALERT** Stop the transfusion by closing the clamp that's nearest the patient. Remove the blood container and tubing. Use a new I.V. administration set and normal saline solution to keep the line open.
- Check the name and blood group on the bag against the recipient's name and blood group to make sure the patient is receiving the correct transfusion.
- Send the blood bag and blood administration tubing as well as the saline solution used with the transfusion and its tubing to the blood bank. Label the unused blood and tubing with "blood transfusion reaction."
- Check the patient's vital signs and repeat every 30 minutes thereafter for the next 4 hours.
- If the patient shows signs of heart failure, raise the head of his bed to enhance lung expansion and facilitate breathing. Assess his oxygen

T

saturation by way of pulse oximetry, and give oxygen, as ordered. Prepare to give a diuretic as well, if ordered.
- If the patient develops anaphylaxis, give epinephrine subcutaneously or by I.V., as ordered.

WHAT TO DO NEXT
Once your patient has stabilized, take these actions:
- Obtain serum samples for direct antiglobulin (Coombs'), hemoglobinemia, bilirubin, complete blood count, creatinine, and coagulation testing.
- Send a urine specimen, preferably the first-voided, to the laboratory. Label the specimen with "blood transfusion reaction."
- If the reaction involves only urticaria and symptoms are mild and transient, give diphenhydramine (Benadryl) and restart the infusion after 15 to 30 minutes, as ordered.
- If the reaction is febrile, administer antipyretics, as prescribed, and provide comfort measures.
- If the reaction is hemolytic, prepare to treat the patient for shock. Give I.V. fluids and diuretics to prevent renal failure, and monitor his vital signs closely. Anticipate insertion of an indwelling urinary catheter and assess his output hourly. Anticipate invasive monitoring to evaluate his hemodynamic status.
- If the patient has hypotension, give dopamine (Intropin) as prescribed.

FOLLOW-UP CARE
- Record your observations and assessments of the patient's reaction, and complete any transfusion reaction forms required by your facility.
- Try to determine what caused the reaction.
- Continue giving fluids and diuretics to maintain diuresis.
- If the patient developed acute renal failure after a hemolytic reaction, anticipate the need for hemodialysis to correct fluid and electrolyte imbalances.
- If bacterial contamination may have caused the reaction, obtain cultures of the patient's blood and the blood container for both aerobic and anaerobic organisms. Give the patient broad-spectrum antibiotics, vasopressors, and corticosteroids, as indicated.

SPECIAL CONSIDERATIONS
- If a patient scheduled to receive blood or blood products has developed urticaria or other signs of mild allergic reaction with previous transfusions, give him prophylactic antihistamine, as ordered.
- If the patient developed fever without hemolysis from previous transfusions, give him prophylactic antipyretic therapy before the next transfusion, as indicated.
- ➡ **NurseALERT** Before administering blood, check the patient's name, number, ABO status, and Rh status; the blood bank identification number; and the expiration date on the blood container's label. Have another nurse or physician verify that the information is correct. Make

sure that both people who check the blood also check the patient's identification bracelet and sign the slip that accompanies the blood.
- Before beginning a transfusion, obtain the patient's baseline vital signs. Then begin to transfuse the blood slowly. Check vital signs again in 10 to 15 minutes, and observe the patient closely for the first hour. If a major incompatibility exists or a severe allergic reaction occurs, it usually appears during infusion of the first 50 ml of blood. If no problems arise during this observation time, adjust the flow rate as ordered and continue to monitor the patient according to your facility's policy.
- Always administer blood within 30 minutes of obtaining it. Use an 18G or 20G I.V. catheter and blood filter. Infuse 1 unit of packed red blood cells or whole blood over about 2 hours. To prevent hemolysis, use only normal saline solution to infuse the blood.
- ➡ **NurseALERT** Taking more than 4 hours to infuse the blood or blood products raises the danger of bacterial growth and contamination. Infusing blood too rapidly can result in circulatory overload, leading to pulmonary edema.

TRAUMA, MULTIPLE

Multiple trauma involves injury to more than one body system. Common causes of multiple trauma include motor vehicle accidents, falls, thermal or electrical burns, and violence.

Depending on their cause, the patient's injuries may or may not be visible. They may involve penetrating wounds, as from a gunshot, a stabbing, or an impalement. Or they may involve blunt trauma, as from a motor vehicle accident, a fall, or an assault. Naturally, nonpenetrating wounds can be much more difficult to detect.

Too much emphasis on the patient's visible injuries is a common and dangerous mistake in trauma evaluation. While you're trying to treat a serious but not life-threatening surface wound, for example, your patient could die as a result of a silent splenic injury. That's largely why visible wounds typically aren't repaired until the patient undergoes a complete assessment.

The key to mounting an efficient, coordinated response to multiple trauma is an understanding of assessment, management, and treatment principles appropriate for these types of injury. In general, you'll want to follow predetermined protocols and launch an organized team effort. By doing so, you can improve your patient's outcomes—possibly save her life.

WHAT TO LOOK FOR
Clinical findings vary with the combination of injuries sustained but may include:
- changes in level of consciousness, such as agitation, disorientation, drowsiness, lethargy, stupor, and coma

T

- swollen or asymmetrical body parts
- closed or open fractures
- lacerations, contusions, and abrasions
- asymmetrical pupils or an abnormal reaction to light
- drainage of clear or bloody fluid from the ears or nose
- nasal flaring and circumoral cyanosis
- cervical deformity, swelling, tenderness, or vein distention
- chest deformity or asymmetry of chest wall movement
- sternal retractions, altered respiratory rate and depth, and adventitious breath sounds
- decreased range of motion
- tenderness to palpation
- abdominal distention, contusions, swelling, and bleeding
- absent bowel sounds
- perineal contusions, swelling, and bleeding
- pelvic instability
- blood in stool or urine
- bleeding from the urinary meatus
- incontinence
- foreign objects in body orifices
- depressed or bulging anterior fontanelle (in an infant).

WHAT TO DO IMMEDIATELY

If your patient sustains multiple trauma, notify the physician and follow these measures:

- Assess the patient's airway, breathing, and circulation; perform cardiopulmonary resuscitation as necessary.
- ➡ **NurseALERT** Until proved otherwise, assume that a traumatic injury affects the cervical spine and immobilize the area.
- If needed, use suction to clear the patient's airway. Prepare for endotracheal intubation and manual ventilation, as necessary. Verify the adequacy of manual ventilations repeatedly as you continue to assess the patient's injuries.
- Remove the patient's clothing by cutting it off. As you do so, assess for vasoconstriction or diaphoresis and for the rate and fullness of the pulse at her wrist or foot.
- Note the motion of the patient's chest wall and the pattern of her breathing. Watch for retractions. Auscultate the patient's breath sounds. Be alert for absent breath sounds, which could indicate lung collapse, or adventitious breath sounds.
- Assess the patient's cardiac function and treat cardiac arrest; begin closed-chest compressions, if necessary.
- Look for open wounds and deformities. If the patient is bleeding, apply direct pressure to control it. Inspect her limbs for lacerations, contusions, and swelling. Check their temperature, pulses, sensation, and tenderness to palpation or range of motion.

- Assess the patient's level of consciousness and the size and reactivity of her pupils.
- Examine the patient's abdomen for contusions, swelling, and bleeding. Using a gentle squeezing motion, assess her pelvis for instability.
- ➡ **NurseALERT** Don't rock the patient's pelvis because you could do further injury to bones or blood vessels.
- Inspect the patient's urinary meatus for bleeding or incontinence. Assist with vaginal and rectal examinations, as needed. If the pelvic and perineal examination shows no obvious injuries, insert an indwelling urinary catheter to assess hourly urine output.
- ➡ **NurseALERT** If the patient might have a urethral injury that isn't readily apparent, delay insertion of the catheter until further radiologic studies rule out the injury.
- Roll the patient onto her side to assess her back for injuries.
- Assess for and take steps to control hypovolemic shock. Establish I.V. access fluid resuscitation; if you can't establish a peripheral venous line, anticipate insertion of a central venous line.
- Be prepared to help apply or manage a pneumatic antishock garment, as indicated.
- Obtain baseline laboratory studies, as ordered.

WHAT TO DO NEXT
When the patient has stabilized, take these steps:
- Prepare her for additional diagnostic tests, such as computed tomographic scanning, magnetic resonance imaging, and ultrasonography, as ordered.
- Splint any possible fractures to stabilize them. Then prepare the patient for X-rays to determine the extent of bony injury.
- Clean and bandage any open wounds. Assist with suturing if time and the patient's condition permit.
- Facilitate specialist consultations, additional tests, and surgical intervention.
- If the patient is at risk for aspiration, such as if her level of consciousness is decreased or her gag reflex is absent, insert a nasogastric tube to decompress the patient's stomach and decrease her risk of vomiting and aspiration.
- ➡ **NurseALERT** If the patient has maxillofacial injuries or a possible basilar skull fracture, use the orogastric route for decompression.
- Obtain additional diagnostic tests, including blood type and crossmatch, complete blood count, coagulation studies, blood urea nitrogen level, and serum amylase, glucose, creatinine, electrolyte, and bilirubin levels.
- ➡ **NurseALERT** Keep in mind that you may need to obtain blood alcohol levels and toxicology tests. If so, take samples during the primary survey when you establish I.V. access.
- Continue to monitor the patient's arterial blood gases; provide respiratory and cardiac support, as needed.

T

DIAGNOSTIC PERITONEAL LAVAGE

If you're caring for a multiple trauma patient who has sustained blunt abdominal injury, be prepared to assist with diagnostic peritoneal lavage. This procedure helps detect signs of significant intra-abdominal injury that might otherwise be missed during a routine abdominal assessment. It's particularly useful if your patient can't provide you with valuable assessment information because she's intoxicated, unconscious, or hemodynamically unstable.

Diagnostic peritoneal lavage may be performed as a closed, open, or semiopen procedure. In the closed procedure, the physician inserts a percutaneous peritoneal catheter into the peritoneal cavity. This approach is somewhat risky because the catheter may penetrate underlying organs and blood vessels.

In the open procedure, the physician opens the abdominal cavity to directly visualize the underlying structures and insert the peritoneal catheter. This procedure takes more time and introduces air into the peritoneal cavity.

In the semiopen approach (see illustration), which is preferable because it's quick, easy, and reliable, the physician makes a small incision around the umbilicus to allow insertion of the peritoneal catheter.

Before the procedure, as ordered, expect to insert a nasogastric tube to decompress the stomach and an indwelling urinary catheter to drain the bladder to prevent injury to those organs. After making the incision, the physician inserts a peritoneal catheter. If he withdraws at least 10 ml of frank blood, the test is considered positive. Depending on her condition, the patient will probably require further diagnostic evaluation, such as computed tomography, or immediate surgery. If no frank blood appears, 1 L of warmed normal saline solution or lactated Ringer's solution is infused into the peritoneal cavity. Then the liter bag is inverted and placed below the patient at floor level to allow the fluid to drain

by gravity. The fluid is sent to the laboratory for analysis. The following test results are considered positive:

- red blood cell count greater than or equal to 100,000 cells/mm^3
- white blood cell count greater than or equal to 500 cells/mm^3
- amylase greater than or equal to 200 milliunits/ml
- bile present
- bacteria present in significant numbers.

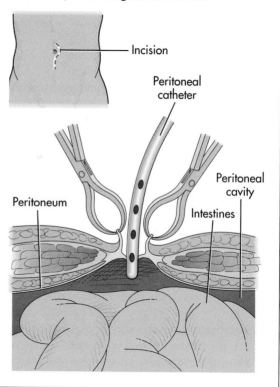

- Obtain a lateral X-ray of the patient's cervical spine (C1 to C7), as ordered, and an anterior view of her chest and abdomen.
- Test the patient's stool, nasogastric aspirate, and urine for blood.
- Update the patient and her family frequently about her status.

FOLLOW-UP CARE
- Provide supportive care, as necessary; assess frequently for changes in the patient's condition.
- Continue to provide support and information to the patient and her family about her progress and treatments.

SPECIAL CONSIDERATIONS

- Because the condition of an injured patient can change rapidly and repeatedly, you'll need to constantly reassess all aspects of the patient's condition, even as you undertake your initial assessment.
- If the patient is unstable and unresponsive to fluid resuscitation, prepare her for diagnostic peritoneal lavage to determine whether she has internal bleeding (which would account for her continued hypovolemia) and needs surgery. She also may undergo this procedure if she could have peritonitis from blunt or penetrating abdominal injury. (See *Diagnostic peritoneal lavage*.)
- Keep in mind that traumatic physical injury can involve traumatic emotional injury as well. Do your best to provide supportive emotional care to the patient and her family throughout her assessment and care.

T-TUBE OCCLUSION

A T-tube is a temporary drain inserted into the biliary drainage system and extended out of the abdomen through a stab wound. It's commonly used in patients with gallbladder disease to help prevent scarring of the common bile duct after duct exploration and to provide controlled postoperative external biliary drainage. A T-tube also permits access to the biliary system for postoperative extraction of residual stones. (See *Visualizing T-tube placement*, page 384.)

If your patient's T-tube becomes occluded by gallstones or gallstone gravel, biliary flow may become obstructed, causing pressure in the common bile duct to rise. This in turn may lead to leakage around the suture line. In some cases, occlusion causes perforation of the duct with subsequent peritonitis, which may imperil your patient's life. An occlusion may occur anywhere along the path of the T-tube—above or below the cross T or within the stem. Your prompt response can improve your patient's outcome.

WHAT TO LOOK FOR

Clinical findings may include:
- decreased or absent drainage of bile from the T-tube, depending on the part of the tube that's occluded
- leakage around the insertion site
- complaints of sudden abdominal pain in the right upper quadrant or epigastric area
- fever.

WHAT TO DO IMMEDIATELY

If you suspect that your patient has an obstructed T-tube, notify the physician. Then carry out these interventions:
- Inspect the drainage tubing for kinking and clamping.
- ➡ **NurseALERT** Don't try to irrigate or aspirate the T-tube because you may worsen the occlusion and raise pressure in the common bile duct.

VISUALIZING T-TUBE PLACEMENT

Your patient may return from cholecystectomy (surgical gallbladder removal) with a T-tube. This illustration shows T-tube placement in relation to the hepatic and common bile ducts and the duodenum. The tube may be placed over a roll of gauze and taped to the skin to prevent it from moving.

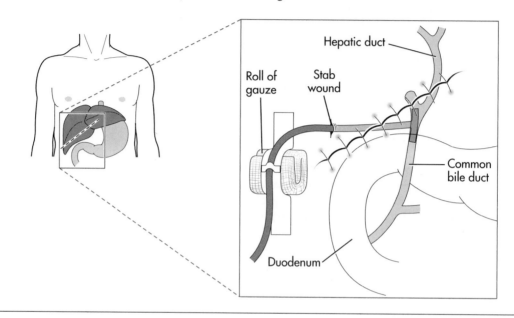

- Obtain your patient's vital signs and regularly monitor for changes that suggest he's developing peritonitis.
- Evaluate the patient's pain for severity, type, and location.
- Assess his abdomen, listening for hypoactive bowel sounds and gently palpating for tenderness and muscle rigidity.
- ➡ **NurseALERT** Don't assess for rebound tenderness or perform deep palpation. Doing so could increase intra-abdominal pressure and, possibly, perforate the common bile duct.
- Assess the T-tube site for leakage. Suspect possible aseptic peritonitis caused by bile irritating the peritoneum or biliary fistula if you notice leakage in a patient who has increased abdominal pain, chills, fever, and decreased tube drainage.

WHAT TO DO NEXT
After taking the initial actions, follow these guidelines:
- Prepare the patient for possible surgical or radiologic correction of the T-tube occlusion.
- Continue to monitor the patient's vital signs, biliary drainage, and complaints of pain every hour. Be sure to evaluate for changes in the nature of his pain.

- If leakage develops around the T-tube insertion site, keep the area clean; bile is highly irritating to the skin.
- Establish I.V. access, and administer fluids and antibiotics, as prescribed.

FOLLOW-UP CARE
- After the T-tube occlusion has been corrected, provide appropriate postprocedure care.
- Continue to monitor T-tube drainage for color and amount.
- ➡ **NurseALERT** Report T-tube drainage that exceeds 1,000 ml/day.
- Frequently inspect the tubing for kinks; ensure adequate slack between the tubing and drainage bag so the patient can move.
- Keep the drainage bag below the level of the patient's waist or common bile duct to prevent reflux of bile.
- Expect T-tube drainage to decrease as bile resumes its normal flow. Observe for reduced drainage and return of stools to their usual color.
- Care for the T-tube site, as ordered. Report signs and symptoms of infection, such as redness, warmth, and inflammation.

SPECIAL CONSIDERATIONS
- Be aware that a T-tube routinely is removed 7 to 10 days after surgery. It may be left in place longer if the patient's at risk for retained stones or if the bile duct remains edematous. The tube can be removed easily in an outpatient setting.
- Before discharge, teach the patient and family members how to care for the T-tube and its site. Instruct them to keep the drainage bag below the level of the T-tube insertion site. Demonstrate how to empty the drainage bag and clean the insertion site. Review which signs and symptoms to report immediately: redness, swelling, and purulent drainage at the insertion site; fever; and recurrence of right upper quadrant pain, bile drainage around the T-tube, nausea, vomiting, and clay-colored stools (signs of obstruction).

TUBE-FEEDING ASPIRATION

A patient who's receiving enteral nutrition through a nasoenteric tube may aspirate the feeding formula—an event that may either cause sudden, obvious signs of respiratory distress or go undetected until the patient develops fever, pulmonary infiltrates, tachypnea, hypoxemia, hypercapnia, or respiratory acidosis.

Aspiration usually results from improper tube placement during insertion, tube migration after insertion, or aspiration during a feeding. (See *Detecting aspirated feeding formula*, page 386.)

Identifying patients at high risk for tube-feeding aspiration can reduce the incidence of this complication. Conditions that increase a patient's risk include:
- impaired cough or gag reflex

T

TIPS AND TECHNIQUES

DETECTING ASPIRATED FEEDING FORMULA

To detect aspiration early in a patient receiving tube feedings, consider using one of these methods.

GLUCOSE OXIDASE REAGENT STRIPS

If your patient receives a glucose-containing formula, you can test his respiratory secretions with a glucose oxidase reagent strip.

Because these strips also detect blood sugar, be sure to use only a bloodless tracheal aspirant. Suspect aspiration of feeding formula—and discontinue feedings—if the patient's secretions repeatedly test above 130 mg/dl of glucose.

FOOD COLORING

Because food coloring alters the appearance of tracheobronchial secretions, you can detect aspiration by observing the patient's respiratory secretions for the color added to the feeding formula. Some manufacturers now supply formulas with a food dye already added.

Be aware, though, that adding food coloring may cause false-positive results when testing stool or gastric fluid for blood, and it may complicate interpretation of results obtained when using reagent strips to estimate the pH of bodily secretions. Also, this method is less reliable than glucose oxidase reagent strip testing.

- decreased level of consciousness
- heavy sedation
- neurologic disorders
- dementia
- administration of neuromuscular blocking agents
- compromised esophageal sphincter (as from hiatal hernia or gastroesophageal reflux disease)
- delayed gastric emptying (common in diabetics)
- ileus.

If your patient has one of these risk factors, the physician may insert the tube under fluoroscopic guidance.

The severity of long-term pulmonary injury after tube-feeding aspiration depends on the pH of aspirated secretions. Acidic secretions cause mechanical damage to lung tissue, whereas alkaline secretions promote pneumonia. In the worst-case scenario, tube-feeding aspiration may be fatal. Clearly, you need to be ready to respond swiftly if your patient shows signs of aspiration.

WHAT TO LOOK FOR

Clinical findings in a patient who has aspirated feeding formula may include:

- cough that produces frothy sputum
- crackles or rhonchi on auscultation
- wheezing
- tachypnea
- tachycardia
- immediate fever (a direct response to aspiration) or later-onset fever (occurring within 72 hours from respiratory infection)
- increased white blood cell count 24 to 72 hours after aspiration
- cyanosis (usually a late sign)

- hypoxemia, as indicated by decreased oxygen saturation and by arterial blood gas (ABG) analysis that reveals decreased partial pressure of arterial oxygen
- hypoxia, manifested by restlessness, anxiety, decreased level of consciousness, and dyspnea.

WHAT TO DO IMMEDIATELY

If you suspect that your patient has aspirated feeding formula, notify the physician. Then take these steps:
- Discontinue the feeding.
- Perform oral and tracheobronchial suctioning, as necessary, to remove aspirated fluid and secretions.
- Obtain the patient's vital signs, and monitor them every 1 to 2 hours for changes.
- Assess his respiratory status, including rate, depth, and character of respirations; also observe for a productive cough with frothy sputum. Auscultate the patient's lungs for adventitious sounds.
- Send blood samples to the laboratory for complete blood count and ABG analysis.
- Assess his oxygen saturation by way of pulse oximetry and ABG values; administer supplemental oxygen, as indicated and prescribed.
- Obtain a bedside chest X-ray, as ordered.
- Establish I.V. access, and begin fluid therapy, as prescribed.

WHAT TO DO NEXT

Once the patient has stabilized, follow these guidelines:
- Do not restart tube feedings until proper tube placement has been verified. (See *Assessing feeding tube placement*, page 388.)
- Continue to keep the patient's airway clear of secretions by suctioning frequently or by encouraging him to cough.
- Monitor serial chest X-rays for progressive changes in pulmonary infiltrates.
- Administer I.V. antibiotics, if prescribed, to prevent or treat aspiration pneumonia.

FOLLOW-UP CARE

- Evaluate the patient's respiratory status closely at least every 4 hours.
- If the physician reinstates tube feedings, establish a plan of care to prevent aspiration from recurring.
- ➡ **NurseALERT** If your patient has a cuffed endotracheal or tracheostomy tube, check the cuff's seal before starting a feeding. Maintain proper cuff inflation pressure, as ordered.
- Monitor gastric residual volume every 4 hours during continuous feeding or before every intermittent feeding; temporarily discontinue feedings if residual is greater than the last hour's infusion or exceeds 100 ml for 2 consecutive hours.
- Monitor the patient's abdomen for gastric distention, and auscultate for bowel sounds at least every 8 hours.

T

ASSESSING FEEDING TUBE PLACEMENT

The best way to verify proper placement of a nasoenteric feeding tube is by X-ray. At the bedside, you can test gastric pH or auscultate for air—especially if your patient is alert and has a large-bore tube for short-term feedings.

TESTING GASTRIC pH
You may test the pH of gastric aspirate through simple reagent paper testing. After feedings have been stopped for at least 1 hour, collect a specimen of gastric aspirate and test it with the reagent paper; a pH less than 4 (or less than 5.5 in a patient receiving gastric acid inhibitors) suggests that the tube is in the stomach.

Be aware, however, that fluid aspirated from the respiratory system may be acidic as well and thus may be misleading. Also, if the patient has a small-bore feeding tube, aspirating a sufficient amount of fluid for testing may prove difficult.

AUSCULTATING FOR AIR
Alternatively, you may assess feeding tube placement by auscultating for a rush of air during insufflation. With the diaphragm of your stethoscope over the patient's epigastric area, instill 10 to 20 cc of air into the feeding tube. A bubbling, gurgling sound suggests that the tube is in the stomach. However, keep in mind that gurgling sounds sometimes occur even if the tube is misplaced into the respiratory tract.

WHAT *NOT* TO DO
Don't check tube placement by putting the end of the feeding tube in water and then observing for bubbling, which would indicate that the tube is in the lungs. You're likely to get a misleading result, especially if the patient has a small-bore feeding tube, because the tube may be lodged in a bronchiole small enough to block the tube's ports, preventing bubbling. Also, if the tube is in the respiratory tract, water may be drawn into the tube—and the airways—as the patient inhales.

- Elevate the head of his bed 30 to 40 degrees during feedings.
- Mark the correctly placed tube where it exits the patient's nose, and then check every 4 hours during continuous feedings or before each intermittent feeding, according to your facility's protocol, to make sure the tube hasn't migrated.

SPECIAL CONSIDERATIONS
- Always administer tube feedings slowly with the patient sitting upright.
- Stay alert for late complications of tube-feeding aspiration, such as pleural effusions, lung abscesses, and diffuse alveolar infiltrates.
- Know that elderly patients are at high risk for tube-feeding aspiration from age-related weakening of the lower esophageal sphincter (which makes reflux more likely) and from a possibly decreased gag reflex.
- A small-bore feeding tube may help prevent aspiration because it's less likely to disrupt the esophageal sphincter and cause reflux. However, this type of tube may become displaced after an episode of coughing or vigorous tracheal or oropharyngeal suctioning. What's more, the patient may not show respiratory symptoms if a small-bore tube is malpositioned.
- For a patient at high risk for aspiration, some clinicians recommend using a transpyloric feeding tube with a weighted tip, inserting a feeding tube into the duodenum or jejunum by the nasal route, or placing one surgically through the abdomen.

V, W

VENTRICULAR FIBRILLATION AND PULSELESS VENTRICULAR TACHYCARDIA

In ventricular fibrillation (VF), many ventricular sites fire at once. As a result, the ventricles quiver rather than contract normally, a situation that effectively reduces cardiac output to nothing. Unless this rhythm is quickly converted, the patient will die.

VF can result from a number of disorders, including acute myocardial infarction or ischemia, coronary artery disease, cardiomyopathy, hypokalemia, and hypoxia. It may arise if a catheter stimulates a ventricle during cardiac catheterization or cardiac pacing, or during coronary artery reperfusion after thrombolytic therapy or percutaneous transluminal coronary angioplasty. And it can result from electric shock. Ventricular tachycardia (VT) can deteriorate into VF; in fact, persistent pulseless VT receives the same treatment as VF. VT with a pulse receives the treatment outlined in "Ventricular tachycardia," on pages 392 to 395.

Clearly, your quick recognition of VF or pulseless VT and your immediate response are required to save your patient's life.

WHAT TO LOOK FOR
Clinical findings for a patient in VF or pulseless VT may include:
- unresponsiveness
- no pulse
- no heart sounds
- loss of consciousness
- apnea
- seizures
- irregular, chaotic baseline rhythm and unmeasurable rate on the ECG. (See *Recognizing ventricular fibrillation*, page 390.)

WHAT TO DO IMMEDIATELY
If your patient develops VF, notify the physician and follow these measures:
- Find out whether the patient is responsive, and quickly assess his airway, breathing, and circulation. If he has no pulse or respirations, start cardiopulmonary resuscitation (CPR) and continue it until he can be connected to a defibrillator.

V

RECOGNIZING VENTRICULAR FIBRILLATION

Ventricular fibrillation, as shown in this illustration, has an irregular rhythm with a chaotic baseline and an unmeasurable rate. You won't be able to distinguish P waves, PR intervals, QRS complexes, or T waves.

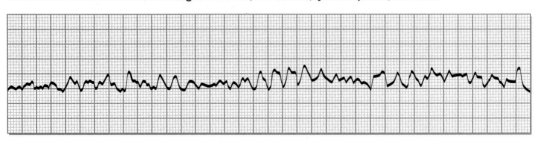

- Connect him to the defibrillator and determine his rhythm. If it confirms VF or pulseless VT, set the defibrillator to 200 joules and deliver a shock. If necessary, follow with a shock at 200 to 300 joules and then one at 360 joules.
- ➡ **NurseALERT** Before delivering the shocks, make sure everyone is clear of the bed. Also remove any nitroglycerin patches from your patient's chest or position the paddles so they aren't touching a patch. (The aluminum backing on some older patches can cause electrical arcing, smoke, explosive noises, and chest burns.)
- Keep the paddles on your patient's chest between shocks, and check his heart rhythm on the monitor while the defibrillator is recharging. Don't take time to check his pulses between shocks.

WHAT TO DO NEXT
After your initial treatment, apply these interventions:
- Continue CPR for persistent or recurrent VF or pulseless VT.
- If necessary, help with endotracheal intubation to support the patient's respirations and maintain a patent airway. Make sure you can see the patient's chest rise and hear bilateral breath sounds.
- Establish I.V. access if your patient doesn't already have a line in place. Then give epinephrine, 1 mg I.V. push, and repeat it every 3 to 5 minutes, as ordered.
- Defibrillate with 360 joules within 30 to 60 seconds.
- ➡ **NurseALERT** Follow the drug-shock, drug-shock pattern. In other words, administer the drug, and then defibrillate with 360 joules within 30 to 60 seconds of drug administration.
- If VF continues or recurs, administer second-line drugs, such as lidocaine (Xylocaine), bretylium (Bretylol), magnesium sulfate, and procainamide (Pronestyl), as ordered. You may give sodium bicarbonate as well, if indicated. Follow all medications with defibrillation at 360 joules within 30 to 60 seconds.

➡ **NurseALERT** When administering I.V. medications during cardiac arrest, follow them with a 20- to 30-ml bolus of normal saline solution. Then raise your patient's arm to speed delivery of the drug to his central circulation.

FOLLOW-UP CARE
- Once your patient regains spontaneous circulation, monitor all his physiologic parameters at least hourly. Continue I.V. administration of whichever antiarrhythmic drug restored his circulation. If defibrillation alone restored his pulse and he hasn't already received lidocaine, give a loading dose of lidocaine (1.0 to 1.5 mg/kg to a total of 3.0 mg/kg) and follow with a continuous infusion at 2 to 4 mg/minute.
- Maintain continuous cardiac monitoring; watch carefully for changes.
- Support your patient's airway and breathing with mechanical ventilation, as necessary.
- Assess his vital signs, heart and breath sounds, level of consciousness, urine output, pulses, capillary refill, skin color and temperature, and oxygen saturation (by pulse oximetry or arterial blood gas values).
- Monitor laboratory results, such as blood urea nitrogen level and serum levels of electrolytes, cardiac enzymes, and creatinine. Report any abnormal results.
- Administer medications, as indicated, to support the patient's blood pressure and heart rate.
- Provide emotional support to the patient and his family. Explain what happened in simple terms and describe the treatments he's receiving.

SPECIAL CONSIDERATIONS
- The most important factor in your patient's survival is early defibrillation. It produces asystole, depolarizing the heart completely and allowing the sinoatrial node to take over. In fact, studies suggest that three successive shocks, one right after the other, are more important to your patient's survival than drug therapy. That's why you should not stop to give drugs or perform CPR between shocks.
- Be sure to leave the defibrillator paddles on the patient's chest and recharge them immediately after each shock. Check the heart rhythm while the defibrillator is recharging. If you see a rhythm other than VF or pulseless VT, remove the paddles, disarm the defibrillator, and check for a pulse.
- If you don't have I.V. access, anticipate giving lidocaine and epinephrine through a long catheter inserted into the endotracheal tube. You'll need to stop chest compressions, inject 2 to 2½ times the usual dose through the catheter, as ordered, and flush with 10 ml of normal saline solution. Then ventilate the patient forcefully three to four times, as ordered.

V

VENTRICULAR TACHYCARDIA

In ventricular tachycardia (VT), one or a number of ventricular sites fire at a rate greater than 100 beats/minute. If that rate lasts longer than 30 seconds, the patient has sustained VT; if it lasts less than 30 seconds, she has nonsustained VT.

A number of disorders are associated with VT, including acute myocardial infarction (MI), coronary artery disease, long-QT syndrome, cardiomyopathy, mitral valve prolapse, and electrolyte imbalances. It also may arise after thrombolytic therapy causes reperfusion. And in some people, it may arise without evidence of heart disease.

No matter what its cause, VT reduces cardiac output by shortening ventricular filling time, which also results in the loss of the atrial contribution to ventricular filling. Consequently, cardiac output is dramatically decreased and your patient may develop reduced cerebral perfusion, pulmonary edema, and shock. Worse, VT can deteriorate into pulseless VT or VF. (For more information, see "Ventricular fibrillation and pulseless ventricular tachycardia," pages 389 – 391.)

WHAT TO LOOK FOR

Unlike with VF, a patient with VT usually has a pulse. Other clinical findings may include the following:

- palpitations
- light-headedness
- chest pain
- dyspnea
- decreased level of consciousness
- hypotension
- shock
- pulmonary congestion
- heart failure
- acute MI
- ECG findings characteristic of VT or torsades de pointes (see *Recognizing ventricular tachycardia and torsades de pointes*).

WHAT TO DO IMMEDIATELY

If your patient develops VT, notify the physician and follow these measures:

- Begin continuous cardiac and automated blood pressure monitoring.
- Assess the patient's oxygen saturation levels by way of pulse oximetry; give supplemental oxygen, as ordered.
- Establish I.V. access, and prepare to administer medications, as ordered.
- Assess your patient's vital signs and cardiovascular status.
- ➡ **Nurse**ALERT If your patient isn't in full cardiac arrest but has a rate above 150 beats/minute and such signs and symptoms as hypoten-

RECOGNIZING VENTRICULAR TACHYCARDIA AND TORSADES DE POINTES

As shown in the top waveform, ventricular tachycardia (VT) produces a regular or slightly irregular rhythm and a rate between 100 and 250 beats per minute. Usually you won't be able to see P waves (they're dissociated from the QRS), PR intervals can't be measured, and QRS complexes are more than 0.12 seconds wide with a bizarre morphology. As shown in the bottom waveform, torsades de pointes is a type of VT in which the QRS complexes seem to twist around the baseline.

Ventricular tachycardia

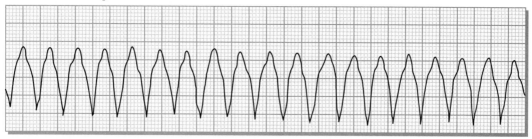

Torsades de pointes

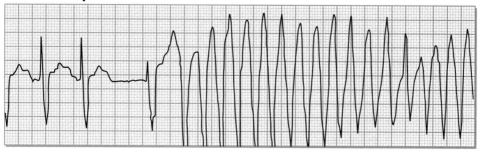

sion, dyspnea, chest pain, decreased level of consciousness, and pulmonary edema, prepare her for immediate cardioversion. (See *Caring for your patient during synchronized cardioversion*, page 39.)

- If the patient is clinically stable, administer lidocaine (Xylocaine)1.0 to 1.5 mg/kg by I.V. push, as ordered, to a total loading dose of 3 mg/kg, if necessary. Then, if the VT converts to normal sinus rhythm, switch to a lidocaine infusion at 2 to 4 mg/minute. Keep in mind that the treatment of choice for torsades de pointes is I.V. magnesium sulfate.

➡ Nurse**ALERT** If at any time your patient loses a pulse or enters full cardiac arrest, immediately begin treating her according to advanced cardiac life support protocols for VF and pulseless VT.

V

WHAT TO DO NEXT

Once the patient's initial crisis has passed, take these actions:

- If she still has VT and is hemodynamically stable, administer procainamide (Pronestyl) as a second-line drug.
- ➡ **NurseALERT** Give procainamide as an infusion, not by bolus, at a rate of 20 to 30 mg/minute to a maximum total dose of 17 mg/kg.
- Monitor her ECG tracing to see if the procainamide converts the VT. If it does, start an infusion at 1 to 4 mg/minute.
- If procainamide doesn't convert the VT, give bretylium (Bretylol) as a third-line drug. Prepare 5 to 10 mg/kg and infuse it over 8 to 10 minutes.
- Monitor her ECG tracing to see if the bretylium converts the VT. If it does, start a continuous infusion at 1 to 2 mg/minute.
- Continue to evaluate her ECG, cardiopulmonary status, and vital signs closely for changes. Track her oxygen saturation levels, and continue giving supplemental oxygen, as needed.

FOLLOW-UP CARE

- Continue to monitor the patient's ECG. Report any recurrence of VT immediately. If the patient develops pulseless VT, follow the protocol for VF.
- If the patient is receiving lidocaine, watch for central nervous system effects, such as twitching, tremors, confusion, paresthesias, and seizures. If they arise, stop the infusion and notify the physician.
- If the patient is receiving procainamide, watch for hypotension and a widening of the QRS complex by more than 50%. If these signs arise, stop the infusion and notify the physician immediately.
- Monitor the patient's blood pressure closely for hypotension while administering bretylium.
- Administer oral antiarrhythmics, as ordered, such as quinidine (Quinora), procainamide, disopyramide (Norpace), propafenone (Rythmol), amiodarone (Cordarone), flecainide (Tambocor), or tocainide (Tonocard).
- Anticipate an order for a pacemaker, an automatic implantable cardioverter/defibrillator, radiofrequency catheter ablation therapy, or such surgeries as endocardial resection, ablation by cryosurgical techniques, or an encircling ventriculotomy (in which the area of myocardium responsible for the arrhythmia is isolated). Prepare the patient, as indicated.
- Monitor her serum electrolyte and drug levels; report any abnormal values.

SPECIAL CONSIDERATIONS

- If your patient is receiving amiodarone, tell her that it may turn her skin a bluish color. Also tell her to use sunscreen and wear protective clothing when she's out in the sun.

- Be aware of the many drug-drug interactions that may occur. For instance, if your patient's taking digoxin (Lanoxin), it's important to decrease the dose of quinidine to reduce the risk of her developing digitalis toxicity.
- Although advanced cardiac life support guidelines specify performing cardioversion first for a hemodynamically unstable patient with VT, you can have other team members prepare and administer lidocaine right away as long as doing so doesn't delay cardioversion.

VIOLENT PATIENT

In all likelihood, no matter what your nursing specialty, you'll encounter a violent patient from time to time. He may use only verbal assault or he may use physical violence. He may use violence against himself, against you or other staff members, or against other patients or visitors.

Useful strategies exist to help keep a patient's agitation from evolving into violence, provided you recognize the early signs that the patient has entered the emotional and behavioral cycle that leads to violence. Although it may seem like an isolated act, violence is a process, characterized by observable behaviors and identifiable risk factors. (See *Risk factors for violence*, page 396.) By responding to them wisely and firmly, you can help ensure your patient's safety—along with your own and that of the other patients, staff, and visitors.

WHAT TO LOOK FOR
Clinical findings for a patient approaching violence may include:
- psychomotor agitation, including pacing, slamming the door, wringing of hands
- irritability
- angry affect and facial expression
- clenched fists
- throwing of objects
- defensiveness
- withdrawal and lack of response to questions
- disorientation
- verbalized fear
- verbalized threats
- profane or obscene language
- repetitious demands
- argumentative demeanor

V

RISK FACTORS FOR VIOLENCE

No set of risk factors can give you a surefire way to predict violence. However, certain risk factors can and should raise your awareness about a patient's potential for violence, as should certain diagnoses and environmental conditions. Consider factors like these when assessing your patient's risk of becoming violent.

HISTORY
- Personal history of perpetrating violence
- History of being a victim of violence, including child abuse, spousal abuse, or other family violence
- History of childhood pyromania or animal cruelty
- Record of criminal activity or weapon possession
- History of substance abuse

MEDICAL DISORDERS
- Evidence of substance abuse during examination
- Delirium
- Dementia
- Head trauma

- Infections, such as viral encephalitis or opportunistic infection, secondary to acquired immunodeficiency syndrome
- Temporal lobe epilepsy

Psychiatric disorders
- Active suicidal or homicidal ideation
- Schizophrenia (especially when actively psychotic)
- Schizoaffective disorder
- Affective disorders, especially manic states
- Antisocial personality disorder
- Borderline personality disorder
- Anxiety disorder

ENVIRONMENTAL FACTORS
- Increased environmental stimulation, such as high noise level or bright artificial light
- Overcrowding
- Extremes in temperature
- Disturbing tone in staff interactions
- Inconsistency among staff

- failure to comply with rules
- active responses to internal stimulation, such as auditory or visual hallucinations.

WHAT TO DO IMMEDIATELY

If you suspect that your patient is becoming violent or has already become violent, notify the physician and follow these measures:
- Stay calm. Your patient will respond to your body language and the tone of your voice.
- Consider whether you need to call for help. If you have any doubt, don't hesitate to summon help. Notify security if the situation warrants it.
- Quickly assess the safety of the environment. Are other patients in the area? Should they be evacuated? Are objects in the area that should be removed? Can you contain your patient without limiting your ability to exit?
- Approach the patient in a nonthreatening manner and call his name.
- Maintain steady eye contact at the same physical level as your patient. In other words, don't approach the patient so you have to look up or down at him. Looking down on a patient who is lying or sitting can seem threatening and may agitate him.
- Ask the patient what's wrong and then listen carefully to his answer. If possible, try to resolve conflict and problem-solve with him.
- Don't crowd your patient's personal space and don't touch him.

➡ **NurseALERT** A violent patient needs up to four times more personal space than normal.

- Set limits by defining unacceptable behaviors. For example, you could say: "Please stop screaming"; "Profanity is not acceptable"; "You don't need to make threats"; or "Put down that vase."
- After setting limits, acknowledge your patient's anger, and again try to problem-solve. Make sure all staff members set consistent limits.
- Administer antianxiety medication, as indicated. If possible, give it early, before the patient loses control. If the patient has a history of psychosis, give an antipsychotic, as prescribed. Using concrete terms, explain that the medication will help him stay in control.
- Communicate in simple terms what you are doing and what you expect from the patient.
- Restrain the patient, as necessary, to protect himself and others until he can regain control. Your objective is to keep yourself and others safe while doing no harm to the patient. In general, you'll want to address verbal threats with a verbal response and use physical measures only to counteract physical aggression.
- Reduce stimulating factors in the patient's environment. Try to distract him by offering food, a beverage, and a quiet place to talk. Turn off the television or radio and eliminate other sources of background noise.
- Avoid arguing with the patient no matter how irrational he may be; instead, acknowledge his anger and allow him to vent his feelings.

WHAT TO DO NEXT
- Continue to assess your patient's mental status. If the prospect of violence continues to escalate, increase your response by involving other members of the team, devising a strategy to help the patient gain control, giving medication as needed, and assessing safety.
- If the patient begins to calm down in response to your interventions, continue to observe him closely. Consider what prompted his violent response, and provide an outlet for the feelings behind it to help him stay calm.
- Document the event carefully, including the patient's threats, issues, fears, and demands. Describe the exact course of the violent episode. Record any medications given and the patient's response to them. Note which actions were successful in calming the patient, along with factors that complicated the situation, such as delirium, recovery from anesthesia, and adverse response to medications.
- If your patient required physical restraint, carefully evaluate his ability to explain the need for restraint and the behavioral limits he's expected to uphold. Gradually reduce the degree of restraint as he adheres to those limits.
- After defusing the situation, you'll need to provide ongoing attention to keep it under control.
- If your patient responds positively to a particular staff member, have that person set limits, give medications, and provide other care.

V

FOLLOW-UP CARE
- Help the patient work through the event in his mind, recognize his anger and frustration, and try to problem-solve.
- Reinforce positive behavior, and reiterate that certain *behaviors* are unacceptable, not the patient himself.
- Arrange for a psychiatric consultation, if indicated, to assess the patient's behavior, maintain his safety, and prevent a recurrence of the episode.
- Continue to give medications, as ordered. Make sure you obtain standing orders for a sedative, antianxiety agent, or other medication, as indicated, to be given immediately if the patient becomes violent again.
- Listen to your patient's concerns, and try to address them as soon as possible rather than allowing him to become frustrated over them.
- If certain family members have a calming influence, encourage them to visit; make exceptions to visiting hours, if possible.
- Allow the patient to retain some control and choices to help decrease defensiveness and the tendency to violence.

SPECIAL CONSIDERATIONS
➡ **NurseALERT** In responding to violence, trust your instincts. If you feel uncomfortable in a situation, get help.
- Always be aware of your own behavior and how it colors your patient's perception of your response to him.
- When more than one staff member must approach the patient together, decide beforehand who will do the talking. Multiple commands and reassurances from several people at the same time will only increase the patient's agitation and could trigger further violence.
- After intervening with a violent patient, allow time for the health care team to evaluate their emotional and procedural responses.
- Place a note in the chart of any potentially violent patient to warn the staff. Also notify security, as necessary.

VISION LOSS, ACUTE

If your patient has an acute loss of vision in one or both eyes, chances are he'll be referred immediately to an ophthalmologist for evaluation. Even so, it's important for you to have a sound understanding of problems that can cause vision loss, along with appropriate responses to them. (See *Possible causes of acute vision loss.*) By doing so, you can help your patient get the information he needs in addition to the treatment he needs.

WHAT TO LOOK FOR
Clinical findings associated with acute vision loss may include:
- irregular corneal light reflex
- corneal abrasion or ulcer (may not be visible until after fluorescein dye is instilled)

POSSIBLE CAUSES OF ACUTE VISION LOSS

Acute vision loss can result from any factor that disrupts transmission of light through the eye, blocks transmission of electrical signals through the retina and optic nerve, or disrupts interpretation of visual stimuli in the brain's visual cortex. A selection of possible disorders follows, along with the mechanisms by which they work.

Cause	Mechanism
Acute cataract	• Proteinaceous changes take place in either the lens cortex or the capsule, causing rapid vision loss
Angle-closure glaucoma	• Blocked aqueous flow causes pressure to build in the eye and, after 2 to 5 days, results in permanent vision loss
Blunt trauma	• A blood vessel may break in the iris, dispersing blood through the aqueous and causing a hyphema • A ruptured globe can disrupt and displace ocular structures • The lens (implanted or natural) may become displaced or subluxated
Corneal abrasions, ulcers, or lacerations	• Lesions in the pupillary area render the cornea unable to refract light, immediately reducing vision
Diabetes mellitus	• In at least one-half of diabetics, proliferative diabetic retinopathy, neovascularization, and spontaneous hemorrhage may develop after about 15 years
Giant cell or temporal arteritis	• Inflammation of the cerebral arteries causes sudden, painless, nonprogressive visual loss that, at least initially, is unilateral
Occlusion of central retinal artery or a branch	• An embolus (usually from an internal carotid artery or vegetations from heart valves) lodges in a retinal artery, blocking blood flow and causing instant loss of vision
Optic neuritis	• Inflammation of the optic nerve causes sudden vision loss in an eye that otherwise looks normal
Retinal detachment	• Separation of the sensory retina from the retinal pigment epithelium causes showers of spots, flashes of light, and visual field loss

- pain, photophobia, tearing, and redness
- discharge (if ulcer is infected)
- hyphema (blood in the anterior chamber blocks your ability to see the color of the patient's iris)
- pupil that looks grayish white instead of black (traumatic cataract)
- intraocular lens that is dislocated into the anterior chamber (seen with a flashlight held temporally at an oblique angle)
- history of trauma, diabetes, or transient vision loss in one eye.

WHAT TO DO IMMEDIATELY

When your patient experiences acute vision loss, notify the physician and follow these measures:

- Anticipate a referral to an ophthalmologist.
- Assess the patient's vision. (See *Assessing the eye*, page 400.) If you have access to a Snellen visual acuity chart, try to obtain a baseline as-

V

ASSESSING THE EYE

Use the guidelines and questions below to enhance your ability to assess a patient with acute vision loss.

- Start by asking the patient if he has any pain associated with the vision loss.
- Examine the cornea and check the corneal light reflex. Is the cornea hazy or the light reflex shattered?
- Check to see if the conjunctiva is red and infected. If so, see whether it's circumcorneal (a sign of associated iridocyclitis) or peripheral.
- Inspect the iris. Can you see all the structures through the cornea? If not, is it because of corneal haze or blood in the anterior chamber?
- Are the pupils round? Do they react to light and accommodation? If the patient has a cataract or vitreous hemorrhage, you can elicit a pupillary light reflex. If he has optic neuritis or temporal arteritis, his pupils will react if you shine a light into the seeing eye but not if you shine the light into the blind eye.
- Check the patient's visual acuity. Darken the room to make the chart easier to see. Remember that some patients say they can't see when, in fact, they can't open their eyes.
- Prepare the patient for measurement of intraocular

pressure with a Tonopen or, preferably, an applanation tonometer.

Performing an ophthalmoscopic examination

- If you've had special training, examine the patient's eye with an ophthalmoscope. Keep in mind that a damaged or hazy cornea will blur the image, a vitreous hemorrhage will block your view of the retina, an artery occlusion will turn the retina grayish white with a cherry red macula. Optic neuritis will cause no visible changes in the fundus.
- Start your ophthalmoscopic examination with the optic disc. Note whether the arteries (the lighter red vessels) emerging from it look full and strong and if the veins (larger, darker vessels) look engorged or beaded.
- Now look at the background retina. Do you see flame-shaped hemorrhages, cotton wool spots, or yellow (lipid) exudates?
- Finally, have the patient look straight ahead so you can see the macula; it should appear as an avascular area in the center of two arched blood vessels. Although a cherry red spot typically indicates an artery occlusion, it also may appear in patients with Tay-Sachs disease.

---

sessment of the patient's visual acuity. If not, shine a flashlight oblique to the patient's eye from the six cardinal positions of gaze, and have him tell you whether he can see the light at all locations. This information tells you whether his retina, the optic nerve, and the visual cortex of the brain are functioning.

➡ **Nurse**ALERT Never try to force the patient's eye open to check visual acuity, especially if he might have a traumatic injury.

- Check to see if the corneal light reflex is a pinpoint or scattered—a finding that reveals disruption of the surface epithelium, probably from a corneal abrasion or ulcer. Note any purulent discharge.

➡ **Nurse**ALERT A patient over age 50 who develops excruciating eye pain, possible nausea, and sudden vision loss may be having an attack of angle-closure glaucoma. Findings include a shallow anterior chamber, a middilated and fixed pupil, corneal hazing, a very red conjunctiva, and history of seeing halos around lights. The patient's intraocular pressure may be as high as 60 mm Hg.

- Find out whether the patient was hammering or using a power tool at the time of the vision loss, especially if he has a cloudy lens—which can result from an intraocular foreign body. If so, ask if he was wearing glasses at the time or if he felt something enter his eye.

- If you suspect a corneal laceration, protect the injured eye with a shield or with a clean paper or Styrofoam cup. Cut and splay the cup's edges, and then tape it over the affected eye.
- If the patient has a visible hyphema, shield the eye and have the patient sit up so the blood can begin settling by gravity, thus improving vision.
- Find out if the patient has had a cataract removed and an intraocular lens implanted in that eye.
- Find out if the patient has a history of diabetes and if he's ever had laser photocoagulation to treat diabetic retinopathy.
- Ask whether the patient has ever had a sudden loss of vision in one eye or has had vision loss that comes and goes.
- Inquire about episodes of tingling in limbs or previous episodes of vision loss that could be associated with multiple sclerosis.
- ➡ **NurseALERT** If your elderly patient complains of headache, muscle and joint pain, weight loss from intermittent jaw pain, reduced appetite, and malaise, be aware that he may have temporal arteritis.

WHAT TO DO NEXT
Your continued care will vary based on the cause of the patient's vision loss, as outlined below.

Corneal abrasion
If the patient has a corneal abrasion:
- Administer cycloplegic eyedrops, such as scopolamine 0.25%, and antibiotic eyedrops, such as tobramycin (Tobrex), as ordered.
- Apply a pressure patch for 12 hours, unless it's contraindicated (because the patient wears contact lens, has an acrylic fingernail scratch, or was injured by vegetable matter [such as a thorn], for example).
- Antibiotics will be continued 4 to 6 times a day after patch removal.

Corneal ulcer
If the patient has a corneal ulcer:
- After a culture has been taken, instill antibiotic eyedrops (such as tobramycin or Polytrim Ophthalmic) or a combination antibiotic (such as fortified bacitracin or vancomycin) anywhere from 4 times daily to once every hour, as ordered. Scopolamine 0.25% reduces iridocyclitis.
- If the ulcer stems from herpes simplex virus, give antiviral drops, such as trifluridine (Viroptic), 5 times daily for up to 7 days.
- Treat fungal ulcers with natamycin 5% (Natacyn) drops every hour, as ordered.

Hyphema
If the vision loss results from hyphema:
- Enforce bed rest with the head of the bed raised 30 degrees for 3 to 5 days. Give aminocaproic acid (Amicar), as ordered, to prevent a secondary bleed. The patient should have daily follow-up with an ophthalmologist.

V

- Give atropine 1% drops 3 or 4 times a day, as prescribed.
- Do not administer any aspirin products.
- Protect the eye with glasses or a shield.
- If intraocular pressure rises, give a beta blocker eyedrop, such as timolol 0.5% (Blocadren), twice daily as ordered.

➡ **NurseALERT** Sharp eye pain suggests rebleeding.

Intraocular foreign body

If you suspect an intraocular foreign body, which can quickly form a traumatic cataract:

- Prepare for ultrasound or computed tomography to identify the object. (Magnetic resonance imaging is contraindicated because metal objects or fragments may migrate under the effects of the magnetic field and cause further eye damage.)
- If an intraocular lens dislocates into the anterior chamber, prepare the patient for surgery to reposition it; otherwise it will damage and cloud the corneal endothelium.
- After corrective surgery for traumatic cataract or intraocular lens exchange or positioning, give antibiotic and steroid drops 4 to 6 times daily, as ordered.

Angle-closure glaucoma

If the patient has acute angle-closure glaucoma:

- Prepare him for a slit-lamp examination, measurement of intraocular pressure, and examination with a gonio lens.
- Instill a topical beta blocker (such as timolol 0.5% or levobunolol [Betagan]) eyedrop and a topical steroid (such as prednisolone acetate 1% [Pred Forte]) every 15 to 30 minutes for four doses and then hourly. Give a carbonic anhydrase inhibitor I.V. (such as acetazolamide [Diamox], 250 to 500 mg in one dose). Then give either an oral osmotic agent (such as isosorbide [Ismotic], 50 to 100 g) or I.V. mannitol 20% (Osmitrol), 1 to 2 g/kg over 45 minutes. Give two doses of pilocarpine 1% to 2% (Pilocar) every 15 minutes if a swollen lens may have caused the attack.

Retinal artery occlusion

If the patient has central retinal artery occlusion:

- Have the patient breath into a paper bag, and transfer him to an ophthalmologist immediately. Treatment includes digital ocular massage. At the slit lamp, anterior chamber paracentesis is performed to remove aqueous humor. Acetazolamide (administered I.V. or orally) and a topical beta blocker, such as timolol, are administered to lower intraocular pressure. This is followed by breathing carbinogen (95% oxygen and 5% carbon dioxide) for 10 minutes every hour for 48 hours. Monitor the patient's blood pressure, pulse rate, and level of consciousness for changes.

- If the patient is suspected of having temporal arteritis (which typically occurs in elderly people), expect that his erythrocyte sedimentation rate (ESR) will be closely monitored.
➡ **NurseALERT** Administer high-dose steroid therapy (1,000 mg in divided I.V. doses for 12 doses), as prescribed, to prevent vision loss in the second eye. The physician may order a temporal artery biopsy on the side on which vision was lost if he suspects giant cell arteritis from the patient's signs and symptoms or from the ESR results.

FOLLOW-UP CARE

- Corneal abrasions heal in 24 to 48 hours; antibiotic drops will continue for the next 4 days. In contrast, corneal ulcers heal slowly; instruct the patient to continue his antibiotic and cycloplegic drops, as prescribed, until the cornea has reepithelialized.
- If the patient has a hyphema, tell him to keep using atropine 1% drops for the next 2 weeks, as ordered. Tell him to wear safety glasses any time he plays contact sports or risks eye injury.
- If a vitreous hemorrhage doesn't absorb on its own, prepare the patient for a surgical pars plana vitrectomy (removal of the vitreous and the hemorrhage, replacing it with a balanced saline solution).
- After an intraocular lens has been repositioned, vision will gradually return to normal (if there isn't underlying retinal disease).
- If the patient has a cataract, prepare him for surgical cataract extraction with an intraocular lens implant to restore his vision. Tell him he'll need steroid and antibiotic eyedrops for 2 to 3 weeks after surgery. He should shield the eye to protect it while sleeping.
- If the patient had an acute glaucoma attack, tell him to use steroid eye drops, oral acetazolamide, and a topical beta blocker, as prescribed. Once the inflammation subsides, prepare him for laser peripheral iridectomy to aid the passage of aqueous humor from the posterior chamber to the anterior chamber. Later, he'll have the procedure on the other eye to prevent another attack.
- If the patient had retinal artery occlusion, prepare him to see an internist for a complete medical workup. Also, if a follow-up eye examination (after 2 to 4 weeks) shows neovascularization, the patient will need to undergo photocoagulation.
- If the patient has optic neuritis, high-dose I.V. steriods followed by oral steroids will be prescribed. Arrange for follow-up by a neuro-ophthalmologist because of the risk of increased intraocular pressure and other neurologic problems.
- If a temporal biopsy confirms giant cell arteritis, give the patient oral steroids for 2 to 4 weeks until his elevated ESR reaches a normal range. Teach him about his drug regimen, and prepare to taper the dose until the smallest dose possible keeps the inflammation in check. The ESR is typically elevated because of the body's inflammatory response.

V

SPECIAL CONSIDERATIONS

- An ulcer-scarred cornea may eventually need to be replaced.
- Urge hyphema patients to wear eye protection when playing sports to help avoid further damage.
- After cataract surgery, an intraocular lens implant or contact lens will restore the patient's distance vision; he'll still need reading glasses.
- Keep in mind that diabetic patients who undergo vitrectomy to remove a vitreous hemorrhage may have clear vision for a while, but they're at risk for recurrent bleeding episodes that need more treatment.
- Warn a patient with optic neuritis that he may never have another episode, or he might have periods of exacerbation and remission.
- Keep in mind that early detection and prompt intervention can prevent loss of vision from temporal arteritis or giant cell arteritis.
- Explain all medications to the patient and his family, and provide them with information about possible adverse reactions.
- Make sure the patient and his family understand the importance of continued eye care and faithful attendance at follow-up appointments.

VOMITING, SEVERE

Virtually everyone experiences vomiting at some time. Typically, it's preceded by nausea—an unpleasant feeling of revulsion usually accompanied by sweating, increased salivation, pallor, tachycardia, dizziness, and light-headedness. Before long, peristalsis reverses, the lower esophageal sphincter relaxes, and strong abdominal muscle contractions expel the upper GI contents through the mouth. (See *The mechanisms of vomiting.*)

When vomiting is repeated and profuse, the patient's fluid volume may become seriously depleted and electrolyte imbalances may arise. Gastric fluids are rich in potassium, sodium, chloride, and hydrogen ions, the loss of which may result in metabolic alkalosis. Vomiting also raises the risk that GI contents could be aspirated into the airways, which can lead to asphyxia, atelectasis, or pneumonitis.

If your patient develops severe vomiting, your prompt response can protect him from potentially harmful complications.

WHAT TO LOOK FOR

Clinical findings associated with severe vomiting may include:
- repeated emesis
- diaphoresis
- increased salivation
- pallor
- tachycardia
- dizziness

- signs and symptoms of dehydration, such as poor skin turgor, dry mucous membranes, decreased urine output, tachycardia, and increased hemoglobin level and hematocrit
- signs and symptoms of metabolic alkalosis, such as nervousness, anxiety, decreased level of consciousness, muscle weakness or twitching, tachycardia, an arterial pH above 7.45, a partial pressure of arterial carbon dioxide above 40 mmHg, and an HCO_3^- above 26 mEq/L.

WHAT TO DO IMMEDIATELY

If your patient experiences severe vomiting, notify the physician and follow these measures:

- Place the patient in a side-lying or semi-Fowler's position to prevent aspiration. If he has dentures, remove them.
- ➡ **NurseALERT** A patient who is comatose, anesthetized, or otherwise impaired may aspirate. Be prepared to remove vomitus from his mouth quickly. Use a washcloth or towel to wipe vomitus from his mouth; suction his oropharynx, if needed, using a tonsil tip catheter to remove vomitus from the back of the throat.
- Assess the character of the vomitus. (See *Assessing vomitus,* page 406.)
- Measure the amount of vomitus, and monitor the patient's intake and output closely.
- Obtain the patient's vital signs. Check his skin turgor and watch for signs and symptoms of dehydration and electrolyte imbalances.
- Auscultate for adventitious breath sounds, a sign of aspiration.
- Establish I.V. access, if the patient doesn't already have a line in place, and begin fluid therapy, as prescribed.
- Withhold oral foods and fluids, and anticipate insertion of a nasoenteric tube.
- Arrange for laboratory tests, including complete blood count, hematocrit, arterial blood gass (ABG) analysis, and serum hemoglobin and electrolyte levels, as ordered.

WHAT TO DO NEXT

Once the patient has stabilized, take these steps:

- Administer antiemetics, as prescribed.
- Continue to withhold oral foods and fluids, and continue to give I.V. fluids, as prescribed.
- Closely monitor all fluid intake and output.
- Monitor laboratory test results, especially serum electrolyte levels.
- As prescribed, discontinue any drugs known to stimulate the chemoreceptor trigger zone (CTZ).

THE MECHANISMS OF VOMITING

Inside the medulla of the brain stem are two areas that influence vomiting: the vomiting center and the chemoreceptor trigger zone (CTZ).

VOMITING CENTER

The vomiting center is stimulated directly by sensory stimuli from the autonomic nervous system in the GI tract and viscera. This stimulation can result from gastric distention, irritants and toxins, injury to the viscera, pain, and even emotional upheaval. It also can be directly stimulated by increased intracranial pressure or by lesions (neoplasms, infarctions) in the brain stem.

CHEMORECEPTOR TRIGGER ZONE

Vomiting also occurs when the CTZ is stimulated by an emetic agent, and the CTZ in turn triggers the vomiting center. Emetic agents include such drugs as morphine, meperidine, ergot derivatives, and digitalis preparations as well as metabolic substances produced by uremia, infection, and radiation. Rapid position changes, which cause motion in the semicircular canals of the inner ear, can also stimulate the CTZ and induce vomiting.

U

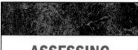

- Administer medications and treatments, as prescribed, to correct metabolic disorders known to produce toxins that stimulate the CTZ.
- Avoid moving the patient suddenly or unnecessarily to prevent indirect stimulation of the vomiting center.
- Tell the patient that taking deep breaths can help reduce nausea.
- Keep the patient's room well ventilated, and remove vomitus and soiled clothing and linens immediately to minimize odors, which may precipitate subsequent episodes of nausea and vomiting.
- Apply cold compresses to the patient's forehead, and help him to rinse and clean his mouth after each episode of vomiting.

FOLLOW-UP CARE

- When the patient resumes oral intake, start with small amounts of water or ginger ale (for example, 20 ml every 30 minutes). If he tolerates this, gradually increase the amount and variety, adding foods like gelatin, tea, and consommé. Progress to small, frequent meals of toast, cereal, chicken, and other bland, easily digested foods.
- Encourage the patient to take fluids an hour before or after a meal but not with it. Fluids with meals distend the stomach and can precipitate vomiting.
- Avoid giving high-fat foods and those known to stimulate peristalsis, such as orange juice, caffeine, and high-fiber foods.
- Monitor the patient for signs and symptoms of hypokalemia.
- If the patient has low potassium levels, anticipate oral or I.V. potassium replacement. Give foods that are high in potassium, as tolerated, including tea, bananas, dry whole milk, and cheese.
- ➡ **NurseALERT** Watch for the possible development of hyperkalemia while treating your patient's hypokalemia.

SPECIAL CONSIDERATIONS

- Keep in mind that elderly patients are particularly susceptible to complications from severe vomiting. They have a decreased fluid reserve, raising their risk of dehydration. They also are more prone to a decreased level of consciousness, increasing the risk for aspiration during a vomiting episode. And they're more likely to have chronic illness, such as cardiac or renal compromise. Consequently, transient electrolyte imbalances associated with vomiting can be life-threatening to elderly patients. Institute continuous cardiac monitoring as indicated to evaluate the effect of hypokalemia on cardiac rhythm. And rehydrate the elderly patient carefully to avoid fluid overload.

WOUND DEHISCENCE AND EVISCERATION

Most wounds—including surgical incisions—progress through a predictable set of stages in the process of healing. In some cases, poor or delayed wound healing can lead to serious complications, such as dehiscence and, possibly, evisceration. (See *Factors that affect wound healing.*)

In dehiscence, the wound edges separate and the wound gapes open, exposing underlying internal tissues to environmental contamination and raising the risk that those tissues could protrude outward through the open wound (evisceration).

Although almost any wound can undergo dehiscence and evisceration, these complications most commonly affect midline abdominal incisions. The risk is especially high for wounds associated with hematoma, seroma, infection, inadequate debridement, foreign bodies, and conditions that predispose the patient to poor healing. Excessive tension on the wound and early suture removal also raise the risk of dehiscence.

Protrusion of the abdominal contents through an open wound can be a serious complication indeed. If your patient develops wound dehiscence with or without evisceration, you'll need to respond quickly.

WHAT TO LOOK FOR
Clinical findings may include:
- complaints of increased pain
- sensation of something "giving way" after coughing, vomiting, or straining
- sudden, profuse drainage of pink, serous fluid
- visible separation of wound edges
- visible protrusion of viscera.

WHAT TO DO IMMEDIATELY
If your patient develops wound dehiscence or evisceration, notify the physician and follow these measures:
- Remain calm to help keep your patient calm.
- If the patient isn't in bed, have her get in bed. Place her in semi-Fowler's position with her knees slightly elevated.
- ➡ **NurseALERT** If the wound hasn't completely opened or eviscerated, this position may prevent further tearing. Call for help and don't leave the patient alone.
- If coils of intestine are protruding from the opening, cover the area with sterile dressings moistened with normal saline solution. If sterile dressings aren't readily available, use clean towels or dressings. Keep the wound covering moist at all times.
- ➡ **NurseALERT** Don't try to push protruding abdominal contents back through the wound. Doing so could cause ischemia and strangulation. It also could raise the risk of infection.
- Check the patient's vital signs and level of consciousness for possible signs and symptoms of shock.
- If the patient doesn't already have I.V. access, insert two large-bore I.V. lines and administer fluids, as prescribed, to support the patient's blood pressure and fluid volume and to prevent shock.
- Give supplemental oxygen, as needed, and continuously monitor her oxygen saturation levels using pulse oximetry.

FACTORS THAT AFFECT WOUND HEALING

Many factors can influence the speed and success with which a wound heals, including:
- presence of wound infection
- preexisting disease, such as diabetes, asthma, bronchitis, emphysema, and anemia
- malnutrition or obesity
- old age
- immunosuppression
- size, shape, and location of the wound
- perfusion of the wound
- techniques and materials used to create, maintain, and close the wound.

W

WHAT TO DO NEXT

Once the patient has stabilized, take these steps:

- Give the patient nothing by mouth because she'll probably need to return to surgery.
- Obtain laboratory tests, as ordered, including preoperative blood work and wound cultures.
- Continue to monitor her vital signs, cardiopulmonary status, and fluid balance frequently for signs and symptoms of shock.
- Premedicate the patient for surgery, as ordered.
- ➡ Nurse**ALERT** Make sure the patient gives written consent for surgery before administering her premedication. Otherwise, consent is legally invalid.

FOLLOW-UP CARE

- Provide routine postoperative care after surgery.
- Give antibiotic therapy, as ordered, because dehiscence and evisceration increase the risk of infection. Monitor the patient's temperature at least every 4 hours. Inspect the wound for redness, swelling, and drainage. Use aseptic technique for wound care.
- Teach the patient to splint her incision when coughing or moving.
- Anticipate the use of an abdominal binder to support weak abdominal muscles and the new suture line.
- Provide adequate nutrition and hydration to promote optimal wound healing.
- After suture removal, assess wound healing frequently and monitor for evidence of recurring dehiscence.

SPECIAL CONSIDERATIONS

- Some patients are discharged with sutures still in place. In these cases, teach the patient how to keep her incision clean and dry and about any special techniques for wound care. Remind the patient about her follow-up visit to have the sutures removed.
- Keep in mind that hematomas or seromas contribute to pain, predispose to infection, and delay primary wound healing. Meticulous hemostasis prevents their formation. If they do develop, they should be evacuated promptly, and measures should be taken to prevent their recurrence.
- If a patient calls the emergency department or physician's office after discharge to report dehiscence or evisceration, tell her to lie down and put a moist (sterile, if possible) dressing or towel over the area. Warn the patient not to walk or sit upright in a car. Instead, tell her to call the emergency medical service in her area as soon as possible for transport to the hospital.
- Dehiscence is most likely to occur 5 to 12 days after the wound was initially sutured. Be sure to monitor patients at risk for dehiscence during this time.

Index

---

i indicates illustration; *t*, table

i indicates illustration; *t*, table

i indicates illustration; t, table

i indicates illustration; *t*, table